Essentials of Orthopaedic Surgery

Second Edition

Essentials of Orthopaedic Surgery

Sam W. Wiesel, M.D.

Professor and Chairman
Department of Orthopaedics
Georgetown University Medical Center
Washington, D.C.

John N. Delahay, M.D.

Professor and Vice Chairman
Department of Orthopaedics
Georgetown University Medical Center
Washington, D.C.

W.B. SAUNDERS COMPANY
A Division of Harcourt Brace & Company
Philadelphia London Toronto Montreal Sydney Tokyo

W.B. SAUNDERS COMPANY
A Division of Harcourt Brace & Company

The Curtis Center
Independence Square West
Philadelphia, Pennsylvania 19106–3399

Library of Congress Cataloging-in-Publication Data

Essentials of orthopaedic surgery / [edited by] Sam W. Wiesel, John N.
  Delahay. — 2nd ed.

    p.   cm.

    Previous ed. entered under Wiesel.

    Includes bibliographical references and index.

    ISBN 0–7216–6671–X

    1. Orthopedics. I. Wiesel, Sam W. II. Delahay, John N.
    [DNLM: 1. Orthopedics—methods. WE 168 E78 1977]
    RD731.W67 1997
    617.3—dc20

    DNLM/DLC   96-41700

ESSENTIALS OF ORTHOPAEDIC SURGERY   ISBN   0-7216-6671-X

Printed in the United States of America.

Last digit is the print number: 9 8 7 6 5 4 3 2

This text is dedicated to
Barbara Wiesel and Cathy Delahay
for all their patience and understanding,
not to mention the liberal use of our services
for problems of their hip, knee, elbow, and neck.

Contributors

Alan D. Aaron, M.D.

Assistant Professor, Department of Orthopaedics, Georgetown University Medical Center, Washington, D.C.
Orthopaedic Infections; Tumors of the Musculoskeletal System

George P. Bogumill, M.D.

Professor, Department of Orthopaedics, Georgetown University Medical Center, Washington, D.C.
Tumors of the Musculoskeletal System; The Hand

John N. Delahay, M.D.

Professor and Vice Chairman, Department of Orthopaedics, Georgetown University Medical Center, Washington, D.C.
Bone Development and Metabolism; Children's Orthopaedics; Skeletal Trauma; The Foot and Ankle

Brian G. Evans, M.D.

Assistant Professor, Department of Orthopaedics, Georgetown University Medical Center, Washington, D.C.
The Hip; The Knee

Peter I. Kenmore, M.D.

Professor Emeritus, Department of Orthopaedics, Georgetown University Medical Center, Washington, D.C.
Fractures; Orthopaedic Infections; The Shoulder; The Elbow; Skeletal Trauma

William C. Lauerman, M.D.

Associate Professor, Department of Orthopaedics, Georgetown University Medical Center, Washington, D.C.
Physical Diagnosis; The Spine

Benjamin S. Shaffer, M.D.

Assistant Professor, Department of Orthopaedics, Georgetown University Medical Center, Washington, D.C.
Sports Medicine; The Shoulder; The Elbow

Sam W. Wiesel, M.D.

Professor and Chairman, Department of Orthopaedics, Georgetown University Medical Center, Washington, D.C.
The Spine

Preface

The goal of the second edition of Essentials of Orthopaedics Surgery continues to be an up-to-date overview of orthopaedics written expressly for the medical student. New chapters for physical diagnosis and for sports medicine, plus a glossary with definitions of common terms have been added. The remaining chapters have been carefully revised keeping to a standardized format as much as possible. Each topic is presented from a practical point of view and the material has been distilled down to its most salient features.

Every chapter has been authored by a subspecialist for that particular topic. In updating each section, the authors have tried to eliminate those areas that are not current and to focus on practical information that is relevant to the medical student. Each topic is covered in enough depth that when confronted with a specific clinical problem, the student should be able to formulate an initial diagnostic and treatment plan.

Finally and most important, it has been a very exciting and stimulating experience to work with all the members of the Orthopaedic Department at Georgetown University Medical Center. Everyone has been enthusiastic. The editors are most appreciative of each contribution and very proud of the final text.

Sam W. Wiesel, M.D.
Jack N. Delahay, M.D.

Contents

Chapter 1

Bone Development and Metabolism

John N. Delahay

NORMAL BONE GROWTH AND DEVELOPMENT

Bone is a biphasic connective tissue consisting of an inorganic mineral phase and an organic matrix phase. The hardness of bone allows it to provide several specialized mechanical functions: the protection of internal organs, the scaffold providing points of attachment for other structural elements, and the levers needed to improve the efficiency of muscle action. In addition, bone serves two biologic functions: a site for hematopoietic activity and a reservoir of minerals needed for metabolic interchange.

Embryology

The major components of the musculoskeletal system originate from the mesoderm layer of the trilaminar embryo. This "middle layer" is populated by mesenchymal cells that are totipotent and capable of differentiating into a number of tissues. The sequence of events important in bone growth and development begins with the appearance of the limb bud around the fifth week of life. It is at that time that a tubular condensation of mesenchyme develops centrally in the limb bud. Discrete areas, called interzones, are seen between these condensations (Fig. 1–1) and represent the primitive joints.

During the sixth week, the mesenchyme differentiates into cartilage through the process of chondrification (Fig. 1–2). Interstitial and appositional growth occurs from within

and from the surface, respectively. In the seventh week, the cartilage model is penetrated by a vascular spindle. This occurs coincidentally with the necrosis of the central cartilage cells. Once this vascular spindle is established, the central portion of the model is populated by osteoblasts. Matrix is secreted and this in turn is ossified, making immature (woven) bone.

Once the central portion of the model is ossified, it is referred to as a primary ossification center (Fig. 1–3). Further ossification of the skeleton occurs via one of two mechanisms: (1) enchondral ossification within a cartilage model (i.e., long bones), and (2) intramembranous ossification within a mesenchymal model (i.e., most flat bones and the clavicle).

From the second through the sixth embryologic months, progressive changes occur in the tubular bones. First the central (medullary) canal cavitates, leaving a hollow tube of bone with a large mass of cartilage persisting at each end (Fig. 1–4). Within these masses of cartilage, the secondary ossification center, or epiphysis, will form (Fig. 1–5). A cartilage plate, the physis or growth plate (Fig. 1–6), persists between the developing epiphysis and metaphysis. This structure is responsible for growth in length, whereas the covering of the bone, the periosteum, is primarily responsible for growth in girth.

Postnatal Development

The physis and the periosteum continue to function postnatally in the growth and development of the infantile skeleton. Numerous

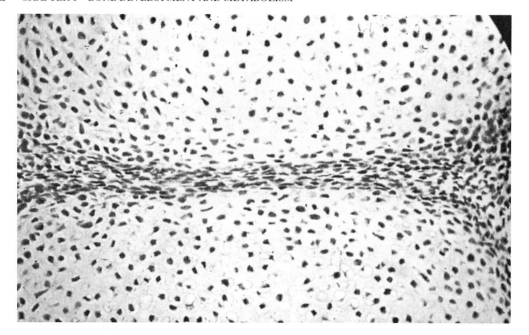

FIGURE 1–1 ■ Histologic study of fetus, approximately 6 weeks' gestation, depicting early joint formation. Note the identifiable cartilage and the condensed mesenchymal tissue of the interzone destined to become the joint.

(From Bogumill GP: Orthopaedic Pathology: A Synopsis with Clinical and Radiographic Correlation. Philadelphia, WB Saunders Company, 1984, p 192; reprinted by permission.)

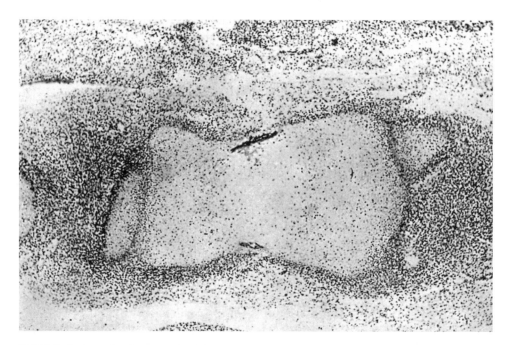

FIGURE 1–2 ■ Histologic study of fetus, approximately 8 weeks' gestation. Earliest ossification is depicted here. A sleeve, or collar, of bone is present on the outer surface of the cartilage model.

(From Bogumill GP: Orthopaedic Pathology: A Synopsis with Clinical and Radiographic Correlation. Philadelphia, WB Saunders Company, 1984, p 5; reprinted by permission.)

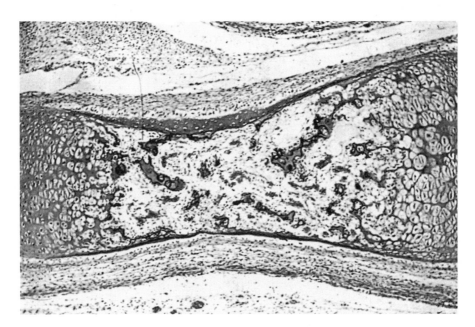

FIGURE 1–3 ■ Primary ossification center of fetus, approximately 14 weeks' gestation. The cartilage cells have been removed almost entirely from the center, leaving remnants of acellular cartilage matrix. Bone deposits on the cartilage remnants will form primary trabeculae. Note that the primary sleeve, or collar, of bone has extended along both margins and is located adjacent to the hypertrophied cartilage at each epiphyseal end.

(From Bogumill GP: Orthopaedic Pathology: A Synopsis with Clinical and Radiographic Correlation. Philadelphia, WB Saunders Company, 1984, p 6; reprinted by permission.)

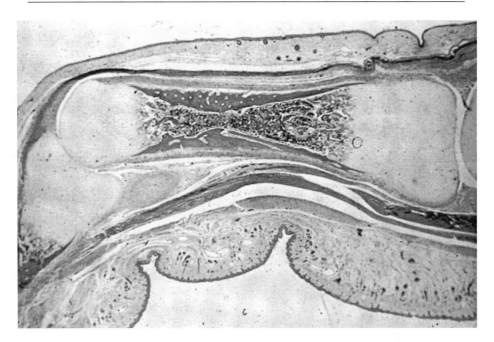

FIGURE 1–4 ■ Primary ossification center, near term. There is complete replacement of cartilage in the diaphyseal portion of the cartilage model. The remaining cartilage is confined to both epiphyseal ends of the model. Note the increasing thickness of the cortical portion of bone, which is a result of conversion of periosteum to bone. A light-staining cambium layer is identifiable. The narrowest portion of the shaft is the site of initial vascular invasion and remains identifiable throughout life in many bones, especially in hands and feet. The eccentric position of this narrowed area indicates the disproportionate contribution to growth in length from each epiphysis.

(From Bogumill GP: Orthopaedic Pathology: A Synopsis with Clinical and Radiographic Correlation. Philadelphia, WB Saunders Company, 1984, p 6; reprinted by permission.)

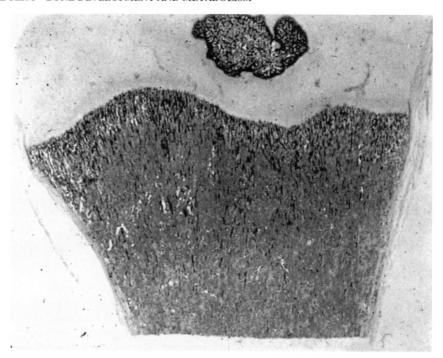

FIGURE 1–5 ■ Early secondary ossification center of mature fetus. The formation of the secondary ossification centers in the lower tibia and upper femur coincide with fetal maturity. The secondary center begins not in the center of the epiphysis, but nearer the growth plate. Expansion, therefore, is eccentric.
(From Bogumill GP: Orthopaedic Pathology: A Synopsis with Clinical and Radiographic Correlation. Philadelphia, WB Saunders Company, 1984, p 9; reprinted by permission.)

local and systemic factors impact on their activity; vascular, hormonal, and genetic effects all play important roles. In essence, the reworking or remodeling of bone that is already present occurs so that the bone can meet the mechanical and biologic demands placed on it.

Bone: The Tissue

Bone, whether it is immature or mature, consists of cells and a biphasic blend of mineral and matrix that coexist in a very exact relationship. The matrix phase consists of collagen and glycosaminoglycans, which are dimeric disaccharides. Both are products of the osteoblast. Calcium hydroxyapatite is the basic mineral crystal in bone. Despite the presence of some less structured amorphous calcium phosphate, the bulk of calcium in the skeletal reservoir is bound in the crystals of hydroxyapatite.

Osteoblasts are bone-forming cells that secrete the matrix components described. As ossification progresses, the osteoblasts become trapped in the matrix they produce and are then referred to as osteocytes. These cells are rather inert but are capable of a small degree of bone resorption. Osteoclasts are those cells whose primary function is the degradation and removal of mineralized bone. It is important to remember that the osteoclasts can remove only mineralized bone and not matrix.

Bone Organization

Microscopically, bone is generally described as mature or immature. Mature bone (Fig. 1–7) has an ordered lamellar arrangement of haversian systems and canalicular communications that give it its classic histologic appearance. Immature bone (Fig. 1–8), in contrast, has a much more random appearance of collagen in a matrix with irregularly spaced cells. It is produced rapidly by osteoblasts and "remodeled" by the cell population until the mature lamellar pattern is achieved. Immature bone is seen in the adult skeleton only under

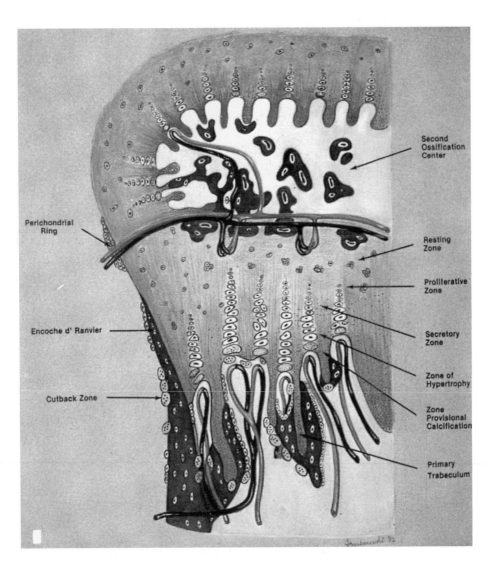

FIGURE 1–6 ■ Schematic diagram of growth plate, consisting of resting zone, proliferative zone, secretory zone, zone of hypertrophy, and zone of calcification. The cross-sectional view helps place events at the growth plate in three-dimensional perspective.

(From Bogumill GP: Orthopaedic Pathology: A Synopsis with Clinical and Radiographic Correlation. Philadelphia, WB Saunders Company, 1984, p 17; reprinted by permission.)

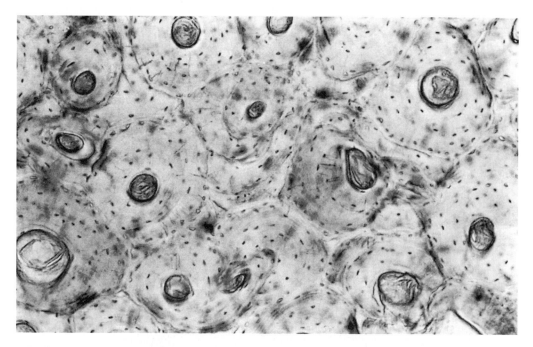

FIGURE 1–7 ■ Mature bone; osteonal structure as seen in undecalcified material. Numerous interstitial fragments (osteonal fragments without an associated haversian canal) are readily observed.

(From Bogumill GP: Orthopaedic Pathology: A Synopsis with Clinical and Radiographic Correlation. Philadelphia, WB Saunders Company, 1984, p 35; reprinted by permission.)

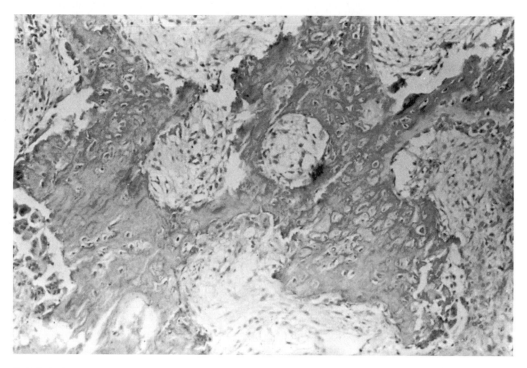

FIGURE 1–8 ■ Immature bone (early callus). Note the large number of osteoblasts and osteocytes.

(From Bogumill GP: Orthopaedic Pathology: A Synopsis with Clinical and Radiographic Correlation. Philadelphia, WB Saunders Company, 1984, p 29; reprinted by permission.)

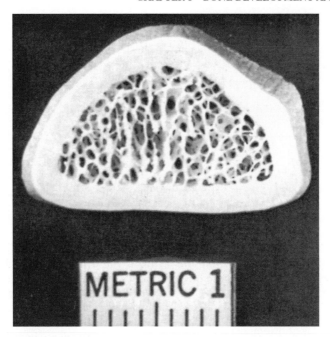

FIGURE 1–9 ■ Cross section of the radius at the distal metaphysis. The majority of bone is cortical bone in which the annual rate of turnover is only 2 per cent.

pathologic conditions (i.e., fracture callus, osteogenic sarcoma). Macroscopically (Fig. 1–9), the lamellar bone is configured either as dense cortical bone or as delicate spicules called trabeculae. In both areas, the cortex and the trabeculae, the bone is the same histologically (i.e., mature lamellar bone).

Turnover and Remodeling

Although the tendency is to think of adult bone as an inert tissue, nothing could be further from the truth. Throughout adult life there is a constant ebb and flow of bone formation and resorption. These two processes are delicately balanced and keep the skeletal mass in a state of equilibrium. A number of authors have popularized the concept of "coupling"; bone formation and bone resorption generally increase or decrease in the same direction. When one process increases, so does the other, and vice versa. It is important, however, to consider the net effect of these rate changes in these two processes. For example, in osteoporosis both bone formation and bone resorption increase, but resorption increases to a much greater degree; so despite a coupled increase in bone formation, the net effect is an overall decrease in bone mass. A number of

factors, systemic and local, affect these processes and hence impact on bone turnover and remodeling. Perhaps the most well-defined factor is mechanical stress, which forms the basis for the classic Wolff's law. Simply stated, trabecular, and to a lesser degree cortical, bone remodels along lines of mechanical stress. Current research indicates that bone functions as a transducer, converting mechanical energy into electrical energy. In turn, the voltage gradients generated modulate cellular differentiation. Osteoblastic activity is stimulated where bone is needed to respond to mechanical load. Osteoclastic activity predominates when the mechanical demands change, and less bone is needed in a specific region. This phenomenon has been called the "piezoelectric effect."

Cartilage

Cartilage, a connective tissue, occurs in three varieties:

1. *Hyaline*–this cartilage covers the ends of long bone articulating in diarthrodial joints.
2. *Fibrocartilage*–this cartilage is located in certain nondiarthrodial joints, such as the symphysis pubis.

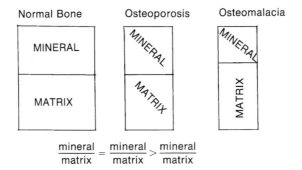

$$\frac{mineral}{matrix} = \frac{mineral}{matrix} > \frac{mineral}{matrix}$$

FIGURE 1–10 ■ Ratio of mineral to matrix in normal and abnormal metabolic states:
normal = osteoporosis > osteomalacia.

3. *Elastic cartilage*–this cartilage may be found in places such as the tip of the nose or lobes of the ears.

In general, hyaline cartilage is a relatively aneural, avascular connective tissue that is essentially 70 per cent water and 30 per cent ground substance and cells. The ground substance is made up of collagen and glycosaminoglycans. The cells, or chondrocytes, are dispersed somewhat randomly in holes called lacunae. The cells are critical to maintaining healthy cartilage by synthesizing new ground substance components. Hyaline cartilage receives the bulk of its nutrition by diffusion from the synovial fluid above and from the vasculature in the subchondral plate below. Normal joint function depends on the presence of normal hyaline cartilage. In its fully hydrated state, hyaline cartilage provides an almost frictionless bearing surface, hence minimizing wear on the articular surface.

AN APPROACH TO EVALUATION OF SKELETAL DISEASES

When a patient with local or systemic skeletal diseases presents for evaluation, the diagnostic

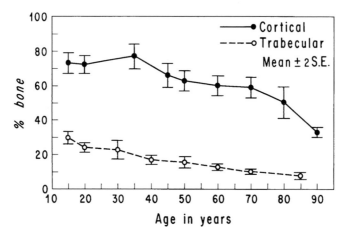

FIGURE 1–11 ■ The relative decrease in cortical and trabecular bone with age in apparently normal persons. Note the relatively rapid loss early in life in trabecular bone and comparatively little loss at this age in cortical bone. The situation is reversed after age 55.

(From Jowsey J: Metabolic Diseases of Bone. Philadelphia, WB Saunders Company, 1977, p 43; reprinted by permission.)

approach should include a history and physical examination, as well as specific diagnostic studies. The standard radiographs provide a unique opportunity to view the affected tissues directly without the need for special stains or dye studies. Armed with these facts, one can then develop a differential diagnosis based on the classic "vitamin" format:

V—vascular diseases

I—infection

T—tumor

A—arthritis

M—metabolic bone diseases

I—injury

N—neurodevelopmental disorders

The remainder of this chapter focuses on those diagnostic groups that affect the skeleton in a more generalized fashion: vascular diseases, metabolic bone diseases, arthritis, and neurodevelopmental disorders. Subsequent individual chapters will consider those diagnostic groups that impact on the skeleton in a localized way: tumor, infection, and injury.

METABOLIC BONE DISEASE

General Concepts

Disease processes affecting bone often can be understood as a change in the relationship of bone formation and bone resorption. It is important to understand the relationship between bone formation and bone resorption as reviewed earlier. Only by doing this can the net effect on the skeleton be appreciated.

The relationship of mineral to matrix may be affected in abnormal metabolic states (Fig. 1–10). For example, osteoporosis is a loss of bone mass, but there is an equivalent loss of matrix and mineral; therefore the ratio remains normal. In contrast, osteomalacia is a relative loss of mineral resulting in a predominance of matrix, hence decreasing the ratio of mineral to matrix. Serum calcium is rarely representative of skeletal activity. Considering that more than 95 per cent of the body's calcium is stored in bone apatite, it is understandable that the 180 mg of ionized plasma calcium represent literally the "tip of the iceberg." Peripheral sampling of the serum calcium provides only a remote clue to the true content of skeletal apatite. It does, however,

provide a convenient way to think about and classify metabolic bone disease.

Eucalcemic States—Osteoporosis

As mentioned, osteoporosis is a predominance of bone resorption over bone formation, with the net effect being bone loss (Fig. 1–11). There is a parallel loss of mineral and matrix, so their ratio remains normal. Essentially, osteoporosis is a decrease in bone mass with an increase in cortical porosity and in diaphyseal bone diameter. This latter phenomenon is an attempt by the organism to use what limited bone there is and to disperse it as far as possible from the neutral axis of the long bone. Mechanically, this increases the torsional rigidity of the bone. Numerous etiologies of osteoporosis have been identified (Table 1–1), but clinically most significant is the postmenopausal type, which occurs shortly after the withdrawal of estrogen (naturally or surgically) from the predisposed female (Table 1–2). The yearly cost in dollars, as well as pain and suffering, is overwhelming. Women with this affliction frequently sustain classic osteoporotic fractures. These fractures typically occur in the vertebrae, about the hip, in the wrist (Colles' fracture), and in the surgical neck of the humerus. In addition to pathologic fractures, there is frequently a loss of height as a result of the cumulative effect of multiple vertebral fractures, as well as the progressive development of a kyphotic deformity in the thoracic spine, which is referred to as a "dowager's hump" (Fig. 1–12).

Patients present with a history of pain and/or repeated fractures. Occasionally they will complain of early satiety because of some abdominal compression resulting from loss of height of the vertebral column, and occasionally they complain of shortness of breath because of the increasing kyphosis in the thoracic region. On examination, typically one finds the prominent dowager's hump, a barrel chest, a protuberant abdomen, and generalized bone pain with percussion tenderness.

One of the most difficult problems in the past has been to determine bone mass. Typically, a crude estimate of bone density determined by plain radiograph has been used to extrapolate to the amount of bone previously lost. Classically, once osteopenia is noticeable radiographically, it has been estimated that the bone density is decreased by 30 to 50 per

TABLE 1–1 ■ *Causes of Osteoporosis*

Primary	Vitamin C deficiency
Involutional (postmenopausal or senile)	Intestinal malabsorption
Idiopathic (juvenile or adult)	*Drug*
Secondary	Heparin
Endocrine	Anticonvulsants
Hypogonadism	Ethanol
Adrenocortical hormone excess (primary	Methotrexate
or iatrogenic)	*Genetic*
Hyperthyroidism	Osteogenesis imperfecta
Hyperparathyroidism	Homocystinuria
Diabetes mellitus	*Miscellaneous*
Growth hormone deficiency	Rheumatoid arthritis
Nutritional	Chronic liver disease
Calcium deficiency	Chronic renal disease
Phosphate deficiency	Immobilization
Phosphate excess	Malignancy (multiple myeloma)
Vitamin D deficiency	Metabolic acidosis
Protein deficiency	Cigarette smoking

From Borenstein D, Wiesel SW: Low Back Pain: Medical Diagnosis and Comprehensive Management. Philadelphia, WB Saunders Company, 1989, p 329; reprinted by permission.

TABLE 1–2 ■ *Types of Involutional Osteoporosis*

	Type 1 (Postmenopausal)	Type 2 (Senile)
Age (yr)	50–75	Over 70
Sex ratio (M/F)	1:6	1:2
Type of bone loss	Trabecular	Trabecular & cortical
Fracture site	Vertebrae (crush)	Vertebrae (multiple wedge)
	Distal radius	Hip
Main causes	Menopause	
Calcium absorption	Decreased	Aging
$1,25\text{-}OH)_2$-vitamin D synthesis from 25-(OH) Vitamin D	Secondary decrease	Primary
Parathyroid function	Decreased	Increased

Modified from Riggs BL, Melton LJ III: Involutional osteoporosis. N Engl J Med 314:1676, 1986.

From Borenstein D, Wiesel SW: Low Back Pain: Medical Diagnosis and Comprehensive Management. Philadelphia, WB Saunders Company, 1989, p 329; reprinted by permission.

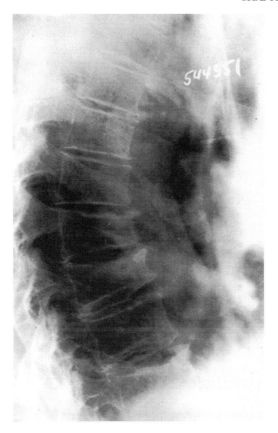

FIGURE 1–12 ■ Radiograph of spine showing osteoporosis. Cortical bone appears accentuated by contrast with osteopenic marrow. Longitudinal trabeculae also appear accentuated because smaller transverse trabeculae are absent. Anterior wedging and end plate compression are present.

(From Bogumill GP: Orthopaedic Pathology: A Synopsis with Clinical and Radiographic Correlation. Philadelphia, WB Saunders Company, 1984, p 244; reprinted by permission.)

cent. Recently, additional diagnostic techniques have become available to more carefully estimate the amount of bone loss and, therefore, the amount of bone that remains. Isotope measurements, specifically single-photon absorptiometry using an iodine compound or dual-photon absorptiometry using a gadolinium compound, have become somewhat popular. Despite their technical limitations, they are clearly better than routine plain radiographs. Quantitative computerized tomographic scanning is useful; however, the amount of radiation has made this a technique of limited use for general application. Without

question, the most definitive diagnostic technique is direct bone biopsy with or without tetracycline labeling. It can clearly give the most reliable information regarding the presence of osteoporosis, its degree, and whether or not a superimposed osteomalacic state exists. Once the diagnosis has been confirmed and the risk analysis carried out, a treatment protocol can be tailored for the individual patient.

Most treatment regimens are considered either prophylactic or therapeutic. Prophylactic regimens include regular weight-bearing exercises such as walking, supplemental calcium, and vitamin D administration with or without the administration of postmenopausal estrogen substitutes. The complications of oral estrogen make its general use somewhat controversial; however, its efficacy in maintaining skeletal mass is beyond question.

Therapeutic regimens, in contrast, are much more debatable. The use of calcitonin, fluoride compounds, and/or diphosphonates has been proposed. At this writing the most up-to-date regimen is the cyclic administration of the diphosphonate in an effort to initially block osteoclastic activity. The diphosphonate is then withdrawn, allowing osteoblastic activity to form more bone. It is hoped that the final net result will be increase in bone mass. The results are clearly still pending.

Hypercalcemic States— Hyperparathyroidism

The effect of parathormone on bone is the same whether it is released as a result of a parathyroid adenoma (primary hyperparathyroidism) or by one of several secondary causes. In essence, parathormone stimulates osteoclastic activity, causing an intense resorption of bone (Fig. 1–13). The cavities resulting from this classic activity fill with vascular fibrous tissue, resulting in the classic osteitis fibrosa cystica. As the cavities coalesce, they form a single large cyst called a "brown tumor" because of the hemosiderin staining one sees within. Clinical and radiographic changes result from this cavitation as well as from the erosive changes occurring under the periosteum.

Hypocalcemic States—Rickets and Osteomalacia

The same underlying mechanism accounts for rickets and osteomalacia: there is a general

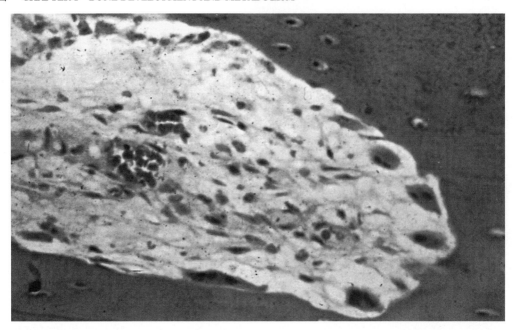

FIGURE 1–13 ■ "Cutting cone." Successive relays of osteoclasts on the right resorb a tunnel of bone, making it longer and wider with each relay. Behind the cutting cone is a "filling cone" of successive relays of osteoblasts secreting osteoid. Resorption is facilitated by high-speed flow of well-oxygenated blood in small vessels, whereas refill is accompanied by dilated sinusoidal vessels with sluggish flow and low oxygen content.
(From Bogumill GP: Orthopaedic Pathology: A Synopsis with Clinical and Radiographic Correlation. Philadelphia, WB Saunders Company, 1984, p 34; reprinted by permission.)

failure to mineralize bony matrix, resulting in the presence of unmineralized osteoid about bony trabeculae. The lack of mineral can be due to a nutritional deficiency, malabsorption, or renal disease (Table 1–3). If this mechanism impacts the skeleton prior to physeal closure, the result is rickets. The child will have bowlegs, frontal bossing, rachitic rosary, and knobby joints (Fig. 1–14) as a result of the presence of these large masses of unmineralized osteoid. In addition, abnormalities of the physis and abnormal physeal growth can be anticipated. If this process occurs after physeal closure, the disease that results is osteomalacia. As noted earlier, the ratio of mineral to matrix is disturbed as a result of a paucity of mineral. In the adult, the area of unmineralized osteoid presents as radiographic lucent areas in the bone, frequently called Looser's lines (Fig. 1–15). In addition, the bones themselves tend to be somewhat malleable and can bow under the load. This is in contradistinction to osteoporotic bone, which is very brittle.

Miscellaneous Metabolic Bone Diseases

Renal Osteodystrophy

Renal osteodystrophy presents with changes in the skeleton that result from chronic acquired renal disease. These changes are truly a collage of metabolic bone diseases. To understand the pathogenesis of renal osteodystrophy is to understand the basis of all of the metabolic afflictions of the skeleton (Fig. 1–16). Chronic uremia allows a twofold drive to depress the serum calcium. First, the kidney is unable to excrete phosphate, hence the serum phosphate level rises. The serum calcium level is then of necessity driven down, to maintain the fixed solubility product. Coincidentally, since the absence of a functional renal parenchyma stops the output of significant amounts of activated vitamin D, intestinal absorption of calcium is retarded, further depressing serum calcium. This dual mechanism profoundly depresses serum calcium and thus in turn mandates a parathormone response. The changes in the bone reflect the metabolic drives. The

TABLE 1–3. ■ *Diseases Associated with Osteomalacia*

Disorder	Metabolic Defect
Vitamin D	Decreased generation of vitamin D_3
Deficiency	
Dietary	
Ultraviolet light exposure	
Malabsorption	Decreased absorption of vitamins D_2 and D_3
Small intestine	
Inadequate bile salts	
Pancreatic insufficiency	
Abnormal metabolism	
Hereditary enzyme deficiency vitamin D–dependent rickets (type I)	Decreased 1-alpha-hydroxylation of 25-(OH)-vitamin D
Chronic renal failure	Decreased 25-hydroxylation of vitamin D
Mesenchymal tumors	
Systemic acidosis	
Hepatic failure	
Anticonvulsant drugs	
Peripheral resistance	Absent or abnormal 1,25-$(OH)_2$-vitamin D receptors
Vitamin D–dependent rickets (type II)	
Phosphate Depletion	
Dietary	Inadequate bone mineralization secondary to low serum concentrations
Malnutrition (rare)?	
Aluminum hydroxide ingestion	
Renal tubular wasting	
Hereditary	Decreased serum phosphate concentrations
X-linked hypophosphatemic osteomalacia	
Acquired	
Hypophosphatemic osteomalacia	
Renal disorders	
Fanconi's syndrome	
Mesenchymal tumors	
Fibrous dysplasia	
Mineralization Defects	
Hereditary	Abnormal alkaline phosphatase activity
Hypophosphatasia	
Acquired	
Sodium fluoride	Inhibition of bone mineralization
Disodium etidronate	
Miscellaneous	
Osteopetrosis	Abnormal osteoclast activity
Fibrogenesis imperfecta	Unknown
Axial osteomalacia	Unknown
Calcium deficiency	Inadequate bone mineralization secondary to low serum calcium concentration

From Borenstein D, Wiesel SW: Low Back Pain: Medical Diagnosis and Comprehensive Management. Philadelphia, WB Saunders Company, 1989, p 339; reprinted by permission.

vitamin D deficiency is demonstrated by the presence of unmineralized osteoid (Fig. 1–17). The elevated levels of parathormone cause osteitis fibrosis cystica. Unique to this syndrome, the hyperphosphatemia results in a diffuse osteosclerosis and some pathognomonic radiographic findings (Fig. 1–18), such as the "rugger jersey" spine.

The "Sick Cell" Syndromes— Osteogenesis Imperfecta, Osteopetrosis

The underlying mechanism seen in these conditions is a qualitative functional deficit in a

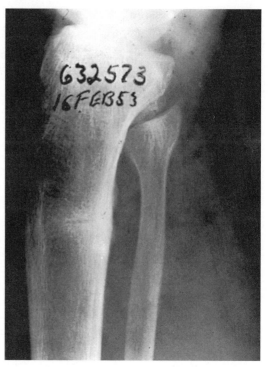

FIGURE 1–15 ■ Radiograph of osteomalacia showing Looser's transformation zone. These lines appear at sites in which stress fractures would occur. Stress of normal use incites remodeling with removal of bone. In normal individuals, the removed bone is replaced by normal osteons. In persons with osteomalacia, the removed bone is replaced with abnormal osteoid, which fails to mineralize and leaves a linear radiolucency that may persist for years.

(From Bogumill GP: Orthopaedic Pathology: A Synopsis with Clinical and Radiographic Correlation. Philadelphia, WB Saunders Company, 1984, p 265; reprinted by permission.)

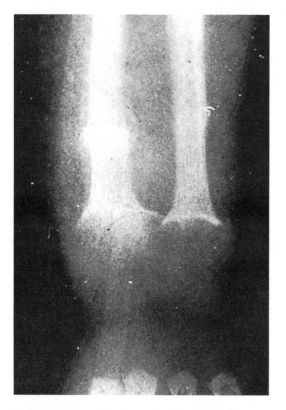

FIGURE 1–14 ■ Radiograph of wrist of child with active rickets exhibiting the irregular widened zone of provisional calcification that is replaced by abnormal osteoid. The cartilage masses are not visible, but the widened epiphyseal growth plate and irregular calcification are readily seen. Note pathologic fracture of radial shaft.

(From Bogumill GP: Orthopaedic Pathology: A Synopsis with Clinical and Radiographic Correlation. Philadelphia, WB Saunders Company, 1984, p 259; reprinted by permission.)

$$\downarrow \begin{array}{c} \text{Vitamin D} \\ \text{Synthesis} \end{array} \longleftarrow \text{Uremia} \xrightarrow[\text{Retention}]{PO_4} \uparrow PO_4 s$$

$$\downarrow \downarrow$$

$$\downarrow \begin{array}{c} \text{Absorption} \\ \text{of Ca} \end{array} \longrightarrow \downarrow\downarrow Ca^{2+}{}_s \longleftarrow \text{(maintain solubility product)}$$

$$\downarrow$$

$$\uparrow \text{PTH}$$

FIGURE 1–16 ■ Pathogenesis of renal osteodystrophy. (P_s, serum phosphate; $Ca^{2+}s$, serum calcium; PTH, parathormone.)

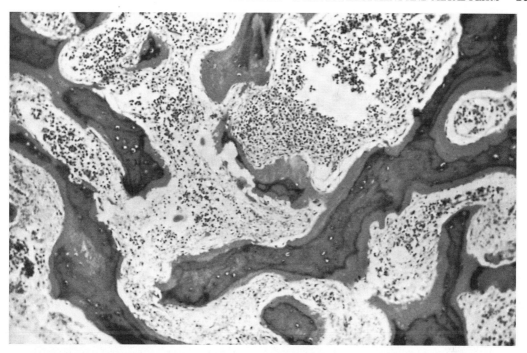

FIGURE 1–17 ■ Renal osteodystrophy. Histologic section of bone exhibiting wide osteoid seams. These are seen in patients with primary renal disease, but they are not present in patients with primary hyperparathyroidism because the osteoid produced in primary hyperparathyroidism is normal.

(From Bogumill GP: Orthopaedic Pathology: A Synopsis with Clinical and Radiographic Correlation. Philadelphia, WB Saunders Company, 1984, p 269; reprinted by permission.)

cellular population—despite the fact that the population is quantitatively normal.

Osteogenesis imperfecta (Fig. 1–19) is typified by the inability of the osteoblasts to secrete normal collagen. Ossification is therefore abnormal and results in marked cortical thinning and a slender skeleton, which is easily fractured (Fig. 1–20). Osteopetrosis is a syndrome in which the end result is the failure of osteoclasts to remove primary spongiosa. This osseous material "piles up" in the skeleton, making it appear very dense radiographically (Fig. 1–21) but also causing it to be mechanically weak. An additional complication is the displacement of marrow elements, necessitating extramedullary hematopoiesis in an effort to compensate for the myelophthisic anemia.

Paget's Disease

Sir James Paget described a syndrome of unknown etiology that bears his name. Strong evidence, specifically the finding of radiodense virus-like particles in the bone cells (Fig. 1–22), points to a slow virus as the cause of Paget's disease. It is basically a disease of bone turnover wherein bone formation and bone resorption dramatically increase. The two processes occur alternatively rather than simultaneously in any given bone, and the net effect is bones of increased density with a marked trabecular thickening (Fig. 1–23). The skull, pelvis, tibia, and femur are favorite targets of this process. Sadly, and not unlike osteopetrosis, the pagetic bones are mechanically weak, making pathologic fracture a frequent complication. Despite the presence of a lot of bone, it is poorly formed and the mineral and matrix are poorly integrated. Bone pain and hearing deficits are frequent problems in these patients. Several different therapeutic approaches have been attempted. Currently, diphosphonates are popular. The rationale is to freeze the skeleton and thereby decrease bone formation and bone resorption. The serum alkaline phosphatase level provides a reliable way of monitoring the response to treatment.

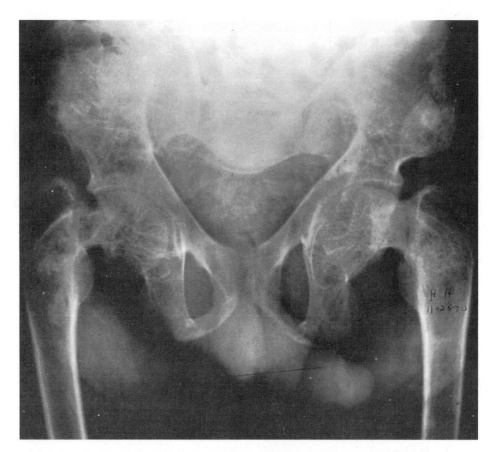

FIGURE 1–18 ■ Radiograph of patient with long-standing renal osteodystrophy. Marked osteoporosis attributable to secondary hyperparathyroidism is evident. There is bowing of the proximal femurs, marked lordosis, and pelvic tilt. The deformity of the pelvis is commonly seen in osteomalacia, but it does not usually occur in primary hyperparathyroidism.

(From Bogumill GP: Orthopaedic Pathology: A Synopsis with Clinical and Radiographic Correlation. Philadelphia, WB Saunders Company, 1984, p 270; reprinted by permission.)

ARTHRITIS

Since any significant discussion of this subject is well beyond the scope of this chapter, it is hoped that presentation of some basic concepts will allow consideration of this diagnosis in the scheme of differential diagnosis. It is important to recall that a diarthrodial joint includes three tissues: bone, cartilage, and synovium. Each of the arthritic diseases tends to impact one of these tissues, with changes in the other two resulting from secondary phenomena. The radiographic and microscopic changes encountered represent a composite of the results of the initial injury and the organism's attempt at repair of that injury.

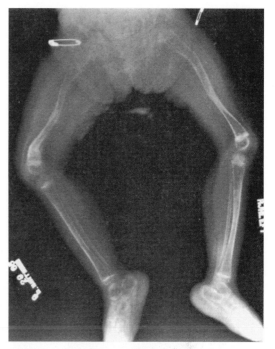

FIGURE 1-20 ■ Radiograph of the lower extremities of a child with osteogenesis imperfecta. The bones are slender and the cortices excessively thin; both femurs have incurred fractures that are partially healed, although deformity still exists.

(From Jowsey J: Metabolic Diseases of Bone. Philadelphia, WB Saunders Company, 1977, p 188; reprinted by permission.)

Noninflammatory Arthritis—Osteoarthritis

Osteoarthritis can be primary or secondary if one considers the degenerative joint disease that can follow trauma or other primary events. The process itself targets the articular cartilage. Whether the initial event is mechanical or biochemical remains controversial. The net result is progressive damage to the articular surface. The secondary bone changes that occur are reparative in nature. Joint space narrowing, subchondral sclerosis, osteophytes, and subchondral cysts, therefore, are the classic radiographic changes. Since this is most typically a disease of weight-bearing joints, the hip and knee oftentimes require orthopaedic care. Total joint arthroplasty has become the mainstay of surgical management in these patients, producing reliable long-term results.

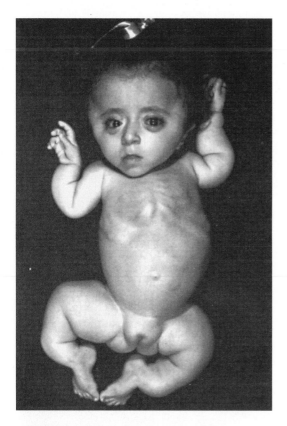

FIGURE 1–19 ■ Deformity in a child with severe osteogenesis imperfecta. Note the prominence of the ribs in the abnormally shaped thoracic cage, the flattening of the skull with frontal bulging, and the malformed ribs.

(From Gertner JM, Root L: Osteogenesis imperfecta. Orthop Clin North Am 21[1]:153, 1990; reprinted by permission.)

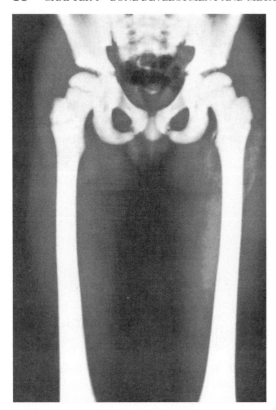

FIGURE 1–21 ■ Radiologic appearance of the femurs and pelvic girdle of a patient with osteopetrosis. There is almost complete absence of the marrow cavity and lack of remodeling of the femoral neck and acetabulum.

(From Jowsey J: Metabolic Diseases of Bone. Philadelphia, WB Saunders Company, 1977, p 173; reprinted by permission.)

Inflammatory Arthritis—Rheumatoid Arthritis

Rheumatoid arthritis, and to some degree its variants, target the synovial membrane as the site for the immunologic process that is the root mechanism of this disease. As the synovium hosts this inflammatory process, it becomes hyperplastic and hypertrophic. The thickened synovium destroys the articular cartilage by enzymatic degradation and destroys the underlying bone by pressure necrosis and erosion (Fig. 1–24). Unlike osteoarthritis, repair changes are, for the most part, abortive. The radiograph reflects this overall atrophic process. Soft tissue swelling, osteopenia on both sides of the joint, and bone erosions are the standard findings (Fig. 1–25). Joint de-

struction is generally symmetric and much more global than with osteoarthritis. Extensive alterations in normal anatomy usually necessitate multiple joint arthroplasties.

Metabolic Arthritides

The common denominator of the metabolic arthritides is the deposition of crystals or metabolic by-products in or around joints. Destructive changes in these joints necessitate rheumatologic and frequently orthopaedic care.

In *gout*, sodium urate crystals are deposited in the joints. Finding these crystals in joint fluid is the diagnostic sine qua non of this metabolic imbalance. An intense chemical synovitis and bony erosions can occur. Typically, the first metatarsophalangeal joint is the classic site, but certainly the process can

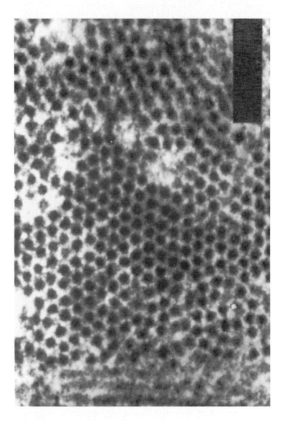

FIGURE 1–22 ■ Viral particles located in osteoclasts within pagetoid bone have been implicated as a causal factor in Paget's disease.

(From Merkow RL, Lane JM: Paget's disease of bone. Orthop Clin North Am 21[1]:172, 1990; reprinted by permission.)

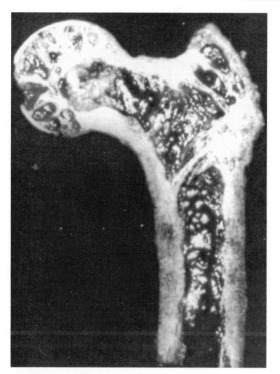

FIGURE 1–23 ■ Example of pagetoid bone demonstrating deformity and thickening of the cortex of the hip. The neck shaft angle has developed varus deformity.

(From Merkow RL, Lane JM: Paget's disease of bone. Orthop Clin North Am 21[1]:173, 1990; reprinted by permission.)

present in any joint, including the spine. The acute onset and signs of acute inflammation should suggest the diagnosis, which is best confirmed by arthrocentesis. The finding of needle-like, negatively birefringent crystals under polarized light confirms the diagnosis. The treatment is usually medical. However, in the presence of late destructive changes, surgical intervention can be considered.

Pseudogout is one of the many causes of chondrocalcinosis and should not be considered synonymous with it. The presence of weakly positively birefringent crystals, rhomboid in shape, attests to the diagnosis. The calcium pyrophosphate crystals are radiopaque and, as such, can be viewed on standard radiographs as calcification of cartilage, including the menisci and articular surfaces. The condition rarely mandates surgical intervention, and treatment frequently revolves around nonsteroidal anti-inflammatory drugs or intra-articular steroid injection.

Ochronosis is an inborn error of metabolism. In this disease entity, the error is absence of homogentisic acid oxidase. As a result, homogentisic acid accumulates and targets articular cartilage for its deposition. The articular cartilage is stiffened by the presence of this by-product and loses its resiliency. The net result is fissuring and fibrillation of the articular surface; these changes radiographically and pathologically mimic osteoarthritis. The unique feature of this condition is the fact that the material pigments and stains the cartilage black (Fig. 1–26), thereby accounting for the blackish tinge of the earlobes and the tips of the nose seen in these patients.

VASCULAR DISEASE

This diagnostic category is a somewhat diverse grouping of clinical entities that are considered under this heading lest they be overlooked.

Circulatory Diseases

Afflictions of the vascular tree, especially the arterial side, tend to produce similar lesions in bone despite the etiology. Bone deprived of a portion of its blood supply becomes necrotic, like all other tissues (Fig. 1–27). Depending on the extent of the vascular involvement, the infarcts can range from small areas of bony necrosis in the metaphysis (Fig. 1–28), which are clinically inconsequential, to extensive involvement at the ends of the long bones that progresses to significant degenerative joint disease.

The radiographic appearance of dead bone is essentially that of sclerosis. In truth, the dead tissue is incapable of changing its density since no viable cells exist. Rather, the viable bone adjacent to the necrotic segment develops a reactive hyperemia and resorbs. The necrotic bone then appears to be more dense on the radiograph. There is also some compaction of dead trabeculae as well as marrow necrosis with subsequent saponification and calcification of fat marrow, to additionally explain the sclerotic changes seen on radiographs.

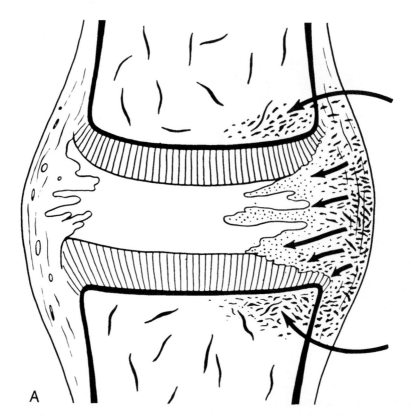

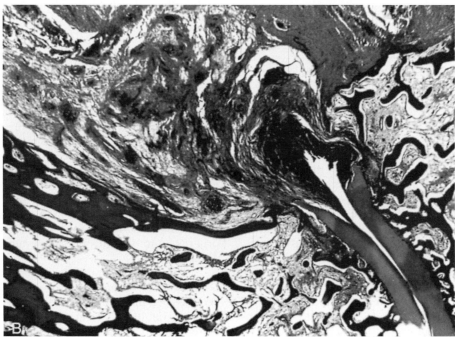

FIGURE 1-24 ■ Diagram *(A)* and section *(B)* of a finger joint of a patient with rheumatoid arthritis. The marked synovitis is evident in the synovial recesses with erosions into the bone on both sides of the articular surface *(long curved arrows)*. The pannus is beginning to encroach on margins of the joint *(short arrows)*. Although the cartilage retains its normal appearance in the center of the joint, the proteoglycan structure is affected by the altered synovial fluid. It is susceptible to rapid removal by wear and tear as well as by the encroaching pannus. Since the pannus grows in from the margins, the earliest radiographic erosions are seen at the margins, and the contact surfaces are spared until relatively late.

(From Bogumill GP: Orthopaedic Pathology: A Synopsis with Clinical and Radiographic Correlation. Philadelphia, WB Saunders Company, 1984, p 231; reprinted by permission.)

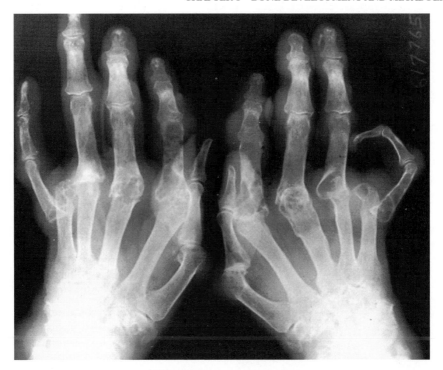

FIGURE 1–25 ■ Radiograph of both hands of a patient with long-standing rheumatic arthritis. Osteoporosis in all bones is marked. The wrist joints show advanced destruction. There is dislocation of the metacarpophalangeal joints of all fingers. Steroid therapy causes expansion of metacarpals and phalanges secondary to changes in the marrow fat (steroid lipomatosis).
(From Bogumill GP: Orthopaedic Pathology: A Synopsis with Clinical and Radiographic Correlation. Philadelphia, WB Saunders Company, 1984, p 223; reprinted by permission.)

A number of occlusive phenomena can cause avascular (aseptic) necrosis. The single most important focus of this process is the femoral head
(Fig. 1–29). Etiologies can be grouped by causation:

1. *Trauma*–damage to vessels supplying the segment of the bone in question (i.e., fractures of the femoral neck and scaphoid).
2. *Occlusive phenomenon*–embolic fat as seen in alcoholism and pancreatitis; embolic nitrogen as seen in Caisson's disease; vasculitis from lupus and diabetes, coagulopathies, and red cell abnormalities.
3. *Storage diseases*–occlusion of the vessel as a result of the increasing pressure of the stored material, as seen in Gaucher's and Fabry's diseases.
4. *Idiopathic*–the causative factor is un-

known, as in steroid-induced osteonecrosis and Chandler's disease.

Hematologic Syndromes

The genetic hemoglobinopathies, although not truly circulatory diseases, are best remembered in this group. Sickle cell disease, and to a lesser degree thalassemia, produce skeletal changes primarily through two mechanisms: myeloid hyperplasia and vaso-occlusive phenomena. Because of the anemia these patients suffer, there is a drive to increase medullary hematopoiesis, and this results in dilation of bony contours to accommodate a marrow driven to produce more blood. Widening of the diploë of the skull, dilation of the small bones of the hands and feet, and increased trabecular markings are all radiographic hallmarks of this process. The vaso-occlusive effect of these distorted red cells

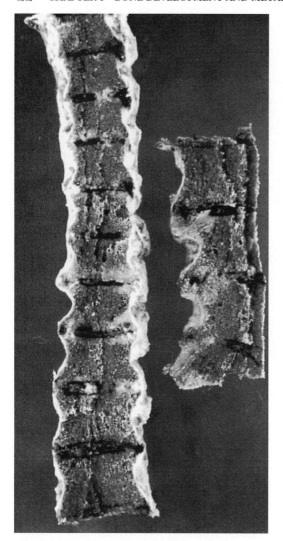

FIGURE 1–26 ■ Gross appearance of vertebral bodies in a patient with ochronosis. Notice the diminution of the intervertebral discs, black discoloration of the cartilage components, virtual disappearance of all joint spaces, and bony bridging.
(From Bogumill GP: Orthopaedic Pathology: A Synopsis with Clinical and Radiographic Correlation. Philadelphia, WB Saunders Company, 1984, p 293; reprinted by permission.)

causes bone infarcts similar to those previously discussed
(Fig. 1–30). However, in a select group of patients the infarcts are frequently painful and a component of the "painful crisis." The stasis, sludging, and dead bone create a comfortable environment for bacterial invasion, account-

ing for the increased incidence of osteomyelitis in these patients.

NEURODEVELOPMENTAL DISORDERS

The final diagnostic category discussed in this chapter is the most heterogeneous of all. There are a few common threads that can be found to tie this eclectic mix of clinical states together. Clearly, they all have an impact on the musculoskeletal system. An attempt is made to describe them generically and use an example in each category to underscore their impact on the skeleton.

Neurologic Diseases

The deficit produced by neurologic diseases can be either sensory, motor, or central in origin. The level of involvement will determine the skeletal changes. Central nervous system deficits are typified by cerebral palsy. Prenatal anoxia can cause damage to the cerebral cortex. This includes damage to neural tissue that normally inhibits or dampens muscular tone and keeps it at an acceptable level. Without normal inhibitory influences, these muscles become spastic. Muscle spasticity existing over a protracted period results in imbalance around joints, contractures, and chronic joint deformities such as subluxations and dislocations. The hip, for example, is of particular concern in the spastic child.

Poliomyelitis is an example of a motor deficit disease. Viral damage to anterior horn cells results in focal motor weakness in various muscle groups in the extremities. Bone deprived of normal muscle loading tends to become osteopenic. In addition, the variable nature of the involvement again causes muscle imbalance around joints, with its subsequent deformities.

Sensory deficits may result in neuropathic arthritis. Joints deprived of proprioception are rapidly destroyed. The aggressive sequence of microtrauma, repeated effusions, ligamentous incompetence, articular damage, and severe degenerative joint disease is the fate of patients with tertiary lues, diabetes, pernicious anemia, leprosy, and heavy metal intoxications. Although proprioception is the initial sensory component lost, pain fiber deficit usually follows, resulting in destroyed but painless joints.

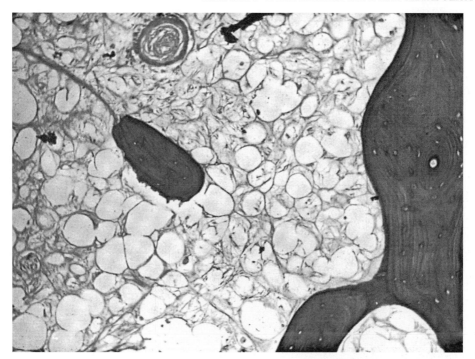

FIGURE 1–27 ■ Bone from central area of infarction, exhibiting infarcted fatty tissue, obliterated vessels, and infarcted bone. Note absence of either osteoclastic or osteoblastic activity. The trabeculae in this zone have retained their original density.

(From Bogumill GP: Orthopaedic Pathology: A Synopsis with Clinical and Radiographic Correlation. Philadelphia, WB Saunders Company, 1984, p 166; reprinted by permission.)

Spina bifida, or myelodysplasia, may result in mixed deficits. This congenital defect combines motor and sensory deficits to produce skeletal changes that parallel both. Osteopenia, joint deformity, and joint destruction may all be found. The joints, as expected, are insensate, a fact that only compounds the clinical problems.

Developmental/Congenital Defects

It is important to remember that congenital defects (present at birth) need not be genetic, and vice versa. However, any process that impacts on the growing skeleton, whether it be congenital or developmental, can be expected to produce changes. These changes can generally be expected to be alterations in the configuration of the bone itself. Shortening, bowing, or angular deformities may be seen. Changes in bone density may or may not be seen.

Achondroplasia is the most common dwarfing syndrome. It follows an autosomal-dominant inheritance pattern (Fig. 1–31).

This syndrome disrupts normal enchondral bone growth and therefore results in shortening of all bones that depend on this mechanism for their growth (Fig. 1–32).

Bone dysplasias (intrinsic defects of bone growth) are, as a general rule, genetic in origin despite the fact that some of the milder (tarda) forms may not be apparent until the child begins growing.

Chromosomal defects such as those seen in Down's syndrome may result in the significant ligamentous laxity seen in these patients. Flat feet, patellar subluxation, bunions, and subluxation of the hips all point to the inability of the ligamentous structure to stabilize joints. Many of the chromosomal abnormalities involve defects in mesoderm development. This accounts for the common coincidence of musculoskeletal, genitourinary, and cardiac abnormalities.

The clubfoot deformity is probably multifactorial in its etiology. The interplay of heredity and environment is accepted, although poorly understood. Clubfoot, like developmental hip disease and scoliosis, is a defect that

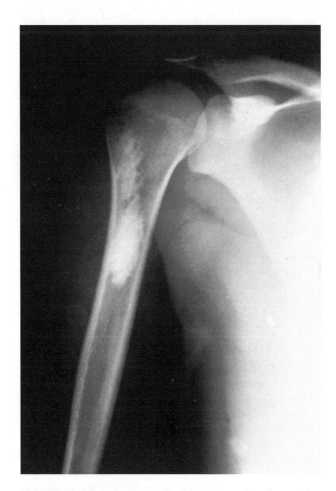

FIGURE 1–28 ■ Radiograph of humerus of patient with history of deep-sea diving. The sclerotic area represents infarction of the marrow cavity with formation of calcium soaps and new bone from the reparative margins.

(From Bogumill GP: Orthopaedic Pathology: A Synopsis with Clinical and Radiographic Correlation. Philadelphia, WB Saunders Company, 1984, p 172; reprinted by permission.)

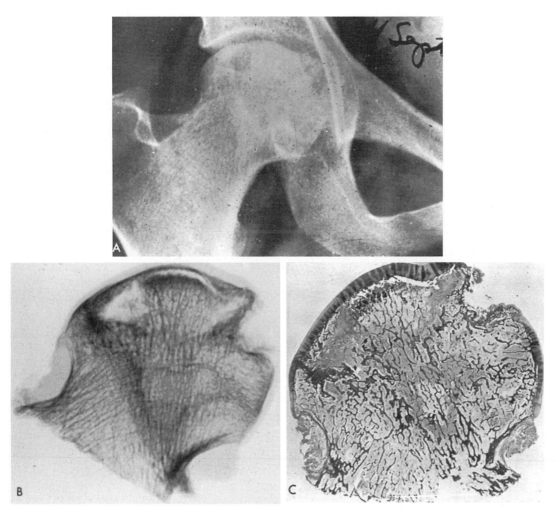

FIGURE 1–29 ■ Clinical radiograph *(A)*, specimen radiograph *(B)*, and corresponding macrospecimen *(C)* of femoral head from a 26-year-old patient on long-term steroid therapy for idiopathic thrombocytopenic purpura with progressive pain and disability of both hips. Note the crescent sign, a cleft beneath the articular cartilage resulting from compression fractures of dead trabeculae. Also note the lytic areas in lateral aspect of the femoral head caused by revascularization with removal of dead trabeculae and replacement with viable fibrous tissue. Zones of increased density are also evident.

(From Bogumill GP: Orthopaedic Pathology: A Synopsis with Clinical and Radiographic Correlation. Philadelphia, WB Saunders Company, 1984, p 164; reprinted by permission.)

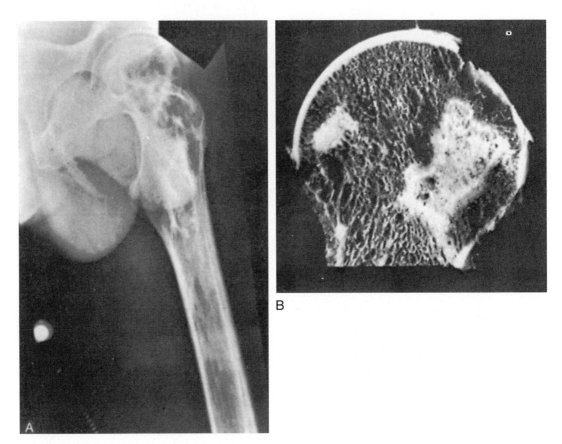

FIGURE 1–30 ■ *A,* Radiograph of hip and proximal femur of a 25-year-old male with sickle cell anemia. Areas of mottling and sclerosis are seen, suggestive of bone infarction. Evidence of sequestrum formation is seen in the lateral femoral cortex (bone within a bone). *B,* Gross specimen of the femoral head taken from the same patient. Light necrotic areas are well demarcated from viable bone.

(From Johanson NA: Musculoskeletal problems in hemoglobinopathy. Orthop Clin North Am 21[1]:196, 1990; reprinted by permission.)

is considered to be a reflection of this interplay. Usually identified at birth, clubfoot is a generalized dysplasia of the mesenchymal structures (bone, ligament, muscle) of the foot and perhaps the entire lower extremity. Genetic as well as environmental (intrauterine position) factors have been implicated, but their exact interaction remains unknown.

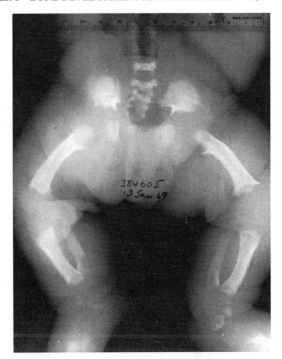

FIGURE 1–32 ■ Radiographic appearance of lower limbs in a patient with achondroplasia. Note the narrow sciatic notch and flat broad acetabulum resulting from inadequate growth of "Y" cartilage in acetabulum. Shortened, thick femurs, fibias, and fibulas are bowed. Bone density is normal. Epiphyses do not yet exhibit secondary ossification centers.

(From Bogumill GP: Orthopaedic Pathology: A Synopsis with Clinical and Radiographic Correlation. Philadelphia, WB Saunders Company, 1984, p 46; reprinted by permission.)

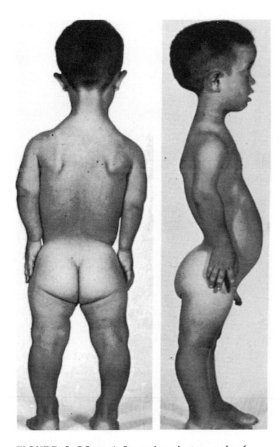

FIGURE 1–31 ■ A, Posterior photograph of achondroplastic dwarf showing distorted growth of long bones. The proximal limb segments are proportionately shorter than the distal, with the hands reaching only to the hip region. The legs are bowed, and the scapulae and pelvis are smaller than normal. Scoliosis is uncommon. B, Lateral photograph of child with achondroplasia. Note marked lumbar lordosis with prominent buttocks as a result of pelvic tilt. The lordosis is due in part to differential growth of vertebral body versus posterior elements.

(From Bogumill GP: Orthopaedic Pathology: A Synopsis with Clinical and Radiographic Correlation. Philadelphia, WB Saunders Company, 1984, p 48; reprinted by permission.)

SUGGESTED READINGS

Bogumill GP: Orthopaedic Pathology: A Synopsis with Clinical and Radiographic Correlation. Philadelphia, WB Saunders Company, 1984.

Lane JM (ed): Pathologic Fractures in Metabolic Bone Disease. 21(1), 1990.

Orthopaedic Knowledge Update for American Academy of Orthopaedic Surg. 1993.

Rodriga J: Orthopaedic Surgery: Basic Science and Clinical Science. Boston, Little, Brown, 1986.

Simon, S: Orthopaedic Basic Science. American Acad. of Ortho. Surg. 1994.

Weissman BNW, Sledge CB: Orthopedic Radiology. Philadelphia, WB Saunders Company, 1986.

Chapter 2

Physical Diagnosis

William C. Lauerman

GENERAL PRINCIPLES

Physical examination of the patient with a suspected disorder of the musculoskeletal system is driven, in large part, by the history given by the patient. The maxim, "listen to the patient," certainly holds true in orthopaedic history taking and physical diagnosis but it is also essential, when evaluating the musculoskeletal system, to be aware of the very real possibility that the underlying source of a patient's symptoms may be well removed from the focus of the patient's complaints. Referred pain, such as hip pathology causing pain on the medial aspect of the knee or a cervical spine disorder causing pain in the area of the scapula and shoulder, is common, as is radicular pain, which extends down the arm or leg due to nerve root compression in the cervical or lumbar spine. Both must be considered as the patient describes his or her symptoms.

With the exception of the hand or foot, examination of the musculoskeletal system cannot be adequately accomplished without having the patient undressed and changed into either a gown or gym shorts, and it cannot be performed with the patient's pants pulled down, or shirt slipped off the shoulder. Establishing a routine practice of having the patient change into an examining gown facilitates thorough physical examination and is encouraged.

With an understanding that distal symptoms in an extremity may be related to pathology more proximally, or even in the spine, it is essential that an examination of any part of an extremity include examination of the entire extremity. Furthermore, many musculoskeletal conditions are best diagnosed by comparing the affected extremity to its unaffected counterpart; one should routinely examine the opposite extremity to determine the significance of abnormal findings such as instability, weakness, or atrophy. Examination of the cervical spine, in the case of upper extremity disorders, and the lumbar spine, for disorders of the lower extremity is frequently necessary to insure that there is no central nervous system explanation for the patient's problem. This is particularly true in the pediatric population, and very thorough inspection and palpation of the thoracolumbar spine should be a routine part of evaluating the infant or child with any disorder of the lower extremity.

A final general principle in the approach to physical diagnosis of the musculoskeletal system is the benefit of observing the function of the affected body part. The musculoskeletal exam should routinely begin with observation of the patient's gait, and it can be quite helpful to observe upper extremity function when evaluating a shoulder, elbow, or hand problem.

The following pages will be devoted to reviewing some of the basic principles of physical diagnosis as they pertain to specific areas of the musculoskeletal system. Further details, as well as correlation of history and physical findings, are discussed in the individual chapters.

PHYSICAL EXAMINATION OF THE UPPER EXTREMITIES

Cervical Spine

Examination of the spine cannot proceed until the patient is changed into an examining gown. Physical findings in both the cervical and lumbar spine are obtained through palpation of the bony and soft tissue structures, determination of the range of motion, neurologic examination, and the performance of special tests. These findings fall into two major categories: (1) nonspecific findings that are present in most patients with a problem in their neck or lower back, but that provide little clue as to the location or source of the problem; and (2) specific findings that are most useful in localizing the exact site of pathology.

Tenderness to deep palpation in the muscles around the neck, such as the trapezius, rhomboids, and the cervical paraspinal muscles, is ubiquitous in individuals with neck pain, but is nonspecific. Midline tenderness is less common and can be helpful in localizing the site of pathology. This is particularly true in acute injuries, and in the emergency department setting careful palpation, from the occiput to the upper thoracic spine, is an important part of the physical examination. Range-of-motion testing of the cervical spine will routinely demonstrate diminished motion in most patients with neck pain. Although this decrease generally provides little useful information regarding the etiology of the problem, range-of-motion testing can be a very helpful way of monitoring the patient's response to treatment.

Careful neurologic examination of the upper extremities is the most important part of physical examination of the cervical spine patient. Characteristic sensory, motor, and reflex changes can be seen in the patient with compression of various cervical nerve roots; while some overlap may occur, it is usually possible to identify a specific nerve root that is compressed or inflamed and to determine the disc level involved (Fig. 2–1). Manual tests to increase or decrease root compression may also aid in the diagnosis.

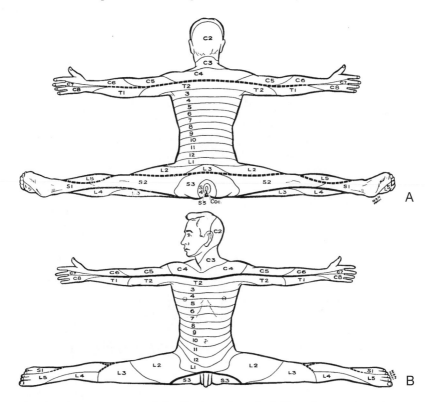

FIGURE 2–1 ■ Dermatomal distribution of cervical *(A)* and upper thoracic nerve roots *(B)*.

(Modified from Haymaker W, Woodhall B: Peripheral Nerve Injuries, ed 2. Philadelphia, WB Saunders Company, 1953, p 19; reprinted by permission.)

Another important part of the neurologic examination is the search for evidence of myelopathy. A broad-based, shuffling gait is characteristic of the individual with cervical spondylotic myelopathy. Upper motor neuron findings such as hyperreflexia, Hoffman's sign (reflex contraction of the thumb interphalangeal (IP) joint with flicking of the distal phalanx of the middle finger), ankle clonus, or Babinski's sign are all important findings that suggest spinal cord dysfunction. Weakness, wasting, and evidence of hand clumsiness, such as the loss of mirror movement (dysdiadochokinesia), also suggest myelopathy.

Reproduction of shoulder and arm pain with extension and lateral bending of the neck toward the painful extremity (Spurling's sign) is a specific special test indicative of cervical radiculopathy. Adson's test is performed by palpating the patient's radial pulse first with him or her in the resting position and then by having the patient hunch the shoulders forward, turn the head toward the effected extremity, and extend the arm backward; diminution of the pulse represents a positive test and may be indicative of thoracic outlet syndrome (Fig. 2–2).

The Shoulder

Evaluation of the shoulder begins with inspection and palpation of the entire shoulder girdle, followed by testing of active and passive ranges of motion, motor and sensory testing, and the evaluation of special tests. The frequent overlap of neck and shoulder pathology, as well as their propensity to coexist in a given patient, make it essential that, as in all other upper extremity complaints, evaluation of the cervical spine be performed.

Inspection and observation are helpful in evaluating patients with shoulder pathology. When modesty allows, viewing patients as they take off their shirt can provide clues as to the function of shoulder girdle mechanics. Inspection for evidence of bony prominences, such as a prominent distal clavicle in patients with a history of acromioclavicular dislocation, or deltoid atrophy is also important. Palpation of the area above the shoulder is frequently a direct way to determine the site of pathology. Localized tenderness over the acromioclavicular (AC) joint, the bicipital tendon, the coracoacromial ligament, or the greater tuberosity may point to such corresponding pathologies

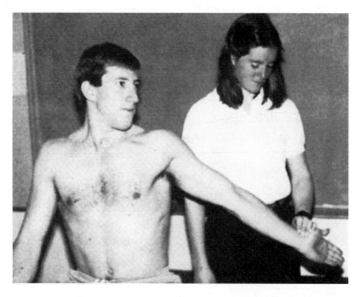

FIGURE 2–2 ■ The Adson test. Diminution of the radial pulse when the patient turns his head, with the arm extended, abducted, and externally rotated *(B)*, suggests compression of the subclavian artery. This may be a cause of thoracic outlet syndrome.

(From Magee DJ: Orthopeadic Physical Assessment, ed 2. Philadelphia, WB Saunders Company, 1992, p 122; reprinted by permission.)

as AC arthritis, bicipital tendinitis, impingement syndrome, and degenerative rotator cuff tendinitis, respectively. Soft tissue palpation of all muscle bellies and their tendinous attachments is also carried out.

Active and passive ranges of motion are then tested. Normal motion at the shoulder includes elevation (combined abduction and forward flexion) of 180 degrees, internal rotation of 55 degrees, external rotation of 45 degrees, and extension of 45 degrees. A significant loss of external rotation, following trauma, should raise the suspicion of posterior dislocation, a shoulder injury that is frequently missed. Markedly limited and painful motion in all planes with both active and passive testing suggests adhesive capsulitis, while active motion that falls short of passive motion may be indicative of a rotator cuff tear. By palpating the scapula, one can differentiate glenohumeral from scapulothoracic motion. Limited motion, occurring entirely at the scapulothoracic articulation, is also typical of adhesive capsulitis. Palpation of crepitus with motion may be suggestive of degenerative arthritis in the shoulder joint, and a rotator cuff tear may result in palpable grinding of the greater tuberosity under the acromion on shoulder elevation.

Shoulder injuries may result in injuries to the brachial plexus, and motor and sensory testing of its five major end branches (axillary, radial, musculocutaneous, ulnar, and median nerves) should be carried out when this is suspected. Atrophy of the deltoid muscle is not uncommon and is usually evidence of a long-standing axillary nerve injury. Sensory loss in the autonomous zone of the axillary nerve, on the lateral aspect of the shoulder over the deltoid, is also evidence of axillary nerve dysfunction.

Several special tests are extremely useful in evaluating the patient with shoulder pathology, including the impingement test, the drop-arm test, and the apprehension test. The impingement sign is elicited by passively flexing the shoulder to 90 degrees with the examiner's opposite hand stabilizing the acromion. Reproduction of pain with this maneuver is evidence of rotator cuff tendinitis, or impingement syndrome (Fig. 2–3), and the sensitivity of this test can be enhanced by internally rotating the shoulder once it has been elevated to 90 degrees (Rockwood sign). The drop-arm sign also indicates rotator cuff pathology. By abducting the arm to 90 degrees, the patient

should be able to slowly lower it to his side. Failure to control the arm as it "drops" to the side is suggestive of a tear in the rotator cuff. Finally, the apprehension test is performed in individuals in whom shoulder instability is suspected. Standing behind the patient, the examiner slowly abducts, extends, and externally rotates the shoulder. Patients with recurrent subluxation or dislocation will, at a certain point, sense recurrence of their instability and resist this maneuver, frequently in a spirited fashion (Fig. 2–4).

The Elbow

Examination of the elbow is facilitated by observation of its use during function of the upper extremity. Inspection of the elbow at rest includes evaluation of the carrying angle, which is the angle subtended by the arm and forearm with the elbow in full extension (Fig. 2–5). This angle is usually five degrees of valgus (the apex or elbow pointing toward the midline) in males and 10 to 15 degrees in females. An abnormal carrying angle can be the result of malunion of a fracture of the distal humerus or a growth injury following a pediatric fracture, and it can result in delayed ulnar nerve symptoms as well as a cosmetically displeasing appearance.

Palpation of the elbow is extremely helpful in determining the source of pathology. Palpable bony landmarks include the medial and lateral epicondyles, the olecranon process, and the radial head. The ulnar nerve, the medial and lateral collateral ligaments, the annular ligament, and the origin of the extensor and flexor muscle groups are soft tissue structures that can be directly palpated and identified as sources of the patient's complaints. The distal tendons of the biceps and triceps should be palpated, and evidence of tendinitis or tendon rupture should be appreciated. In addition, palpation of the olecranon bursa, and observation of an enlarged, fluctuant, or erythematous mass can be made in individuals with olecranon bursitis (Fig. 2–6).

The elbow is a highly mobile joint, and stiffness or loss of motion is a frequent complaint of individuals with disorders in this region. Normal flexion of the elbow is in excess of 135 degrees and an individual can usually flex his elbow far enough to be able to touch his shoulder. Normal extension is to 0 degrees (arm and forearm form a straight line). This

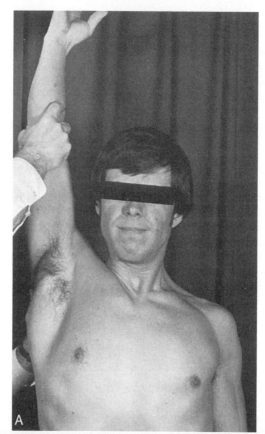

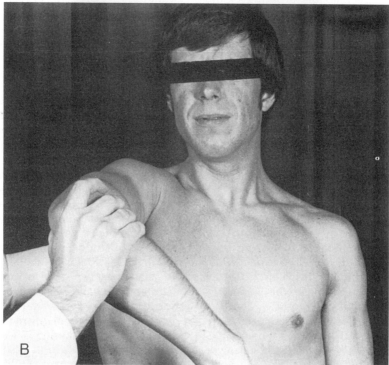

FIGURE 2–3 ■ The impingement sign is elicited by forward elevation of the shoulder *(A)*, compressing the greater tuberosity against the anterior acromion. Further internal rotation *(B)* brings the greater tuberosity under the coracoacromial ligament, increasing the sensitivity of this test.

(Modified from Hawkins RJ, Kennedy JC: The impingement syndrome in athletes. Am J Sports Med 8:57, 1980; reprinted by permission.)

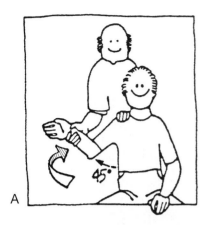
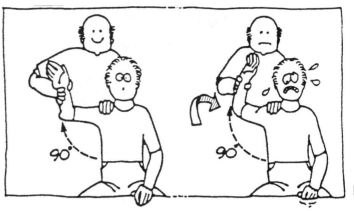

A   B

FIGURE 2–4 ■ The apprehension test. With the arm abducted beyond 90 degrees, and with external rotation *(B)*, the patient senses impending instability and resists or complains, constituting a positive test.

(Modified from Rockwood CA, Green DP, Bucholz RW: Fractures in Adults, ed 3. Philadelphia, JB Lippincott Company, 1991, p 1058; reprinted by permission.)

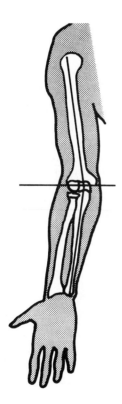

FIGURE 2–5 ■ The carrying angle, measured clinically as the angle formed by the arm and the forearm, with the elbow extended.

(Modified from Morrey BF: The Elbow and Its Disorders, ed 2. Philadelphia, WB Saunders Company, 1993, p 74; reprinted by permission.)

may be exceeded in females, although it is not uncommon for heavily muscled males to lack several degrees of full extension. Normal pronation and supination are 90 degrees each. This is most easily measured by comparing one side to the other and asking the patient to hold a pen or pencil while rotating the forearm. It can be quite helpful, when examining the elbow, to palpate for crepitus or irregular motion as the extremity is passively taken through a full range of flexion, extension, pronation, and supination.

Manual motor testing of the flexors, extensors, pronators, and supinators of the elbow is carried out. Of note, the biceps functions as both a flexor and supinator of the elbow. Sensory testing in the dermatomal and peripheral nerve distributions is also carried out.

Special tests about the elbow include the tennis elbow test, Tinel's test, and tests for ligamentous stability. Individuals with tennis elbow (lateral epicondylitis) have reproduction of their lateral elbow pain with resisted active extension of the wrist (Mill's sign) (Fig. 2–7). Tinel's sign refers to the production of pain and radiating paraesthesias when tapping over an injured peripheral nerve or neuroma. The ulnar nerve, as it passes between the olecranon and the medical epicondyle, is a frequent source of pathology, with pain on the medial aspect of the elbow and pain and paraesthesias down the medial forearm into the ulnar aspect of the hand. Tinel's sign confirms the ulnar nerve at the elbow as the source of pathology. Finally, the medial and

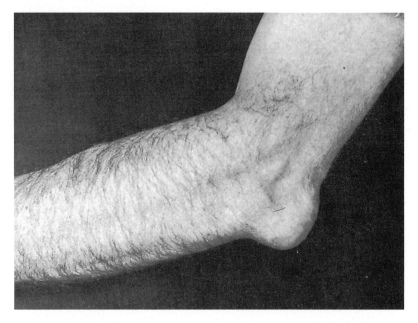

FIGURE 2–6 ■ Olecranon bursitis in a patient with tophaceous gout.

(Modified from Polley HF, Hunder GG: Rheumatologic Interviewing and Physical Examination of the Joints, ed 2. Philadelphia, WB Saunders Company, 1978, p 83; reprinted by permission.)

lateral collateral ligaments of the elbow can be tested with the elbow slightly flexed and a varus or valgus force is applied. The examiner's hand can stabilize the elbow, act as a fulcrum, and palpate for gapping on the involved side, and the results should be compared to the uninvolved elbow.

Wrist and Hand

Because of the complexity of the involved anatomy, the high functional demand, and the significance of the disability related to any loss of function, physical examination of the wrist and hand is the most complex area in

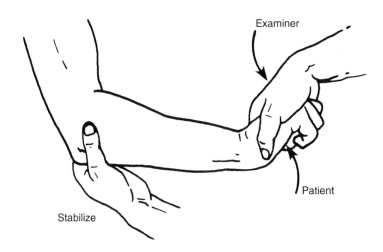

Examiner

Patient

Stabilize

FIGURE 2–7 ■ The Mill's test for tennis elbow syndrome.

(From Magee DJ: Orthopaedic Physical Assessment, ed 2. Philadelphia, WB Saunders Company, 1992, p 153; reprinted by permission.)

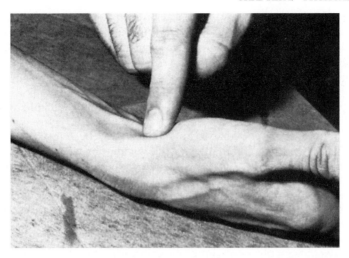

FIGURE 2–8 ■ Tenderness to palpation over the anatomical snuff box may indicate injury to the scaphoid.

(From Tubiana R. (ed): The Hand, vol 3. Philadelphia, WB Saunders Company, 1984; Reprinted by permission.)

physical diagnosis of the musculoskeletal system. Thorough documentation of a thorough physical examination, including region by region testing for tenderness, swelling, range of motion, and neurologic function is tedious but is essential in determining diagnosis and response to treatment. Since injuries to the hand are frequently associated with medicolegal or workers' compensation claims, a detailed and well-documented examination, performed soon after the injury occurred is essential.

Inspection of the hand includes inspection of the patient's hands during function. Routine activities such as grip, the ability to shake hands, and the ability to use a pen or pencil are quite helpful. Determining that a patient is protecting or not using an injured digit, either through observation, lack of uniform callus formation, or other means, is informative. Inspection of both the palmar and dorsal surfaces of the hand and wrist includes identifying changes in the general condition and color of the skin and fingernails. Identifying scars can be very helpful in determining potential disruption of tendons deep to the skin, as well as possible sources of contracture or neuroma formation. The intrinsic musculature of the hand should be carefully evaluated and wasting of the intrinsic muscles, including the muscles of the thenar or hypothenar eminences, is suggestive of significant dysfunction

of either the ulnar nerve or the anterior horn cells of the spinal cord. In addition, clubbing of the fingertips is an important sign of significant pulmonary pathology and should not be overlooked.

Palpation of the skin, particularly on the palmar surface, can reveal pathology. Thickening of the palmar fascia, with associated contracture of the digits (Dupuytren's disease), is common on the ulnar side of the hand in men. Bony palpation, including palpation of the radial styloid and the bones of the carpus, yields specific information regarding disorders of the wrist. In particular, palpation of the scaphoid in the anatomical snuffbox is an important sign of potential injury, particularly a non-displaced fracture (Fig. 2–8). Careful palpation of the hook of the hamate, on the ulnar boarder of the palmar surface of the hand, may suggest injury to this structure. Other important sources of pathology, which may be tender on palpation, include the carpometacarpal joint of the thumb, the ulnar styloid process, the flexor carpi radialis tendon, and the tendons of the extensor pollicis brevis and abductor pollicis longus.

Range of motion of the wrist in flexion, extension, and radial and ulnar deviation should be measured and recorded. Ranges of motion of the fingers at the metacarpophalangeal as well as the distal and proximal interphalangeal joints is also checked. Differences between active and passive ranges of motion may be found and may serve as clues to tendon injuries. In addition, differences in the range of motion of the proximal interphalangeal (PIP) joint, with flexion and extension of the metacarpophalangeal (MP) joint (Bunnell-Littler test), can result from intrinsic contracture.

Other special tests for the hand and wrist include Phalen's test, Tinel's test, the Allen test, and tests for competence of the long finger flexors. Phalen's sign is elicited by having the patient flex the wrist to 45 degrees and wrist is left in this position for about 60 seconds. Reproduction of paraesthesias into the thumb, index, and long fingers is a sensitive but relatively non-specific sign of carpal tunnel syndrome. Tinel's sign is elicited at the wrist by tapping over the median nerve as it enters the carpal tunnel, just proximal to the wrist crease. Radiating pain and paresthesias along the distribution of the median nerve constitutes a positive test. The Allen test is performed by having the patient hold the hand above the level of the heart. The examiner manually exsanguinates the hand or asks the patient to open and close his fist tightly several times, and then manually occludes the ulnar and radial arteries. First one artery and then the other is released and the opposite hand checked for comparison. Delayed or incomplete reperfu-

sion of the hand represents partial obstruction of flow in the involved artery. This test should always be checked before drawing an arterial blood gas from the radial artery. A similar version of the Allen test can also be performed on individual digits.

The status of the flexor digitorum superficialis and the flexor digitorum profundus tendons can be determined for each digit. The flexor digitorum superficialis tendon can be isolated and tested by holding the other fingers in full extension at the distal interphalangeal (DIP) joints. This blocks excursion of the flexor digitorum profundus for the involved digit and leaves only the superficialis to perform flexion of the PIP joint. Only by blocking profundus function can one be certain that the superficialis is functioning; isolated lacerations or ruptures of this tendon are relatively common. The flexor digitorum profundus is tested by holding the PIP joint of the involved digit in full extension. Active flexion of the DIP joint signifies a functioning profundus tendon in that finger (Fig. 2–9).

Careful neurologic examination of the hand involves motor and sensory testing. Sensory testing in the autonomous zones of the median (radial aspect of the volar distal phalanx of the index finger), ulnar (ulnar aspect of the volar distal phalanx of the little finger), and radial (dorsal aspect of the web space between

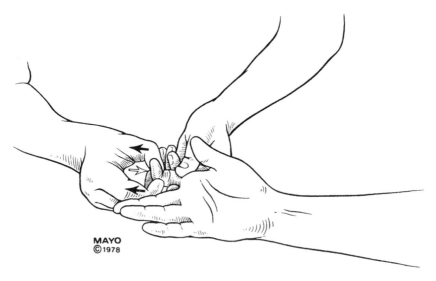

MAYO
©1978

FIGURE 2–9 ■ The integrity of the flexor digitorum profundus is tested by active flexion of the distal interphalangeal joint with the proximal interphalangeal joint held in extension by the examiner.

(Modified from Polley HF, Hunder GG: Rheumatologic Interviewing and Physical Examination of the Joints, ed 2. Philadelphia, WB Saunders Company, 1978, p 142; reprinted by permission.)

the thumb and index finger) nerves is carried out. Two-point discrimination should also be tested whenever a digital nerve injury is suspected. Motor strength testing of the intrinsic muscles of the hand, including the lumbricals, interossei, thenar, and hypothenar groups, as well as the extrinsic wrist and finger flexors and extensors is carried out and recorded. Resisting the temptation to explore lacerations, the experienced clinician can define the structures injured or disrupted in a laceration by carefully evaluating the function of the parts distal to the site of the open wound. Treatment decisions can be based accordingly, rather than on the unreliable identification of proximal and distal nerve and tendon stumps viewed in a field of blood.

PHYSICAL EXAMINATION OF THE LOWER EXTREMITIES

Lumbar Spine

Examination of the low back, as in the neck, elicits findings that are either nonspecific but quite common or very specific for certain conditions or levels of nerve root involvement. Palpation of the lumbar spine commonly reveals areas of tenderness along the lumbar paraspinal muscles or over the posterior superior iliac spine, but does not point to a specific diagnosis. Tenderness directly over the spinous processes, in the trauma patient, may be evidence of a bony fracture. Tenderness to percussion, along the mid-line, is sometimes indicative of an infection of the spine. Tenderness over the buttocks or in the gluteal notch is a relatively common finding in patients with nerve root compression and sciatica. Finally, the trochanteric bursa should be palpated because trochanteric bursitis can sometime coexist with, or mimic, lumbar radiculopathy.

Decrease in the range of motion of the lumbar spine is most easy to elicit in flexion and extension and is a relatively nonspecific finding. Patients with lumbar spinal stenosis frequently have loss of lordosis and have pain on extension of the low back, but often a normal range of forward flexion. Isthmic spondylolisthesis often causes a painful limitation of extension as well. Segmental instability of the lumbar spine may be characterized by a "torturous return from forward flexion," wherein patients have full forward flexion but have difficulty returning from the flexed posi-

tion and may use their hands on their thighs to aid their return to neutral.

A thorough neurologic examination of the lower extremities is essential in evaluating the patient with lumbar spine pathology. Prior to this, however, it is important to evaluate the hip and consider this as a possible source of the patient's complaints. In addition, careful palpation of the distal pulses and evaluation of the quality of the skin for dysvascular changes should be undertaken in the patient with a history of claudication or lumbar radiculopathy. Because intraabdominal and pelvic pathology can cause back pain, the examiner should also be aware that problems such as pancreatitis, abdominal aortic aneurysm, peptic ulcer disease, and ovarian cyst should be considered.

Neurologic examination of the lower extremities begins with evaluation of the patient's gait, and asking the patient to walk on the toes and heels can help elicit subtle weakness in the gastroc-soleus complex and ankle dorsiflexors, respectively. Light touch and pinprick testing for dermatomal sensory loss is carried out. Manual motor testing and testing of the deep tendon reflexes is also performed. Because the presence of a neurologic abnormality is such an important part of the diagnosis of herniated nucleus pulposus, it is important to perform and document a complete neurologic exam and to be careful to pick up subtle abnormalities, particularly in motor strength. In the author's experience, mild weakness of the extensor hallucis longus is the most common neurologic abnormality seen, followed by asymmetry of the ankle jerks.

Nerve root compression caused by disc herniation frequently results in a positive "tension sign." The relevant tension signs are the straight leg raising test and the femoral nerve stretch test. The straight leg raising test is performed with the patient in either the seated or supine position: with the knee extended, the leg is elevated by the examiner. The sciatic nerve does not realize tension until 30 to 35 degrees of elevation of the leg, but between 35 and 70 degrees there is an increasing stretch of the nerve, with increasing hip flexion. The reproduction of leg pain, radiating distal to the knee, and/or paresthesias represents a positive straight leg raising sign and is an important component in the clinical diagnosis of a herniated disc at L4-5 or L5-S1 (Fig. 2–10). The sensitivity of the test can be augmented by dorsiflexing the ankle at the point at which the patient has difficulty with further leg elevation. The femoral nerve stretch test is performed by

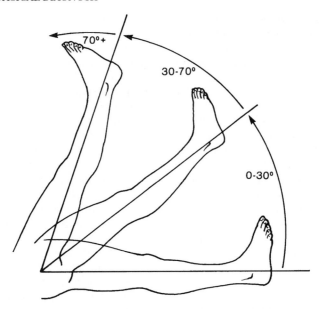

70°+

30-70°

0-30°

FIGURE 2–10 ■ Dynamics of the straight leg raising test. Maximal tension is applied between 30 to 70 degrees of hip flexion, with the knee extended.
(Modified from Borenstein DG, Wiesel SW: Low Back Pain: Medical Diagnosis and Comprehensive Management. Philadelphia, WB Saunders Company, 1989, p 71; reprinted by permission.)

simultaneously extending the hip and flexing the knee. Reproduction of the patient's pain down the anterior thigh is seen in patients with radiculopathy secondary to a herniated disc at L2-3 or L3-4. It is important to note that production of back pain with straight-leg raising is universal in patients with lumbar spine disorders, is non-specific, and does not constitute a positive tension sign.

The Hip

Physical examination of the hip begins with observation of the patient's gait, which should occur on a level surface and with enough room for the patient to take at least 10 to 12 steps. Two common abnormalities of gait seen with hip pathology are an antalgic gait and a Trendelenburg (or gluteal) lurch. In single stance phase the hip abductors maintain the pelvis level, against the force of gravity. If the patient places the hands against a wall and stands on one leg, a normal hip will be able to prevent the pelvis from drooping. Abnormal function of the hip abductors, which may be secondary to mechanical or neurologic causes, will result in

drooping of the contralateral pelvis; this is a positive Trendelenburg sign. Because normal contraction of the hip abductors on single-leg stance results in an increase in the joint reactive force across the hip, the resulting pain can be another reason for a positive Trendelenburg sign. When a patient with a positive Trendelenburg sign walks, the tendency for the contralateral pelvis to droop is countered by swaying the torso over the involved (ipsilateral) hip to prevent contralateral pelvic drooping. This gait pattern is referred to as a "Trendelenburg gait" (Fig. 2–11). "Antalgic gait" refers to the patient's unconscious attempt to shorten the stance phase in order to reduce pain and is nonspecific for hip pathology. Trendelenburg and antalgic gait patterns can coexist.

The most specific finding on palpation of the hip is tenderness directly over the greater trochanter. Between the greater trochanter and the fascia lata is the trochanteric bursa, which is a common source of lateral hip pain. Trochanteric bursitis is usually easily diagnosed by identifying tenderness about the greater trochanter.

Range of motion of the hip is best tested

in the supine position. Normal ranges of motion of the hip include at least 120 degrees of flexion, full extension, 40 to 45 degrees of abduction, 10 to 30 degrees of internal rotation, and 30 to 40 degrees of external rotation. Loss of internal rotation, particularly when accompanied by pain, is a very sensitive indicator of hip pathology, usually degenerative arthritis of the hip. Flexion contracture of the hip, or loss of full extension, often cannot be appreciated unless the lumbar lordosis is eliminated. The Thomas test involves flexion of the contralateral hip and knee to flatten the lordosis, followed by attempting to fully extend the hip; if this test is not performed, a flexion contracture of the hip can be masked by an increase in compensatory lumbar lordosis, thereby allowing the patient to appear to fully extend both hips when supine (Fig. 2–12).

Sensory and manual motor testing of the lower extremity is carried out, and it is essential to remember, in the patient with a complaint of hip pain, that the lumbar spine can be the source of referred or radicular pain. This is particularly true in patients with buttock and posterior thigh complaints, which they frequently describe as "hip" pain.

The Knee

Evaluation of the knee begins with observation of gait and inspection and proceeds to palpation of the bony and soft tissue structures. Testing of active and passive ranges of motion and joint stability is followed by neurologic examination. A number of special tests to identify sources of pathology, such as the menisci, ligaments, and the patella, are then performed.

Gait observation is best performed with the patient wearing a pair of gym shorts and in bare feet. Joint alignment should be observed during gait and in double-leg stance. Varus (bowlegged) and valgus (knock-kneed) malalignment should be identified as well as any tendency toward hyperextension (recurvatum), giving way, or lateral thrusting on stance phase. Palpation of the knee should be performed in both the flexed and extended position, and the knee should be palpated as it is taken through a range of active motion. Retropatellar crepitus is easily appreciated during active or passive knee flexion with the hand over the patella. With the knee extended the suprapatellar pouch is "milked" down to in-

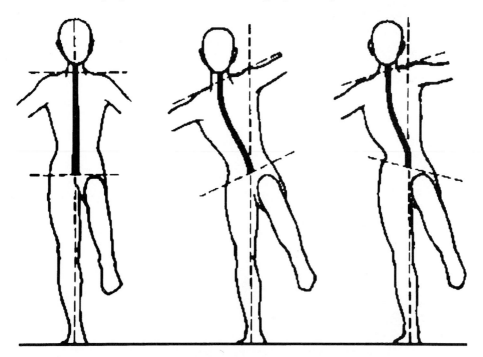

FIGURE 2–11 ■ Diagramatic representation of the Trendelenburg sign and Trendelenburg lurch. *A,* negative Trendelenburg sign, normal gait. *B,* Trendelenburg lurch, but negative Trendelenburg sign. *C,* positive Trendelenburg sign and lurch.
(Modified from Johnston RC, Fitzgerald RH Jr, Harris WH, et al: Clinical and radiographic evaluation of total hip replacement. J Bone Joint Surg 72–A:165, 1990; reprinted by permission.)

crease the volume of any fluid in the main joint space. A transmissible fluid wave between the medial and lateral parapatellar spaces is usually the most sensitive sign of a joint effusion (Fig. 2–13). A ballottable patella is usually not present unless there is a large joint effusion.

Palpation of the medial and lateral joint lines with the knee extended and flexed is performed, and tenderness suggests injury to the menisci. Ecchymosis or tenderness to palpation along the medial or lateral collateral ligaments suggests injury to these structures. Tenderness along the patellar tendon is found in patients with patellar tendinitis or tendon disruption. Pressure over the patella, with the knee extended, is performed, and grinding

A.

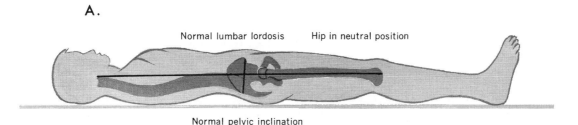

Normal lumbar lordosis   Hip in neutral position

Normal pelvic inclination

B.   Note increased pelvic inclination

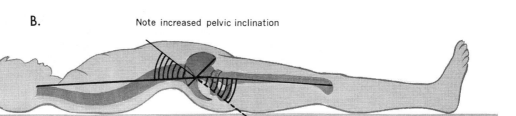

Compensatory lumbar lordosis in flexion contracture of the hip

C.

Opposite hip and knee
are maximally flexed

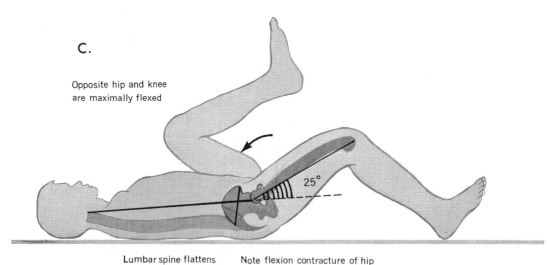

25°

Lumbar spine flattens   Note flexion contracture of hip

FIGURE 2–12 ■ The Thomas test for hip flexion contracture, demonstrating how increased lumbar lordosis can mask a flexion contracture of the hip.

(Modified from Tachdjian MO: Pediatric Orthopedics, ed 2. Philadelphia, WB Saunders Company, 1990, p 28; reprinted by permission.)

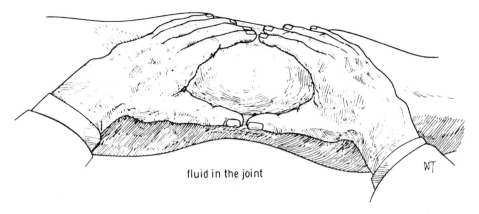

fluid in the joint

FIGURE 2–13 ■ Palpation of a fluid thrill by alternately compressing medial and lateral to the patella, to demonstrate a joint effusion in the knee.

(Modified from Insall JN, Windsor RE, et al: Surgery of the Knee, ed 2. New York, Churchill Livingstone, 1993, p 67; reprinted by permission.)

and pain suggests patellofemoral pathology (Fig. 2–14). The examiner should also attempt to force the patella laterally out of the trochlea of the femur with the knee extended; apprehension and pain suggests a history of recurrent patellar subluxation or dislocation. Palpation about the knee also includes palpation over the subcutaneous bursae, including the prepatellar bursa, the pes anserine bursa, and the superficial infrapatellar bursa—common sources of inflammation and pain.

The collateral and cruciate ligaments are then tested for stability. The results are best compared to those of the opposite knee, as a modest amount of laxity is frequently seen and may not have significance unless it is clearly different from the findings on the opposite side. The medial and lateral collateral ligaments are tested by applying a valgus or varus stress, with the knee flexed to 30 degrees. The most specific test for anterior cruciate ligament (ACL) injury is the Lachman test. With

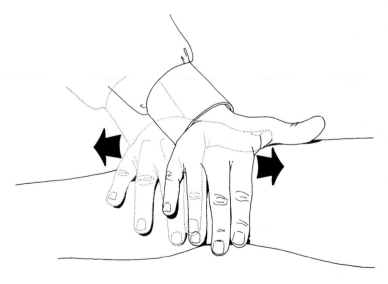

FIGURE 2–14 ■ Compressing the patella against the femoral trochlea will elicit pain and/or crepitation in patients with patellofemoral disorders.

(Modified from Hughston JC, Walsh WM, Puddu G: Patellar Subluxation and Dislocation. Philadelphia, WB Saunders, 1984, p 27; reprinted by permission.)

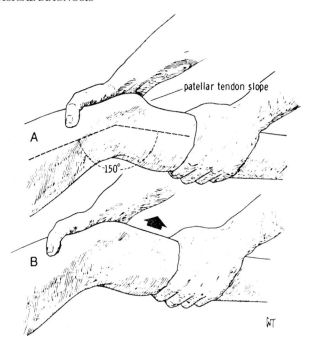

FIGURE 2–15 ■ The Lachman test, performed with the knee in 20 to 30 degrees of flexion.
(Modified from Insall JN, Windsor RE, et al: Surgery of the Knee, ed 2. New York, Churchill Livingstone, 1993, p 75; reprinted by permission.)

the knee flexed to 20 degrees the examiner holds the distal thigh in one hand and applies an anterior stress to the proximal leg with the other. Anterior translation, exceeding that of the other knee, particularly if there is no discrete end point suggests insufficiency of the ACL (Fig. 2–15). The anterior drawer sign, performed by applying an anterior stress to the knee when flexed to 90 degrees, is less sensitive due to the stabilizing effect of the posterior horns of the menisci. The pivot-shift test is a more specific, but less sensitive maneuver for ACL insufficiency. With the leg internally rotated and a mild valgus force applied, the knee is flexed and extended between 0 and 45 degrees. Subluxation of the lateral compartment of the tibia in full extension, which reduces with flexion beyond 20 to 30 degrees and recurs with return to full extension, is diagnostic of anterolateral rotatory instability caused by insufficiency of the anterior cruciate ligament.

Posterior cruciate ligament (PCL) insufficiency is characterized by a posterior drawer sign or by a positive "sag sign." The posterior drawer test is performed with the patient supine and the knee bent to 90 degrees. Appli-cation of a posterior force resulting in posterior translation of the tibia suggests injury to the PCL. A positive sag sign is elicited by flexing the hip and knee to 90 degrees with the patient supine. By holding the foot and allowing gravity to act on the leg, subluxation of the tibial tubercle beyond that seen on the opposite side is a very specific sign for PCL injury.

Measurement of any muscle atrophy and testing of active and passive range of motion is then carried out. Normal individuals have full extension with a very distinct "bounce home" at the extreme of extension, and they have flexion to at least 135 degrees. Loss of a distinct end point on full extension suggests an intra-articular block, commonly a displaced bucket-handle tear of the medial meniscus. Flexion contracture of the knee is common and can be due to many causes. The presence of a flexion contracture should be distinctly sought and recorded. Passive extension that exceeds active range of motion (extensor lag) suggests disruption of the extensor mechanism of the knee, such as rupture of the quadriceps or patellar tendon. Pain on hyperflexion of the knee, particularly in the area of the posterior medial or posterior lateral joint lines, suggests injury to the meniscus, particularly when associated with tenderness to palpation.

Several special tests about the knee are performed to further identify sources of pathology. The apprehension test for patellar dislocation and the patellofemoral grind test have been described. McMurray's test is performed by hyperflexing the knee and applying a valgus stress and external rotation. A palpable or audible click over the medial joint line suggests injury to the medial meniscus, most commonly in its posterior half.

Other helpful tests include the Apley compression and distraction test. The compression test also aids in the diagnosis of a torn meniscus. With the patient prone on the examining table the knee is flexed to 90 degrees. Downward compression on the heel with internal and external rotation increases the force on the meniscus and, if pain is reproduced, suggests a meniscal injury. This test can be simulated by asking the patient to "duckwalk," which, when painful, also suggests a meniscal injury. The distraction test is also performed with the patient prone and the knee flexed to 90 degrees. Stabilizing the thigh with the examiner's knee, the foot is distracted and the leg internally and externally rotated. Pain with this maneuver over the medial or lateral joint line suggests injury to the respective collateral ligament. These two tests, performed in sequence, are designed to help differentiate meniscal from ligamentous pathology.

Foot and Ankle

No other structure in the musculoskeletal system is subjected to the repetitive forces experienced by the foot. These forces are applied—and can create pathology—in every component of the foot, including the skin, subcutaneous tissue, muscles, tendons and ligaments, and bones. Disorders of the foot and ankle are common sequelae of many general medical conditions, the most notorious being diabetes mellitus, and are experienced by individuals of all ages.

Examination of the foot begins with evaluation of the patient's gait. Inspection includes inspection not only of the foot itself, but of the patient's shoes. Many patients, from runners to grandmothers, will report to the doctor with a shopping bag full of shoes and evaluation of these shoes provides, at times, very useful information about abnormal wear patterns and pathology in the foot or leg. Any orthoses routinely worn by the patient should also be evaluated. Palpation, careful neurologic examination, testing for stability, and testing for range of motion are also important parts of the examination.

Evaluation of gait should be performed with the patient shod and then barefoot. Abnormal gait patterns, deformities of the foot that change through the gait cycle, as well as changes in gait with shoeing should be noted.

Inspection of the foot begins with inspection of the shoes. Abnormal patterns of wear are especially important. It is also important to identify shoe types that predispose to pain or deformity of the foot; the relationship between high-heel wear and the development of bunions is only the most obvious of these. Inspection of the foot is perhaps the most important part of the entire examination. Many deformities can be appreciated with inspection alone, including hallux valgus (bunions), bunionette deformity, hammertoes and claw toes, and excessive inversion or eversion of the foot. The foot should be inspected in both the non-weightbearing and weightbearing posture, and differences, specifically in inversion of the heel should be noted. Careful inspection of the skin, particularly in middle-aged and older adults, is essential. Peripheral vascular insufficiency and diabetic neuropathy are common causes of foot complaints and may be misinterpreted by the patient as causing foot pain of a mechanical nature. The dorsalis pedis and posterior tibial pulses should be carefully palpated and recorded. Equally important is inspection and palpation of the skin, color, and temperature, and the presence of hair on the dorsum of the foot and toes should all be assessed. It is helpful at the time of inspection of the foot and skin to proceed to sensory testing. Pinprick and light touch sensation are routinely tested, but it is important to realize that the first sensory modality lost in many patients with diabetes mellitus and peripheral neuropathy is position sense. It is important, therefore, to note that retention of light touch sensation does not by itself constitute a normal sensory examination in the patient with diabetes.

Evaluation of the longitudinal arches is especially important and should be carried out in the weightbearing and non-weightbearing position. A supple flatfoot is characterized by contact of the medial border of the foot with the floor on weightbearing, with restitution of a normal longitudinal arch in the nonweightbearing position. This supple flatfoot is a common developmental condition and is usually

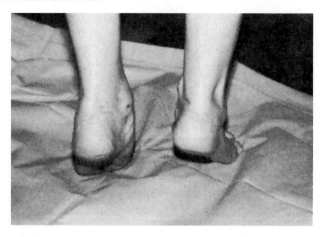

FIGURE 2–16 ■ Loss of active heel inversion, with the patient standing on tiptoes, suggests a rupture of the posterior tibial tendon.

(Modified from Mann RA: Surgery of the Foot, ed 5. St. Louis, CV Mosby Company, 1986, p 477; reprinted by permission.)

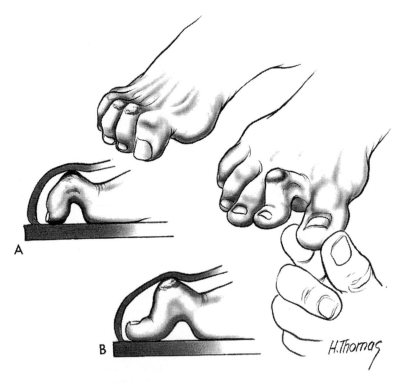

FIGURE 2–17 ■ Claw toes with associated hard corns *(A)* and hammer toes with associated hard corns *(B)*.

(Modified from Jahss MH: Disorders of the Foot. Philadelphia, WB Saunders, 1982, p 113; reprinted by permission.)

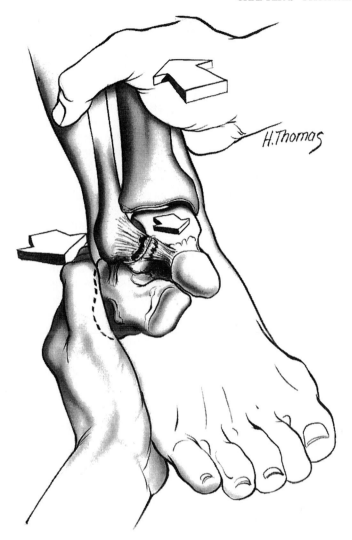

H.Thomas

FIGURE 2–18 ■ The anterior draw test for ankle instability.
(Modified from Jahss MH: Disorders of the Foot. Philadelphia, WB
Saunders, 1982, p 108; reprinted by permission.)

bilateral. New onset or acquired flatfoot in the middle-aged or older adult, particularly with a history of posterior and medial ankle pain in the area of the medial malleolus and posterior tibial tendon, may be evidence of posterior tibial tendon rupture and is important to diagnose as early as possible. Other findings consistent with this diagnosis include loss of active heel inversion when the patient stands on his or her tiptoes (Fig. 2–16) and asymmetrical splaying of the affected foot when viewed from behind, compared to the opposite "too many toes sign."

Bony and soft tissue palpation is carried out. Careful bony palpation allows the examiner to localize the source of pain, which may

be quite vague based solely on the patient's history. Knowledge of the underlying anatomy and careful inspection and palpation of the foot frequently allows one to very accurately arrive at a clinical diagnosis without further testing. Palpation of the malleoli, the head of the talus, the base of the fifth metatarsal, the shafts of each of each of the metatarsals, and the area of the heel pad and plantar fascia is carried out. Fixed deformities, particularly of the forefoot, are assessed, and the presence of skin changes such as corns and calluses or crowding or overlapping of the toes is identified (Fig. 2–17).

Range-of-motion testing of the foot and ankle can be readily carried out, and the results should be compared to the opposite side. Normal ankle dorsiflexion extends to 20 degrees beyond neutral and plantar flexion to 50 degrees. Inversion and eversion occur at the subtalar joint and extend 5 to 10 degrees in each direction. The normal forefoot can adduct 20 degrees and abduct 10 degrees. Motion of the great and lesser toes should also be noted, and fixed deformities such as hammertoes identified. It is important to be aware of the mobility present in the normal great toe metatarsophalangeal (MTP) joint, because loss of this motion is a common source of pain and gait alteration. The first MTP joint has a normal range of flexion of 45 degrees and can dorsiflex from 70 to 90 degrees. The IP joint of the great toe, on the other hand, cannot dorsiflex beyond neutral but is routinely capable of 80 to 90 degrees of plantar flexion. The lesser toes have slightly less motion at the MTP and PIP joints, and loss of motion of the lesser toes is tolerated somewhat better than loss of motion of the great toe.

The final part of the examination is testing for ankle joint stability. The anterior drawer test is designed to test the competence of the anterior talofibular ligament. It is performed by stabilizing the patient's leg, just above the malleoli, with the examiner's hand and applying an anterior stress with the opposite hand, cupping the patient's heel (Fig. 2–18). Any significant anterior translation is usually an abnormal finding, although, as with all stress testing, comparison to the opposite side is mandatory. Straight inversion of the foot and ankle can be performed, with the examiner's thumb placed over the calcaneofibular ligament to test the combined integrity of the anterior talofibular and calcaneofibular ligament. Finally, deltoid ligament instability can be determined, on occasion, by the presence of excessive motion over the deltoid with the application of an eversion stress.

CONCLUSION

Several principles have been stressed in the examination of the patient with a musculoskeletal injury or complaint. The interplay between the patient's history and the physical examination is common to all areas of physical diagnosis, but the musculoskeletal system is unique in the ability of the examiner, in many cases, to look directly at, and palpate, the affected body part. The need to expose the area in question and its contralateral control cannot be overemphasized, as is true for the benefit of observing function of the extremity, particularly gait. Finally, the examiner must bear in mind the possibility that pain in a given area (e.g., shoulder, knee) may be related to pathology in a more proximal region.

The remainder of this text will deal with a variety of conditions; some are relatively trivial, but some are serious or even life threatening. Patients with slipped capital femoral epiphysis presenting as medial knee pain or with metastatic disease at C5 presenting as shoulder pain are seen in emergency rooms and primary care settings on a daily basis. A careful approach to physical examination adhering to the above principles will facilitate accurate diagnosis and appropriate treatment.

SUGGESTED READINGS

Tachdjian MO: Pediatric Orthopaedics. The Orthopaedic Examination, pp 4–58. Philadelphia, WB Saunders, 1990.

Hopperfeld S: Physical Examination of the Spine and Extremities. New York, Appleton-Century-Crofts, 1976.

Hopperfeld S: Orthopaedic Neurology. A Diagnostic Guide to Neurologic Levels. Philadelphia, JB Lippincott Company, 1997.

Ritchie Jr. Miller, Harner CD: History and Physical Examinations in Knee Surgery, pp 253–274. Fu FH, Harner CD, Vince KG (eds.) Baltimore, Williams & Wilkins, 1996.

Boyes JH: Bunnell's Surgery of the Hand. Examination of the Hand, pp 108–129. Philadelphia, JB Lippincott Company, 1970.

Jahss MH: Examinations in Disorders of the Foot, pp 81–102. Jahss MH (ed). Philadelphia, WB Saunders, 1982.

Chapter 3

Skeletal Trauma

Peter I. Kenmore and John N. Delahay

Skeletal trauma, for the subject of discussion, can be divided into three major groups of injuries to the musculoskeletal system:

> Fractures
> Dislocations
> Fracture/Dislocations

A *fracture,* by definition, is a disruption in the continuity of cortical and/or cancellous bone. A *dislocation* is a disruption of the normal articulating anatomy of a joint. Dislocations can either be a complete disruption of the normal anatomy or a partial dislocation, in which case the term *subluxation* is used. A *fracture/dislocation* is a fracture occurring in a periarticular location that results in a subluxation or dislocation of the adjacent joint.

FRACTURES

Fracture Descriptors

A number of different terms can be used to more accurately describe the configuration and features of any given fracture. These descriptors are as follows:

1. *Open versus closed.* A closed fracture is one in which the skin is intact over the fracture site and an open fracture is one in which the skin is not intact.
2. *Simple versus comminuted.* A simple fracture is one in which there are only two major fragments and one fracture line. A comminuted fracture is one in which

there are multiple fragments of bone and multiple fracture lines.
3. *Complete versus incomplete.* "Complete" essentially means that the fracture line goes completely across the bone. Incomplete fractures, most typically seen in children, have a fracture line that only crosses one cortex of the bone involved.

Fracture Deformities

A fracture can be deformed in any one of three possible planes. Classic deformations are described as follows (Fig. 3–1):

1. *Displacement.* Translation of the two fragments in relation to each other in one or more planes. Traditionally, displacement refers to the position of the distal fragment in relation to the assumed stationary proximal fragment. Specific types of displacement include *overriding,* where the two fragments are shortened in relation to one another and *distraction* where essentially the bone ends are pulled apart.
2. *Angulation.* This occurs when the two fracture fragments are not aligned and an angular deformity is present. Alignment means that the axes of the proximal and distal fragments are parallel to each other and the joint above and below are in the normal (parallel) relationship. Angulation is typically defined by the direction in which the apex of the angle points—medial, lateral, dorsal, volar, etc.

Types of Displacement

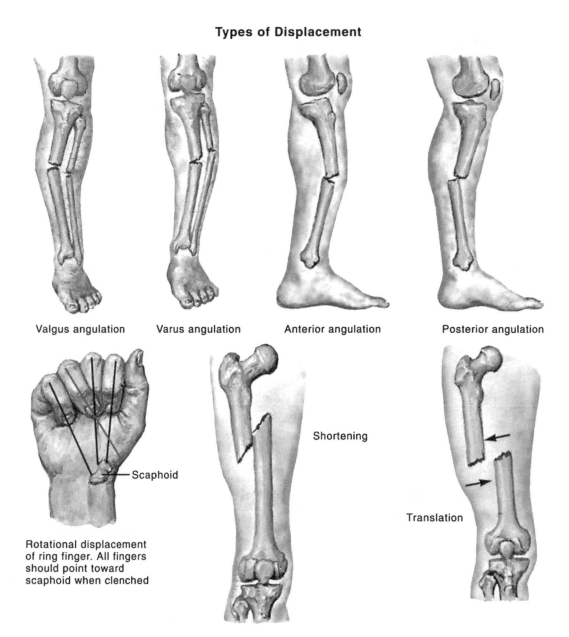

FIGURE 3–1 ■ *A,* Angulation is described by the direction in which the apex of the fracture is pointing. *B,* Displacement is defined as the position of the distal fragment in relation to the proximal fragment. *C,* Rotation is particularly problematic in the hand.

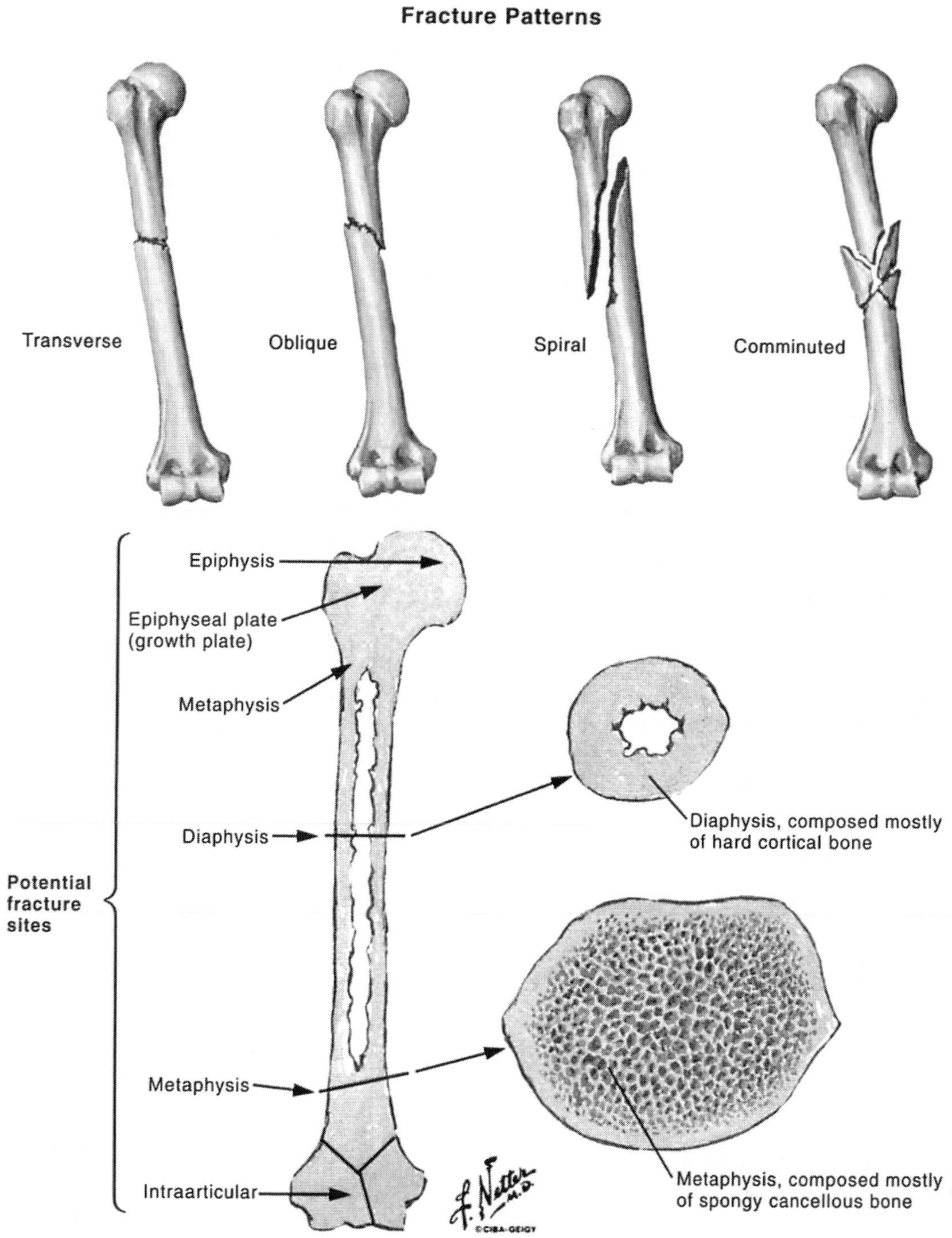
Fracture Patterns
Transverse
Oblique
Spiral
Comminuted
Epiphysis
Epiphyseal plate
(growth plate)
Metaphysis
Diaphysis
Potential
fracture
sites
Metaphysis
Intraarticular
Diaphysis, composed mostly
of hard cortical bone
Metaphysis, composed mostly
of spongy cancellous bone
F. Netter M.D.
©CIBA-GEIGY

FIGURE 3–2 ■ *Top,* Fracture patterns. *Bottom,* Characteristics of long bone at various fracture sites. (From Heckman JD: Fractures: Emergency care and complications. Clin Symp 43(3):4, 1991; © Copyright 1996. CIBA–GEIGY Corporation. Reprinted with permission from the Clinical Symposia illustrated by Frank Netter, MD. All rights reserved.)

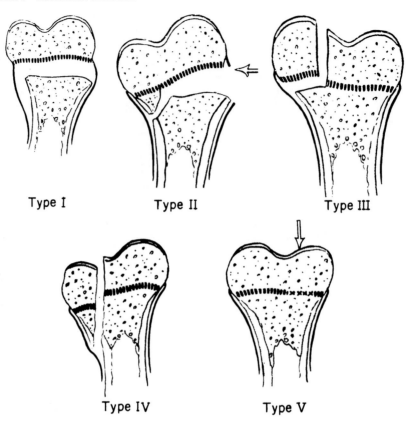

Type I   Type II   Type III

Type IV   Type V

FIGURE 3–3 ■ Salter classification of epiphyseal plate fractures. Type I: separation of epiphysis. Type II: fracture-separation of epiphysis. Type III: fracture of part of epiphysis. Type IV: *A,* fracture of epiphysis and epiphyseal plate; *B,* bony union causing premature closure of plate. Type V: *C,* crushing of epiphyseal plate; *D,* premature closure of plate on one side with resultant angular deformity.

(From Gartland J: Fundamentals of Orthopaedics, ed 3, Philadelphia, WB Saunders Company, 1987, p 90, reprinted by permission.)

3. *Rotation.* This is present when there is a torsional relationship between the two fracture fragments.

Fracture Patterns

A number of different fracture patterns have been described. (Figs. 3–2 to 3–4). They include:

1. *Transverse*
2. *Spiral*
3. *Oblique*
4. *Impacted or compressed*
5. *Avulsion*
6. *Complex*

Fracture Mode of Loading

The mechanical environment creating a fracture offers a great deal of information as to the mechanism of injury and the extent of that injury. For that reason, biomechanical analyses have been performed to more clearly elucidate the fracture pattern and such specific modes of loading as:

1. *Bending loading* produces a transverse fracture
2. *Torsional loading* produces a spiral fracture
3. *Axial loading* produces a compression or impacted fracture
4. *Tensile loading* produces an avulsion fracture

5. *Combined loading* such as bending and axial loading, which together produce an oblique fracture.

The significance of fracture patterns is that they suggest the amount of force that was applied; hence, an extrapolation can be made to the amount of soft tissue damage to be anticipated.

Soft Tissues

As mentioned above, a number of soft tissues can be damaged. They include the periosteum, the vascular tree, nerves, muscles, tendons,

and ligaments, and the types of injury involving them are delineated as follows:

1. *Vascular injury.* A relatively uncommon event when associated with fractures. When it occurs, it is always an emergent situation. The most common vascular injury is a compartment syndrome. Increased pressure within a fascial compartment can cause myonecrosis in a relatively short period of time. In the front of the leg, for example, a compartment with the following boundaries exists: the tibia, the syndesmotic membrane, the fibula, and the fascia overlying the tibialis anterior muscle. Since

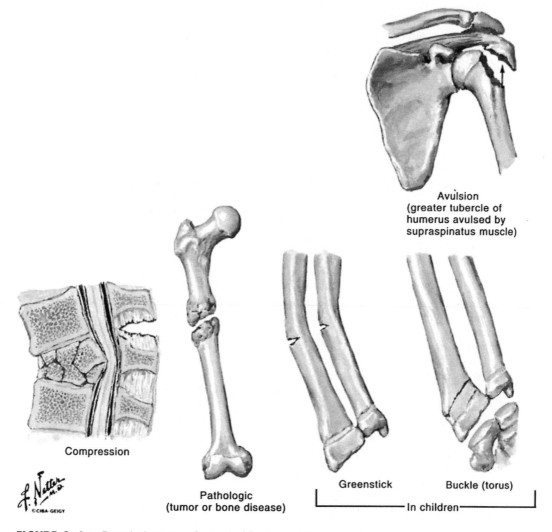

Avulsion
(greater tubercle of humerus avulsed by supraspinatus muscle)

Compression

Pathologic
(tumor or bone disease)

Greenstick   Buckle (torus)

In children

FIGURE 3–4 ■ Descriptive terms for typical fracture patterns.

(From Heckman JD: Fractures: Emergency care and complications. Clin Symp 43(3):7, 1991; © Copyright 1996. CIBA–GEIGY Corporation. Reprinted with permission from the Clinical Symposia illustrated by Frank Netter, MD. All rights reserved.)

none of these four boundaries can be stretched, the contents of the compartment—that is, the tibialis anterior muscle among others—will necrose from increased pressure due to an increase in fluid content, occurring after trauma. This can cause myonecrosis in a relatively short period of time. The diagnosis of this syndrome is mandatory. Clinical findings and evaluation methods such as tenderness, pain with passive stretch, and compartmental pressure monitoring assist in diagnosis. Once the diagnosis is confirmed, immediate fasciotomy of the compartment in question is required.

2. *Arterial injury.* Because the vessels are elastic and are able to get "out of the way" of the oncoming bone this is even less common. The vessels can be damaged when they are either inelastic or fixed by soft tissue structures. The most frequent injury is an intramural hematoma in which the classic signs of arterial injury are usually present. Because of the irreparable damage to the vessel wall, a vein graft or prosthesis is usually required for repair. Injury to the artery is classically associated with several specific fractures involving such sites as the clavicle, the supracondylar region of the elbow (especially in children), the femoral shaft, and the area around the knee.

3. *Nerve damage.* Similarly, a nerve can be damaged in association with a fracture or dislocation. Typically, the nerve is either compressed, contused, or stretched. Classic examples include radial nerve injury secondary to fractures of the distal humerus and sciatic nerve injury following posterior fracture dislocations of the hip. The classic grades of neural injury are:

a. *Neuropraxia.* Death of the axon does not occur. The condition is generally due to pressure or contusion and usually improves by itself in a few weeks. The nerve is anatomically intact and physiologically nonfunctional.

b. *Axonotmesis.* An anatomic disruption of the axon in its sheath. Improvement follows regeneration, the axon growing at a slow rate of 1 mm a day along the existing axonal sheath.

c. *Neurotmesis.* An anatomic disruption of the nerve itself. Surgical repair is required if recovery is to be anticipated.

4. *Muscle and tendon.* It goes without saying that with any fracture or dislocation there is always some associated muscle damage. The extent of this damage and the results will vary depending on the site in question. Myositis ossificans is a specific complication of muscle damage in which heterotopic bone forms within the damaged muscle. The quadriceps and brachialis are specifically predisposed to develop this complication.

5. *Ligament.* The strength of ligaments is constant throughout life. Certain injuries occurring about the joints can damage the ligaments supporting the joints.

Considering the multiplicity of tissues involved in skeletal trauma, age has been shown to be an important determinant in the results of load application. At any given age, the "weak link"—the first structure to fail—varies; it could be bone, ligament, or cartilage growth plates. Once the growth plate closes, however, the ligament is the most likely structure to fail. Ligamentous strength, it has already been noted, is constant throughout life. With aging, there is a decrease in cancellous bone volume and an increase in cortical bone porosity. With increasing age, therefore, bone becomes weaker; hence, cartilage and ligamentous injury are less likely and bone injury more likely. This means that the same mode of loading can produce a different injury pattern depending on the age of the patient. The same force, such as a tackle in football or a blow by an automobile on the outer side of the knee, is likely to cause a fracture through the distal femoral growth plate in a 12-year-old, a tear of the medial and anterior cruciate ligaments in a college football player, and a compression fracture of the lateral tibial plateau in a 70-year-old man.

Fractures: Special Types

A number of "special" fractures have been described in the literature. They are defined as follows:

1. *Incomplete fractures.* An incomplete fracture, typical in a child, is one that traverses only a portion of the bone. Two variations have been described:
   a. *Greenstick fracture.* This occurs on the tension side of the bone and involves the diaphysis or cortical bone.
   b. *Torus or buckle fracture.* Known by either name, this occurs on the compression side of bending and involves cancellous bone.
2. *Stress fractures.* These are fractures resulting from repetitive loading—each load being below the endurance limit, but summated to produce a level of force that indeed causes a fracture. These injuries are typical in the proximal tibia, the second metatarsal, and the femoral neck. They may heal well if the cause of the force ceases soon enough—that is, if the patient stops running for a period of time.
3. *Pathologic fractures.* These are fractures that occur through abnormal or diseased bone. Among the more common examples are those that occur due to tumor or metastatic sites in bone, due to previously infected bone, or due to metabolically involved bone such as that resulting from osteoporosis.
4. *Physeal fractures.* In children, a fracture through the cartilaginous growth plate is a common event. Thanks to the Salter-Harris classification system, such injuries have been more precisely characterized. It is important to remember that physeal fractures heal very rapidly, but they may be complicated by complete or incomplete growth arrest, producing shortening or angular deformity of the limb.
5. *Intra-articular fractures.* These enter a joint and disrupt the joint surface and its articular cartilage. Intra-articular fractures can specifically be complicated by joint stiffness and/or the development of premature arthritis.
6. *Pediatric fractures.* These have a number of special features, which are discussed in Chapter 6.

Fracture Healing

The biology of fracture healing is not particularly complex and parallels that of any nonossified tissue. Essentially, fracture healing occurs in three phases (Fig. 3–5):

1. *Vascular phase* This begins at the time of insult and proceeds through the development of a hematoma. This hematoma will then be infiltrated by cellular elements, which in turn lay down collagen and cause hematoma organization. This is followed by a vascularization step, when the organized hematoma is vascularized by small arterial twigs. The end result of the vascular phase is the development of a soft callous.
2. *Metabolic phase.* This stage begins about 4 to 6 weeks after the injury. During this period, the soft callous is reworked by a number of specific cellular elements to produce a firm, hard callous satisfactory for meeting the mechanical demands placed upon the fracture in the early phase. There are certain biochemical changes specifically in pH and oxygen tension that manipulate the environment during this phase of fracture healing.
3. *Mechanical phase.* This phase begins once a hard callous is present, which is then manipulated according to the rules of Wolff's law. Essentially, mechanical stress is required to produce skeletal remodeling during this phase and ultimately to produce a solid, mechanically strong bone.

Evaluation of the Patient with Skeletal Trauma

A great deal can be said about the evaluation of any surgical patient—much more than the scope of this chapter will allow. A number of specific points relative to the orthopedic patient are listed as follows:

1. *History of injury.* The mechanism of injury and the mode of application are frequently important to determine additional injury.
2. *Occupation of the patient.* Taking this into account is frequently helpful in planning rehabilitation and recuperative efforts once the fracture has been managed.
3. *Activity level prior to injury.* This will frequently mandate the type of treatment given for a specific injury.

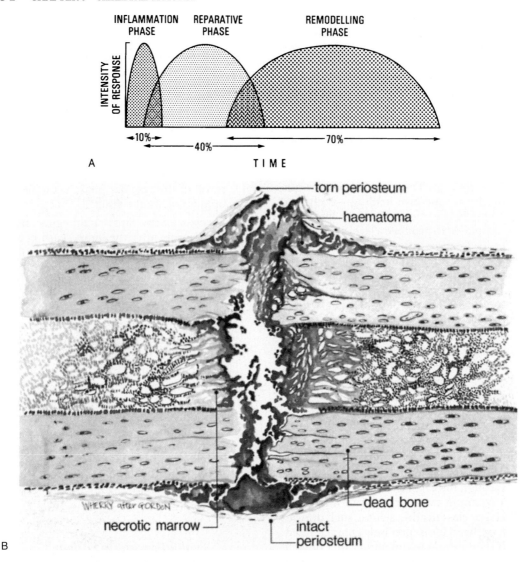

FIGURE 3–5 ■ Phases of fracture healing. *A,* An approximation of the relative amounts of time devoted to inflammation, reparative, and remodelling phases in fracture healing. *B,* The initial events involved in fracture healing of long bone. The periosteum is torn opposite the point of impact and, in many instances, is intact on the other side. There is an accumulation of hematoma beneath the periosteum and between the fracture ends. There is necrotic marrow and dead bone close to the fracture line. *Illustration continued on opposite page.*

(From Cruess RL: Healing of bone, tendon, and ligament. *In* Rockwood CA Jr, Green DP [eds]: Fractures in Adults, ed 2, vol 1. Philadelphia, JB Lippincott, 1984, pp 148-150; reprinted by permission.)

4. *Deformity and swelling.* These must be carefully evaluated physically so that complications can be avoided.

5. *Neurovascular status.* It is imperative that the neurovascular status of the extremity be carefully evaluated, such that

long-term or permanent sequelae can be avoided. Similarly, it is critical that the neurovascular integrity of the extremity—or lack thereof—be documented.

6. *Integrity of the skin.* This is an absolute.

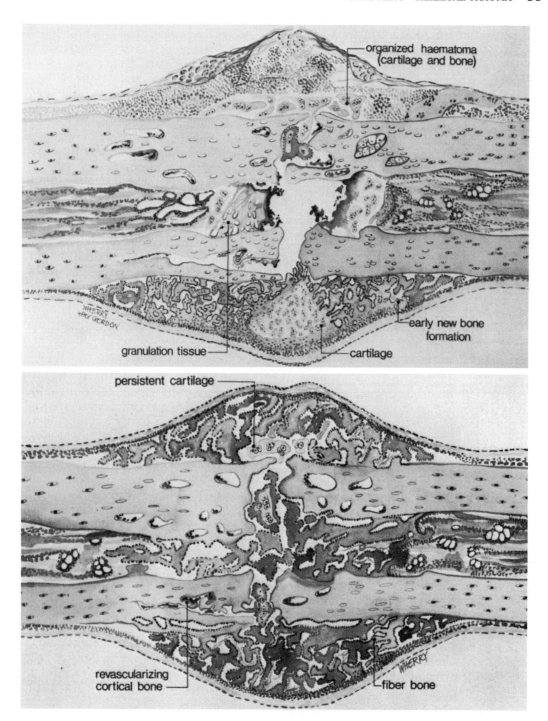

organized haematoma
(cartilage and bone)

early new bone
formation

granulation tissue

cartilage

persistent cartilage

revascularizing
cortical bone

fiber bone

FIGURE 3–5 ■ *Continued. C,* Early repair. There is organization of the hematoma, early primary new bone formation in subperiosteal regions, and cartilage formation in other areas. *D,* At a later stage in the repair, early immature fiber bone is bridging the fracture gap. Persistent cartilage is seen at points most distant from ingrowing capillary buds. In many instances, these are surrounded by young new bone.

(From Cruess RL: Healing of bone, tendon, and ligament. *In* Rockwood CA Jr, Green DP [eds]: Fractures in Adults, ed 2, vol 1. Philadelphia, JB Lippincott, 1984, pp 148-150; reprinted by permission.)

Great care needs to be taken to be sure that there is no violation of the skin in the area of the fracture site.

Fractures: The Principles of Treatment

All fractures essentially mandate that two basic goals be accomplished in their treatment: (1) reduction and (2) maintenance of that reduction. Different techniques may be used for achieving these two goals. First, the reduction of a fracture can be accomplished by closed manipulative methods, by surgical open reduction, or through the application of traction. Following reduction, the fracture site must be immobilized so that the fracture will heal in the optimum position. Immobilization can be achieved with external methods such as casts, splints, and external fixators; with internal methods, using various devices such as screws, plates, and intramedullary rods; or through the maintenance of the patient in traction (Fig. 3–6).

Orthopedic Emergencies

There are relatively few orthopedic problems that mandate immediate intervention. However, those that do exist, truly represent emergent situations. They are open fractures, dislocations of major joints, and fractures associated with vascular injury.

Complications of Fractures

There are a number of complications that can occur following fractures and joint dislocations. These include:

1. *Problems of union*
   a. *Malunion.* Defined as healing in poor position for function.
   b. *Delayed union.* A fracture that has not healed in the usual statistical time frame.
   c. *Nonunion.* A fracture that has not healed and will not heal because it has lost its "biologic drive" (pseudarthrosis).
      A number of reasons can be found for why fractures do not heal. Excessive motion, infection, steroids, radiation, age, nutritional status, and devascularization locally have all been implicated in the delay of healing.

The worst case scenario typically involves skeletal nonunion. If a bone fails to heal, surgical intervention for stabilization is frequently required. In addition to stabilization, biological stimulation will be necessary to make the fracture heal. Usually this is accomplished through the application of bone graft material; however, there are several centers that use electrical stimulation techniques. Most physicians have discarded these techniques as ineffective.

2. *Stiffness and loss of motion.* These commonly occur following many types of fractures—especially intra-articular fractures, in which arthrofibrosis is known to occur. Additional problems such as bony blocks, "joint mice," nerve palsies, and posttraumatic arthritis may only add to this problem.

3. *Infection.* Open fractures are most vulnerable to subsequent sepsis. Closed fractures that have been treated operatively are certainly at risk. The use of implants increases the risk of infection simply because they provide a substrate for the microcolonization of certain bacteria. These bacteria have the unique ability to sequester themselves under a slime layer called the "glycocalyx," which essentially makes them inaccessible both to culture and antimicrobial agents. In addition, the presence of necrotic bone only heightens the risk.

4. *Myositis ossificans.* This problem, previously mentioned under the heading of "Muscle and tendon" trauma, typically is the development of heterotopic bone in certain muscle groups.

5. *Avascular necrosis.* Because of the tenuous and frequently retrograde blood flow in certain regional areas, several specific types of fractures are complicated by necrosis of bone. Bone segments at risk are the head of the femur, the dome of the talus, and the proximal pole of the scaphoid.

6. *Implant failure.* The use of many metallic implants places certain fractures at risk. Because of the high fatigue loading of these implants, their use establishes a "race"—between the fracture healing and the implant failing. If the implant fails, salvage is frequently a significant clinical problem.

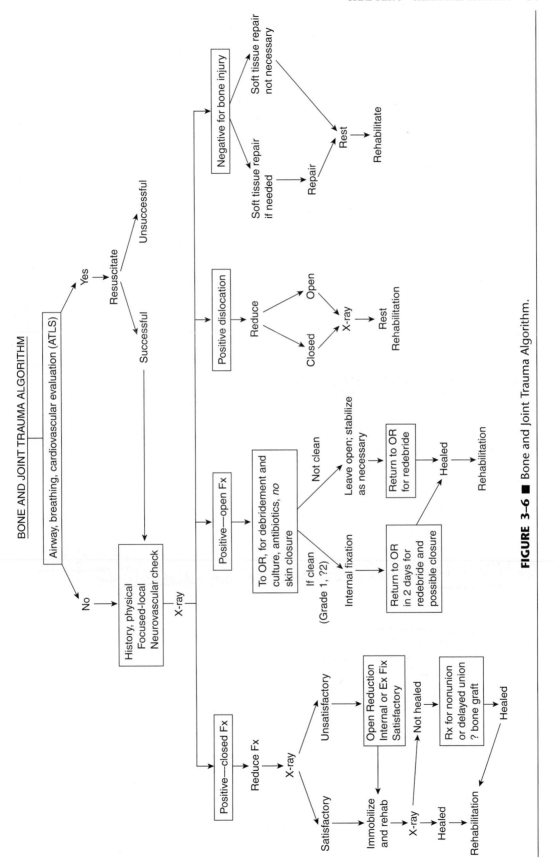

FIGURE 3–6 ■ Bone and Joint Trauma Algorithm.

7. *Reflex sympathetic dystrophy.* This unusual and disastrous complication is typically seen following trivial trauma in a predisposed patient, who then develops abnormal sympathetic tone. The mechanism for the development of symptoms may be associated with a partial nerve injury or contusion. The patients develop an exquisitely painful tender extremity and present a management disaster. Prognosis depends on early recognition of the syndrome and timely initiation of countermeasures such as sympathetic blocks. Stellate ganglion blocks are used for involvement of the upper extremity, whereas epidural blocks and lumbar sympathetic blocks are used in the lower extremity. Early aggressive physical therapy and return to normal function are key to the rehabilitation of patients with these difficult complications.

FRACTURES AND DISLOCATIONS BY REGION: THE UPPER EXTREMITY

The Shoulder Region

The physician must keep in mind that the purpose of the bones and joints of the upper extremity is primarily that of putting the hand where the patient needs it—that is, allowing the hand to do its work.

1. *Fractures of the clavicle.* The clavicle is the first bone to ossify, and it does so by intramembranous ossification. Fractures of the clavicle are very common in children and occur either by direct trauma or a fall on the outstretched hand. Fractures of the clavicle in children heal well. The usual treatment consists of a figure-of-eight brace or bandage that holds the shoulders back and tends to reduce the clavicle. Anatomic reduction is absolutely unnecessary and not practical. If a sling gives the child sufficient comfort, that is perfectly good treatment. In a child, a callous sufficient to provide immobilization and relieve pain will be present in 2 to 3 weeks; shortly thereafter, normal activities are generally possible. The biggest dangers are overtreatment or a rigid type of bandage that interferes with the circulation of the extremity.

   In the adult, fractures of the clavicle require more force than they do in children. Therefore, soft tissue injuries may simultaneously occur. Because of the proximity of the subclavian vessel behind the clavicle and the proximity of the brachial plexus, a careful neurovascular evaluation is imperative. Treatment usually is conservative, using the figure-of-eight brace or perhaps only a sling. The patient must be told at the time of the fracture that a "bump" or swelling may be noticed after healing has occurred; the treatment is usually not influenced by this anticipated event. Not all clavicular fractures heal primarily. Rarely, due to nonunion, it becomes necessary to perform an open reduction and internal fixation employing either a plate or an intramedullary rod. In these cases, bone graft is often added. The indications for surgical treatment are few. The physician must remember that complete healing of a fractured clavicle in the adult will frequently take 3 months or more. An open fracture will require operative debridement. Occasionally, the skin is "tented" over a spike of bone, and an open reduction, just before the skin is pierced by the underlying bone, is warranted. Distal fractures of the clavicle—that is, lateral to the coracoclavicular ligaments—will require an open reduction internal fixation, if displaced (Fig. 3–7).

2. *Fractures of the proximal humerus.* Fractures just distal the head of the humerus—the so-called "surgical neck" of the humerus—are extremely common in elderly osteoporotic bone. Healing of these fractures, even with some displacement, is rarely a problem, but the resulting shoulder stiffness may severely impair the older patient. This stiff and painful shoulder is often referred to as an "adhesive capsulitis." Therefore, treatment of the elderly, with this type of fracture, is directed toward early mobilization after a short period of immobilization; several days is usually adequate for initial pain relief. Codman's exercises are usually begun after the first week. These simple pendulum exercises are done with the arm held in what is referred to as a "collar and cuff" or sling, using the weight of the arm itself as a quasitraction mechanism. Codman's exercises are performed by the patient

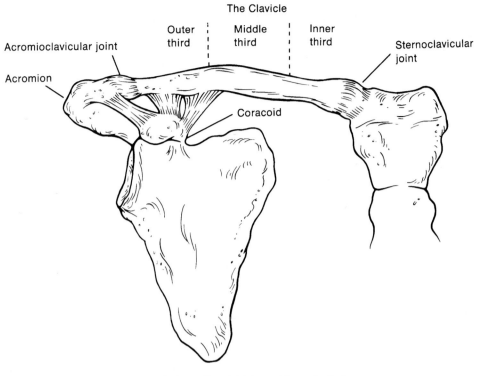

FIGURE 3–7 ■ The clavicle and its articulations.

holding on to a table or other steady object with the good hand, and bending 90 degrees at the waist while allowing the injured extremity to hang straight down—hence, employing the pull of gravity. This maneuver alone is frequently adequate to minimize shoulder stiffness.

An entirely different injury is seen in the younger patient. Although the pattern may be the same, the mechanism and force vary greatly. The high-energy fracture of the head of the humerus seen mostly in younger adults is frequently due to vigorous sports or motor vehicle accidents and high-velocity falls. These injuries are often combined with dislocations of the shoulder (described below). Intra-articular fractures of the head of the humerus present a significant problem. The Neer classification (Fig. 3–8), while not perfect, is nevertheless the best guide we have for treatment of these injuries. Neer pointed out that there are four segments of the proximal humerus: (1) the actual articular cartilage covered head, (2) the shaft, (3) the greater tuberosity, and (4) the lesser tuberosity. Any of these fragments that are separated a cen-

timeter or more from the others, or that are tilted by 40 degrees are considered as a separate Neer fragment. Generally speaking, if conservative treatment is not productive of an adequate reduction in a two- or three-part fracture, internal fixation by means of a wire suture or pin is often elected. A four-part fracture, or one in which the head fragment is actually split, is often treated by the insertion of a humeral head prosthesis replacing the broken segments (Fig. 3–9). Inherent to all treatment protocols is an aggressive rehabilitation program to regain shoulder motion. Therefore, fixation should be strong enough and rigid enough to allow early motion to begin.

3. *Glenohumeral dislocation.* Dislocation of the shoulder is a common event. Typically, the vast majority of these dislocations are anterior, with the humeral head moving anterior to the genoid. They result when the arm is forcefully abducted and externally rotated—a frequent position, unfortunately, in contact sports. This is an extremely painful condition requiring early reduction of the dislocation. If a fracture, such as of the

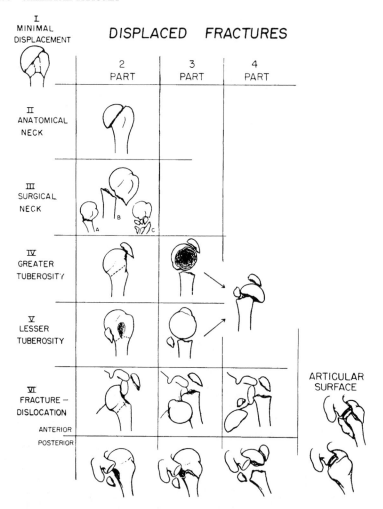

FIGURE 3–8 ■ The Neer classification of proximal humeral fractures.
(From Neer CS II: Displaced proximal humeral fractures. I. Classification and evaluation. J Bone Joint Surg 52-A:1077-1089, 1970; reprinted by permission.)

greater tuberosity, coexists with the dislocation, reduction is even more urgent. The patient presents in the emergency room with an obvious "squared" silhouette of the upper arm (the normal roundness of the humeral head being absent). A careful neurological and vascular exam should be performed, with the appropriate x-rays taken; the anteroposterior and the axillary are the requisite views. Reduction is then accomplished by one of several techniques, most of which employ traction and countertraction with the patient relaxed. Relaxation is usually obtained in the emergency room by the intravenous administration of Valium or Versed, in addition to a narcotic analgesic. Of course, medication must be available in the event it is necessary to reverse the effect of these narcotics. The neurological and vascular exams are then repeated. It must be stated that even before reduction, the so-called "autonomous zone" of the axillary nerve, lateral to the shoulder, must be included in this neurological check. The immediate decrease in pain is striking once the shoulder is reduced. A sling and swathe are generally adequate to immobilize and rest the shoulder; a postreduction x-ray should be taken.

If a couple of students, for example,

should find themselves on a mountain-climbing adventure and one of them were to sustain a shoulder dislocation in a fall, it would be quite reasonable with civilization being several hours away, for the other student to reduce the shoulder without the assistance of an x-ray.

Posterior shoulder dislocations account for only four percent of all dislocations and usually occur in patients during seizures, though occasionally they may occur in such sporting events as wrestling.

The duration of immobilization is not generally agreed upon. The classic thought, that a month of immobilization will decrease the likelihood of a recurrent dislocation, has, unfortunately, not proven to be the case. The percentage of shoulder dislocations that recur after the first dislocation essentially depends on the age at which the first event occurs. In the late teens and early twenties the likelihood of a recurrence is very high (80% to 90%). In patients over 50 years old, the likelihood of a recurrence is

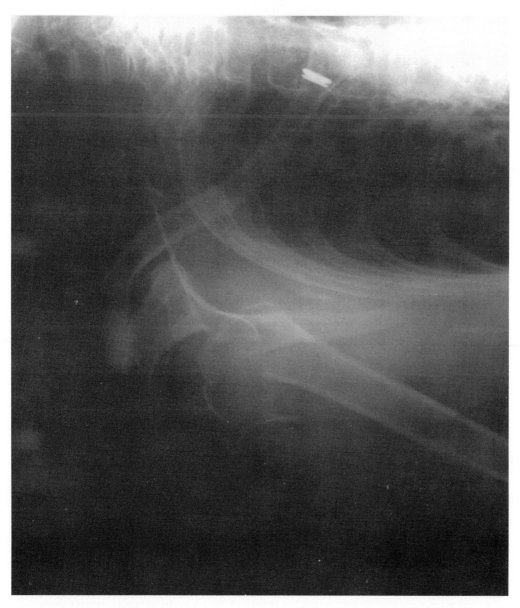

FIGURE 3–9 ■ Four-part humeral fracture. *Illustration continued on following page.*

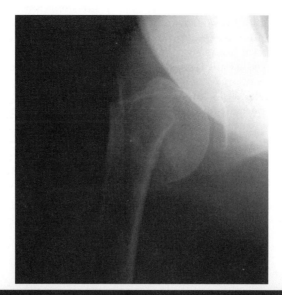

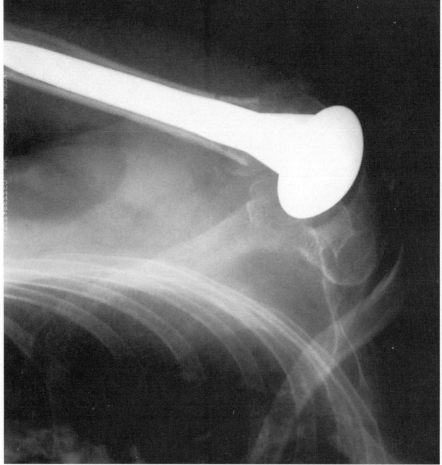

FIGURE 3–9 ■ *Continued*

lower (30% to 40%); however, shoulder stiffness is a concern and therefore shoulder motion should be instituted early.

In the case of recurrent dislocations in a young person, surgical reconstruction is best performed on an elective basis. Repair of the anterior shoulder capsule and glenoid labrum is usually required.

Rotator cuff tears may occur as part of the dislocation or fracture/ dislocation of the shoulder. Rotator cuff structural integrity is imperative for good shoulder function. More will be discussed on the rotator cuff in the chapter on the shoulder.

4. *Acromioclavicular separation.* Also called "separated shoulder" or "acromioclavicular dislocation." It is essentially a ligamentous injury involving the distal clavicle and the acromion. Such separations are frequently sports injuries sustained in a fall on the "point of the shoulder" and can be divided into three classes. Grade I is a sprain of the acromioclavicular ligaments. There is tenderness in that joint on heavy palpation and the treatment is rest until the pain resolves. A Grade II injury is a more pronounced deformity of the joint with some prominence of the distal clavicle felt above the level of the acromion. A complete rupture of the acromioclavicular ligament is seen. The x-ray, taken with the patient standing and the arm hanging down, with or without weight on it, shows the clavicle to be riding higher, but still in some contact with the acromion. Treatment is almost always conservative. Immobilization, as long as it is needed for pain control, and then gentle active motion are appropriate. Full function is usually restored in about two months. Grade III acromioclavicular separations result from a tear, not only of the acromioclavicular ligaments, but also the coracoclavicular ligaments (conoid and trapezoid ligaments). The muscles that insert on the clavicle tend to pull it up superiorly, resulting in an obvious deformity. This injury may be quite painful but, relatively speaking, is nowhere near as painful, dangerous, or requiring of any emergent treatment as a dislocated shoulder. Many of these injuries are treated conservatively, and one can assure the patient that in two months the pain will be gone; the bump, however, will remain permanently. Function, by 2 months, should be quite normal. Open reduction and internal fixation may be appropriate for selected patients to eliminate deformity and possibly improve throwing strength (Fig. 3–10).

5. *Fractures of the shaft of the humerus.* Humeral shaft fractures are common, and their patterns vary. Displacement is generally due to eccentric muscular pull with action of the supraspinatus, pectoralis major, and the deltoid determining the displacement of the proximal fragment (Fig. 3–11). The long muscles determine the displacement if the fracture is below the deltoid insertion. Treatment of the humeral shaft fractures has traditionally been conservative; options include coaptation plaster splints, which serve as a functional brace, as popularized by Sarmiento. The brace is a plastic, prefabricated device, usually worn 6 to 10 weeks. Its use permits excellent function of the hand while healing progresses.

In fractures at the junction of the middle and distal third of the humerus, the radial nerve is vulnerable to injury. Radial nerve function must be documented. Fortunately, most of these nerve injuries are neuropraxias; hence, excellent recovery can be expected. In more comminuted fractures of the humeral shaft, open reduction and internal fixation are currently popular. The use of plates versus intramedullary locked rods is a current controversy.

Elbow and Forearm

1. *Supracondylar fractures in children.* This notorious fracture in children presents a "mine field" for the orthopaedic surgeon. Typically, in the early stages, one must be vigilant in evaluating the child for vascular compromise, specifically compartment syndromes. Later these can result in a Volkmann's contracture. Angular deformity resulting from growth plate damage occasionally may be seen. In an effort to minimize these disastrous complications, aggressive early closed reduction and percutaneous pinning currently form the treatment of choice. Alternatives such as open reduction or

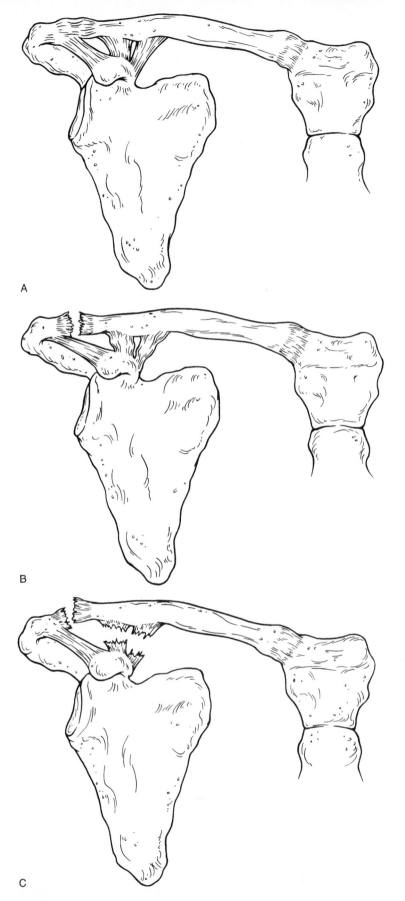

FIGURE 3–10 ■ Acromioclavicular (AC) separations. *A*, Grade I: the AC joint is sprained. *B*, Grade II: the AC joint is disrupted (coracoclavicular sprain). *C*, Grade III: disruption of AC joint and coracoclavicular ligament.

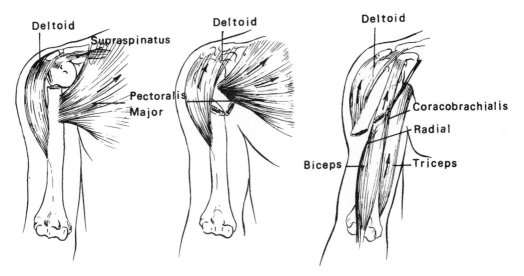

FIGURE 3–11 ■ The deformity of a humeral shaft fracture is dependent on the muscles that insert above and below the fracture.

(From Epps CH Jr: Fractures of the shaft of the humerus. *In* Rockwood CA Jr, Green DP [eds]: Fractures in Adults, ed 2, vol 1. Philadelphia, JB Lippincott, 1984, p 654; reprinted by permission.)

overhead traction are, nevertheless, available.

Closed reduction is best accomplished in the operating room with adequate anesthesia. Considering the risk of vascular compromise, these should be treated emergently. With the C-arm (fluoroscopy) in place, a closed reduction is performed and two Kirschner wires are driven across the fracture site percutaneously. A plaster splint is then used to hold the elbow initially, with cast application in several days. In 3 weeks the pins are generally removed, and in 3 more weeks the cast is discontinued. It is normal for there to be a good deal of stiffness after such an event occurs in a child. The key to postoperative management is to emphatically tell the parents not to make the child move the elbow. In other words, if the child is left alone, in a reasonably short time a good deal of motion is automatically regained. There is absolutely no place for any passive manipulation of the child's elbow. Because of the cartilaginous growth centers (physes, epiphyses, and apophyses) around the child's elbow, diagnosis may be difficult. The inexperienced may benefit from review of comparison views of the normal elbow.

2. *Distal humeral fractures in adults.* These intra-articular fractures are difficult to treat and are often followed by stiffness and arthritis. Therefore, an early open reduction and anatomic restoration of the articular surfaces with rigid fixation of the fragments to the shaft of the humerus give the best result. The ulnar nerve, because of its location, is at risk and generally has to be moved from the cubital tunnel and transported anteriorly out of harms way. The goal of treatment is to restore function by an anatomic restoration of the fragments and initiation of early motion. It is generally agreed that if a traumatized elbow is immobilized for three weeks or more a poor result will follow. Functional elbow motion is approximately 30 to 100 degrees. This will allow the hand to reach the mouth (Fig. 3–12).

3. *Dislocation of the elbow.* Most elbow dislocations occur in a fall on the extremity, and the ulna is pushed posterior to the humerus. Reduction of a posterior elbow dislocation is easily accomplished for the most part by closed means using manual traction and manipulation. Intravenous sedation and often augmentation with local infiltration of Xylocaine into the joint is usually adequate for manipulation. X-rays must confirm the reduction. Short-term immobilization for comfort is all that is required. Following this, active flexion and extension are essential

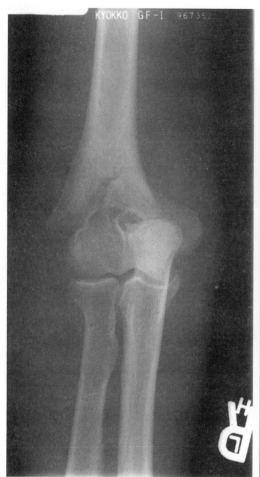

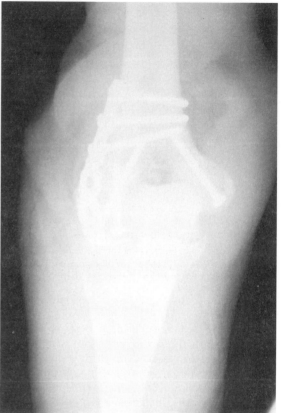

FIGURE 3–12 ■ Distal humerus fracture.

to regain motion. Any elbow trauma in the adult should be accompanied by warning the patient of the likelihood that a few degrees of full extension are normally lost, but that this loss will present no functional disability.

There are two specific forearm/elbow injuries that must be mentioned. The Monteggia fracture-dislocation, a fracture of the proximal ulna with a dislocation of the radial head, requires not only treatment of the ulna, but also reduction of the radial head. While closed reduction is possible in children, in adults the ulna is almost always treated by open reduction and internal fixation with a plate and screws. Radial head position must be assured with x-rays (Fig. 3–13). The Galeazzi fracture-dislocation includes a fracture of the more distal radius with a dislocation of the distal radioulnar joint. This radial fracture is treated by open reduction and internal fixation with plate and screws. The ulnar dislocation usually requires positioning

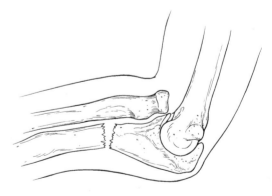

FIGURE 3–13 ■ The Monteggia fracture-dislocation (type 1, anterior).

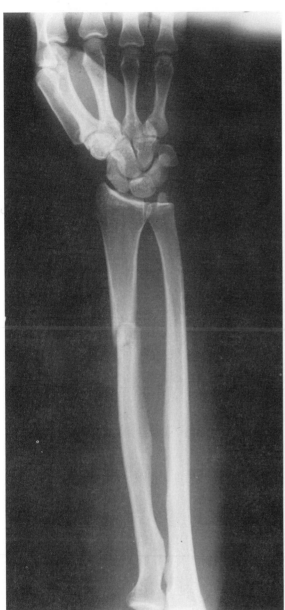
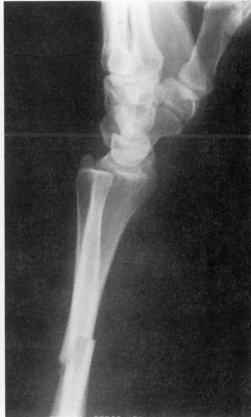

FIGURE 3–14 ■ The Galeazzi fracture.

of the forearm in supination to achieve reduction (Fig. 3–14).

4. *Fracture of both bones of the forearm.* In children this fracture is almost always treated by closed reduction and immobilization in the long arm cast. Anatomic reduction is not necessary because of the excellent remodeling potential in children. Six to 8 weeks of immobilization is necessary in a child. In adults, because of the concern over loss of pronation and supination and delayed union, operative

treatment consisting of open reduction of both the radius and the ulna, done through two separate incisions and fixation with plates, is generally employed.

5. *Fractures of the olecranon.* The triceps muscle inserts into the olecranon process, providing an extensor for the elbow joint. While undisplaced fractures of the olecranon may be treated closed, displaced fractures are routinely opened and fixed by means of a tension band technique. Early motion is allowed after

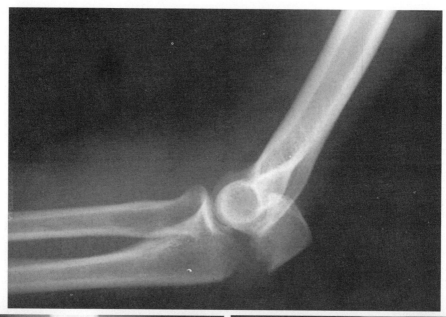

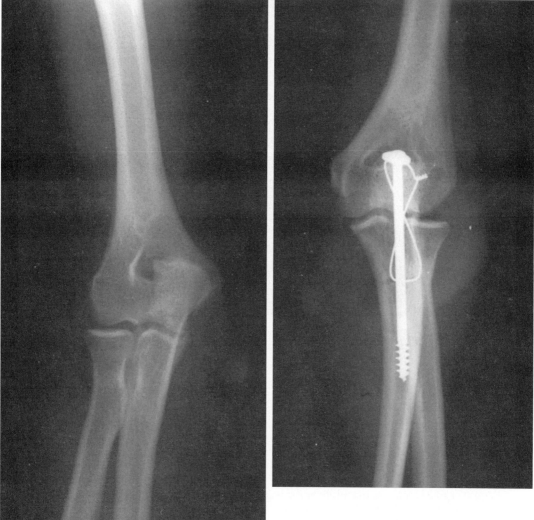

FIGURE 3–15 ■ Olecranon fracture. *Illustration continued on opposite page.*

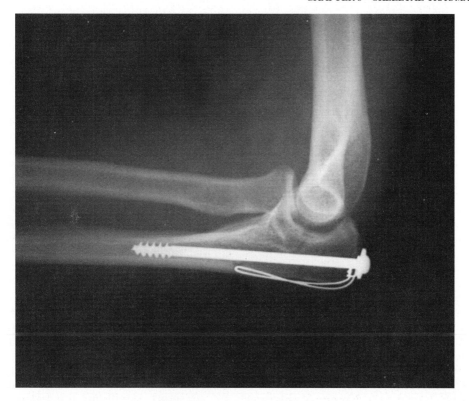

FIGURE 3–15 ■ *Continued*

such a procedure, but heavy work, of course, must await bony consolidation, which takes at least 6 weeks (Fig. 3–15).

6. *Fracture of the head of the radius (elbow).* This common intra-articular injury usually occurs from a fall on the outstretched hand. If displacement is small, conservative treatment will provide a good result. This consists of immobilization for comfort for a short time, 3 to 5 days, then institution of several 10-minute periods of active motion consisting of flexion, extension, supination, and pronation. Each exercise may be followed by splint or sling immobilization for comfort in the first 7 to 10 days. The patient must be cautioned against passive motion, which may cause bleeding and stiffness. If more than one third of the head of the radius articular surface is involved, and more than a 3-mm depression or significant angulation occurs, open reduction and internal fixation with a small screw are occasionally performed. In a very comminuted, displaced fracture, removal of the head of the radius will give a good result, with or without a silastic spacer.

Wrists and Hands

1. *Wrist Fractures (Distal Radius).* Wrist fractures in children are commonly of the torus or buckle type. Reduction is rarely necessary; cast immobilization for 4 to 6 weeks, depending on the age of the child, is suggested. Another frequent fracture, usually occurring in a slightly older child, transverses the open and actively growing physis. Typically, this is a Salter II fracture (Fig. 3–3). Reduction by closed means can be readily accomplished, and a cast is applied until healing has been accomplished. Fractures of both bones of the distal forearm, within an inch of the distal end of the bone, are fairly common. Closed reduction under local hematoma block anesthesia, plus systemic medication such as Phenergan and Demerol, usually work well. Perfect reduction is not needed because of the excellent remodeling potential of the child.

   In the adult, the most frequent fracture about the wrist is the classic Colles fracture. The description in 1894 by Abraham Colles of Ireland predated the discovery of x-rays. This is a fracture of the distal radius usually seen in elderly patients, in whom osteoporosis is common. The three classic deformities are (1) dorsal displacement of the distal fragment, (2) volar angulation, and (3) radial shortening. It is the latter that presents the most significant functional problem if not corrected. Although, traditionally, closed reduction and cast application was the treatment of choice, and is frequently still employed, both patients and their orthopaedic surgeons in many cases have not been willing to accept less than perfect results. Therefore, a good deal of individualization has become necessary. Since these fractures usually occur with a fall on the outstretched hand, comminution, in addition to these three classic deformities, is frequently encountered. A particular type of comminution is the so-called "die-punch" injury. Here the lunate impresses a fragment of distal radius proximally. This requires an open reduction and fixation. The means of fixation range from the use of multiple pins to an external fixator, which consists of two pins in a metacarpal and two pins in the radius with an outside metal adjustable bar. This device holds the fragments out to length. Actual open operation and fixation of the fragments, using a buttress plate after elevation of the depressed fragment, and the application of a bone graft may also be employed. Because many older adults request the best possible wrist they can get, such procedures will be necessary. It is, however, quite usual for people in their upper 70s and 80s to prefer not to have an extensive operation. They will usually be satisfied with a simple closed reduction and cast immobilization. Even though the cosmetic result may not be perfect, the functional result is quite good.

2. *Scaphoid (navicular) fractures.* Vigorous young adults are vulnerable to scaphoid injury. This fracture, like so many others, results from a fall on the outstretched hand. Any patient, who gives this history and has tenderness in the so-called "anatomic snuffbox" of the wrist, should be considered to have a scaphoid fracture and treated in a thumb spica cast. The anatomic snuffbox is the area just distal

to the radial styloid and bordered by the extensor pollicis longus dorsally and by the extensor pollicis brevis and abductor pollicis longus volarly. X-rays of the wrist taken soon after the injury frequently fail to reveal a fractured scaphoid. Because of the danger of nonunion at that site, it is generally accepted to treat such a patient with a thumb spica cast and remove this cast 10 to 14 days later. At that time, clinical examination and new x-ray examination usually reveal whether this is indeed a fracture or not. A bone scan or magnetic resonance image occasionally may be needed. Patients often feel that they have had a sprained wrist, but a true "sprained" wrist is very rare. Because of the risk of nonunion and avascular necrosis of the proximal pole of the scaphoid, open reduction is recommended for displaced fractures. Other carpal bones are usually treated simply by immobilization in a cast and generally do well.

Lunate dislocation and perilunate dislocation are uncommon injuries and require significant trauma. Aggressive operative treatment is usually required to produce a satisfactory result.

3. *Phalangeal fractures.* It is critical to remember to evaluate the patient for rotational malalignment. This deformity is frequently subtle unless the fingers are examined in the flexed position. Once reduced the fracture should be immobilized in the position of function (flexed), never in full extension. Fractures involving articular surfaces must be openly reduced and internally fixed if any displacement is present. Otherwise severe stiffness and arthritis will likely result.

4. *Gamekeeper's thumb.* This is a common and frequently missed injury. The injury is a tear of the ulnar collateral ligament of the metacarpophalangeal joint at the base of the thumb. Typically, it occurs during a fall as a valgus stress is applied to the thumb. This frequently follows falling with a ski pole in the hand. The result, if overlooked, can be significant instability and impairment in use of the thumb for pinching. While partial injuries are treated with a thumb spica cast, complete injuries are best treated by surgical repair.

FRACTURES AND DISLOCATIONS BY REGION: THE SPINE

Injuries to the spine are best understood by considering the anatomy of the spine. For descriptive purposes, the spinal column is divided into the anterior, middle, and posterior columns. The anterior column includes the anterior half of the body of the vertebrae and the anterior longitudinal ligament. The middle column includes the posterior half of the body and the posterior longitudinal ligament. The posterior column includes the pedicles and the lamina (Fig. 3–16). If only one

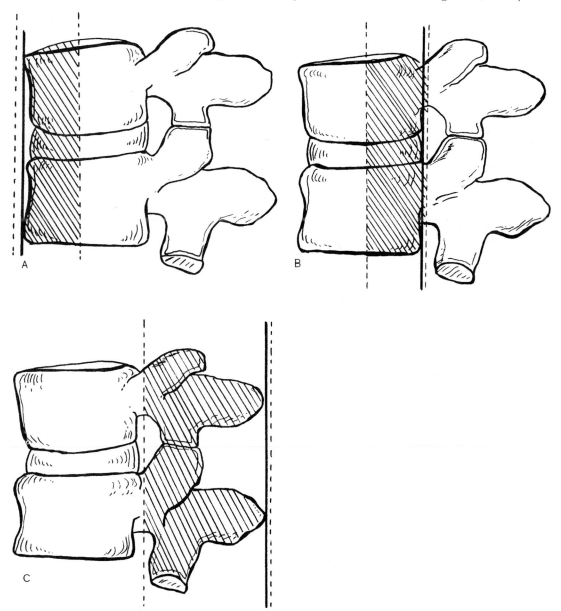

FIGURE 3–16 ■ Schematic diagrams of the components of the three columns of the thoracolumbar spine. *A,* Anterior column: anterior longitudinal ligament, anterior half of the body, and anterior half of the disk. *B,* Middle column: posterior longitudinal ligament, posterior half of the body, and posterior half of the disk. *C,* Posterior column: neural arch, ligamentum flavum, facet joint capsules, and the interspinous ligament.

(From Bucholz RW, Gill K: Classification of injuries of the thoracolumbar spine. Orthop Clin North Am 17[1]:70, 1986; reprinted by permission.)

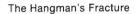

The Jefferson Fracture   The Hangman's Fracture   Odontoid Fractures

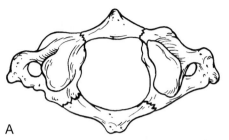
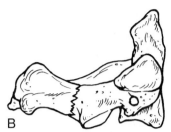
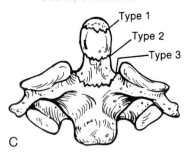

A   B   C

FIGURE 3–17 ■ Fractures of the atlas and axis. *A,* the Jefferson fracture. *B,* The hangman's fracture. *C,* Odontoid fractures.

column is involved, the injury usually can be considered stable and is often treated conservatively. If two or more columns are involved, then the injury is considered unstable. Injury includes bony as well as ligamentous structures. Another consideration that obviously must be determined is the presence of neurologic compromise. X-rays will reveal much of the bony damage of the spine and the computed tomography (CT) scan reveals bony fragments that may be encroaching the spinal canal. It must be remembered that the spinal cord ends at the upper border of the second lumbar vertebra, and below it only the cauda equina inhabits the spinal canal. Magnetic resonance imaging is best used to study additional soft tissue injury.

Simple compression fractures of the anterior portion of the body of the vertebra are usually considered stable if they are less than 50 percent of the height of the vertebral body. If they are more than 50 percent, it is felt that the next column (the middle) is involved, which makes the fractures unstable. Similarly, burst fractures characterized by fragments of the vertebral body being displaced posteriorly may well encroach on the spinal canal. A CT scan will show the extent of encroachment. While patients without neurological symptoms may be treated by prolonged bed rest, modern treatment of spinal trauma with positive neurological findings generally consists of removal of the bony fragments from the neural elements and stabilization by either posterior or anterior instrumentation. Fractures of the facets and dislocations of the facets are also encountered. Generally speaking, these are reduced and, if unstable, fixed. External fixation by means of casts and braces are not very efficient in immobilizing the spine. Halo fixation is sometimes used and, as modern surgical techniques are advanced rapidly, internal fixa-

tion is frequently the most efficient method. The first and second cervical vertebrae have particular anatomic structures. Certain specific types of injuries—the Jefferson fracture, the Hangman's fracture, and the various odontoid fractures (Fig. 3–17)—involve the C1/C2 complex. Aggressive immobilization is required for satisfactory results. Treatment may be closed with a halo application or open employing various techniques.

FRACTURES AND DISLOCATIONS BY REGION: PELVIS

The unique anatomy of the pelvis presents a challenge in management when it is disrupted. The pelvis is a ring structure of three bones: two innominate bones and, posteriorly, the sacrum. They are joined by dense, extremely strong ligamentous structures. Each innominate bone is formed from three bones: an ilium, an ischium, and the pubis, together circumscribing the acetabulum. The juncture between the two hemi-pelves anteriorly is called the "symphysis pubis," and posteriorly there are two sacroiliac joints surrounded by dense sacroiliac ligaments.

There exist two completely different types of pelvic fractures. In elderly and osteoporotic patients, minor trauma such as a minor fall, may cause a crack of the ischium or pubis. This may be the only fracture and, therefore, the fracture is considered stable. Bed rest for a few days or until the pain eases up, followed by mobilization, will allow the patient to become asymptomatic and fully functional in a matter of 6 to 8 weeks.

The other type of pelvic fracture is one following a severe traumatic force. In these injuries, blood loss is often excessive and should be anticipated. Great care in evaluating the patient is essential. A rectal and vaginal examination are required to assure that the fracture is not open through those soft tissue structures. An open fracture of the pelvis with injury to the bowel and the urogenital system still carries with it a mortality rate of 50 percent. Early treatment in these severe life-threatening pelvic injuries usually mandates the application of an external pelvic fixator: three pins in each ilium, with a device in front to hold the fragments together. This seems to be the most effective way of stemming the devastating bleeding. While embolization has its place, it is not always effective. If the bowel is involved, a diverting colostomy is mandatory to prevent fatal sepsis. Thorough exploration, cleaning, and debridement must be done. Then open reduction and internal fixation, often using pelvic reconstruction plates, may become necessary. This is best performed by a surgeon familiar with the operative treatment of pelvic fractures. Fractures through the acetabulum causing articular disruption and, hence, a fracture-dislocation of the hip are best managed by surgical acetabular reconstruction. With the onset of late osteoarthritis, total hip replacement might be necessary.

FRACTURES AND DISLOCATIONS BY REGION: THE LOWER EXTREMITY

1. *Femoral neck fractures.* The neck of the femur is situated *within* the capsule of the hip joint. This makes fractures of the neck of the femur subject to two problems with regard to the aftermath of trauma: avascular necrosis and nonunion. The blood supply is precarious. It originates from the medial and lateral femoral circumflex arteries at the base of the femoral neck and the extracapsular arterial ring. These vessels nourish the head of the femur. Any disruption of the femoral neck is likely to interfere with the blood supply of the head of the femur—hence, causing avascular necrosis. This occurs in more than one third of displaced femoral neck fractures. Nonunion, the other complication of femoral neck trauma, is related to the presence of synovial fluid, which bathes the fracture site. It is more difficult for the bone to heal in this environment, and it is difficult to reduce the fragments anatomically. No displaced femoral neck fracture, therefore, can heal when treated nonoperatively. Fractures of the neck of the femur are classified into nondisplaced and displaced (Fig. 3–18). Nondisplaced (so-called impacted valgus fractures) are inherently stable and may heal without surgery. However, they are generally treated by open reduction and internal fixation (ORIF) using compression screw placed up the neck. This may be done percutaneously or through a small incision and is a relatively minimal procedure. These fractures, undisplaced or valgus impacted, will normally heal,

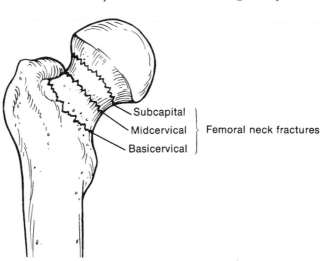

Subcapital
Midcervical } Femoral neck fractures
Basicervical

FIGURE 3–18 ■ Locations of femoral neck fractures. Displacement is important to note.

and the patient is allowed to get up and move about with partial weight-bearing until healing takes place. Usually this occurs in 6 to 8 weeks. When a fracture of the neck of the femur is displaced, an effort may be made to do a closed reduction in the operating room, which must be confirmed radiographically. Then, similar screws may be put across the fracture site for stabilization. In patients generally under age 60 years and those with a vigorous lifestyle, ORIF is the preferred treatment. In the older and frail patient, it may be more advantageous to avoid the possibility of nonunion, avascular necrosis, and an invalid life for several months by removing the head of the femur and replacing it with an endoprosthesis. This device enables patients to walk the day after the operation bearing most of their body weight. These prostheses can last anywhere from 10 to 15 years, and, therefore, in a young person every effort should be made to save the native femoral head. If a reduction of the fracture is performed and avascular necrosis or a nonunion occurs, a total hip replacement is the usual solution.

2. *Intertrochanteric fractures.* These occur at or below the line between the greater and lesser trochanter and lie *outside* the capsule (Fig. 3–19). The blood supply, therefore, is not jeopardized by the fracture.

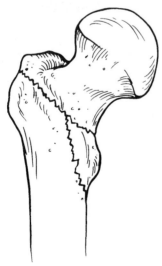

FIGURE 3–19 ■ Intertrochanteric femoral fracture. Involvement of the lesser trochanter defines an unstable fracture pattern.

On physical examination in the emergency room, these patients, similar to those with the displaced femoral neck fractures, will manifest shortening and external rotation. If an attempt were made to treat such a fracture without operative intervention, the patient would likely not survive protracted bed rest. Such a patient is likely to die from pneumonia, pulmonary emboli, bedsores, urinary tract infections, or the emotional damage that occurs in an old person when bedridden. Therefore, surgery is the norm. The compression hip screw with side plate is generally used as shown in the illustration (Fig. 3–20). Review of the x-rays allows one to determine whether the fracture is stable or unstable. When the proximal femur is fractured into three or four separate fragments, and especially if the lesser trochanter with its posteromedial cortex is one of these fragments, the fracture is unstable. In these cases, fixation must be rigid and full weight-bearing often cannot be allowed for quite a few months. Due to the high incidence of implant failure seen with the unstable fractures, other solutions have been sought—one of them being a prosthetic replacement of all the fragments that are damaged. This is a larger operation than the endoprosthesis for a femoral neck fracture and, therefore, is not often done. Healing in the intertrochanteric fracture usually proceeds well, assuming the fixation is adequate.

3. *Subtrochanteric fractures.* These fractures occur through an area below the lesser trochanter and are not quite as rapid to heal as the intertrochanteric injuries. In the younger population, subtrochanteric fractures usually follow the severe trauma of motor vehicle accidents. In the elderly, they are due to severe osteoporosis or a pathologic process in the subtrochanteric area. Fixation is either by a standard hip screw, as described for the intertrochanteric fracture, but with a longer side plate or, even better, an intramedullary nail with proximal and distal locking screws.

In children intertrochanteric and subtrochanteric fractures are generally treated in traction, while the very rare fracture of the femoral neck, even in a child, must be surgically treated in an

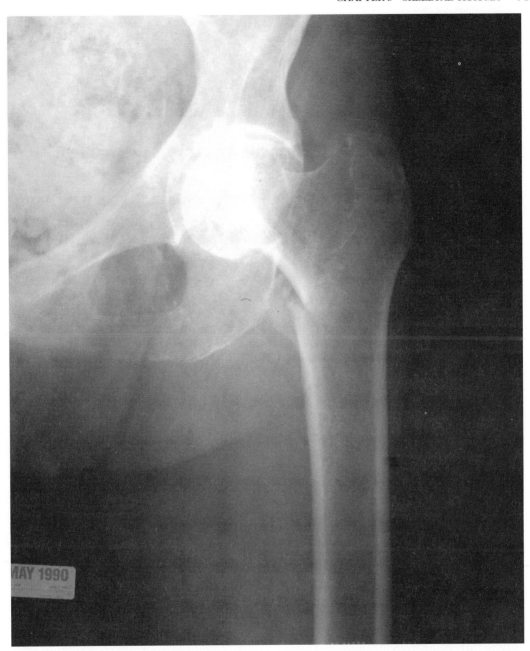

FIGURE 3–20 ■ Intertrochanteric fracture. *Illustration continued on following page.*

effort to achieve union and avoid avascular necrosis.

4. *Femoral shaft fractures.* These injuries usually follow significant trauma. In children, they are treated by skeletal traction with a pin placed in the distal femur, followed by a spica cast. Currently there is an increased interest in fixation of pediatric fractures. In adults, these fractures are almost always treated by intramedullary rods that are locked at both ends. These are inserted using closed techniques. While the fractures do not heal faster with this treatment, the patient is able to walk and function, at first with crutches, and soon without crutches, while the fracture heals. This approach markedly decreases the length of the hospital stay. (Fig. 3–21).

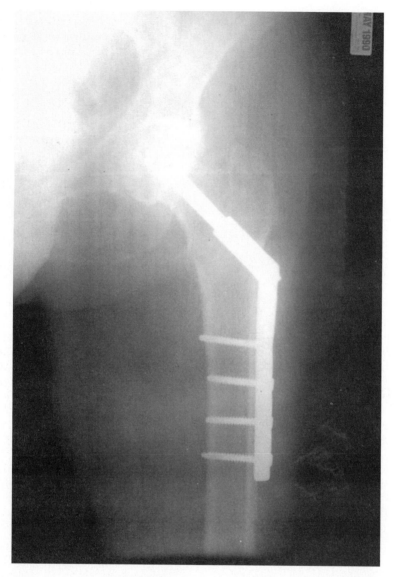

FIGURE 3–20 ■ *Continued*

Dislocation of the Hip

Typically, this occurs from the impact between the dashboard and the knee in a motor vehicle accident. This impact drives the hip out posteriorly and as expected will often damage the blood supply to the head of the femur as well as the sciatic nerve. The latter happens to lie immediately in the path of the oncoming head of the femur. Most dislocations of the hip are posterior and early reduction will decrease the incidence of avascular necrosis. Reduction under six to eight hours is thought to be essential to reduce this risk. A hip that has been dislocated for over 24 hours, almost assuredly will undergo necrosis.

Fractures About the Knee

1. *Distal Femoral Fractures.* Fractures of the lower end of the femur in the region of the condyles may be supracondylar or Y- or T-shaped, the latter types entering the joint. If displaced, these fractures are generally treated surgically and an effort is made to obtain an anatomic reduction of the articular surfaces. The reconstructed articular surface is then affixed to the distal femoral shaft. Anatomic restoration is necessary to prevent significant traumatic arthritis of the knee. Fixation to the shaft is necessary to allow early motion. Generally speaking, weight-

bearing is delayed for three months, but early motion begins within a couple of days of the fixation process. Frequently, a continuous passive motion machine is valuable in the early stages to maximize motion.

2. *Fractures of the tibial plateau.* These intra-articular fractures typically occur on the lateral side of the tibia when the patient is struck, for example, by the bumper of a car. A large hemarthrosis can be antici-

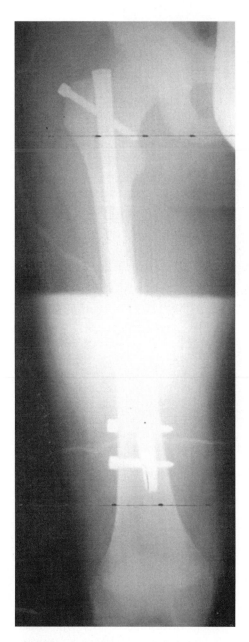

FIGURE 3–21 ■ Femoral shaft fracture.

pated and on aspiration, fat globules floating on the aspirated blood, indicate that the bone marrow of the metaphyses has extravasated. Treatment is similar to that of the lower end of the femur and depends on the degree of displacement and comminution. Nondisplaced fractures may be treated by relieving the patient of both weight-bearing and initiating early motion. Displaced fractures are best treated surgically, including anatomic reduction of the fracture fragments, the placement of bone grafts under the fracture fragments if the bone has been compressed down, and fixation by means of a plate and screws. Early motion is begun immediately, but full weight-bearing should be delayed for 12 weeks, since the cancellous bone is compressible before that time.

3. *Fractures of the patella.* The patella is a sesamoid bone that gives the quadriceps mechanism a mechanical advantage in extending the knee. If the fracture is nondisplaced, closed treatment for up to 6 weeks is preferred. However, there usually is displacement and then an open reduction and internal fixation is the treatment of choice. As we have seen in the fracture of the olecranon (Fig. 3–22), a tension-banding procedure works well. Rarely, in extremely comminuted fractures, a patellectomy may be the only option to avoid irregular patellar fragments causing painful traumatic arthritis of the patellofemoral joint.

4. *Dislocation of the knee.* This injury is the result of very severe trauma. When a patient gives a history that the "knee came out of place," 99 percent of the time they mean that either the patella dislocated (or subluxed) or that a piece of meniscus or loose body of cartilage was caught in the knee joint. True dislocation of the knee is a very serious injury notable for producing arterial damage to the popliteal vessels. The popliteal artery is fixed anatomically at the level of the proximal tibia by the interosseous membrane, and therefore is placed at great risk when the knee dislocates. Routine arteriography has been recommended following immediate closed reduction of the dislocation. The results of arteriography will then determine whether arterial repair will become necessary. Late liga-

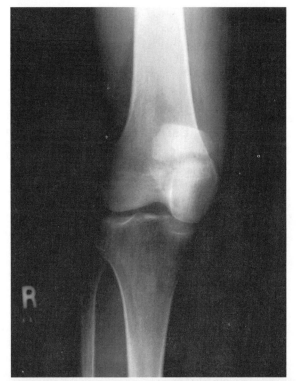

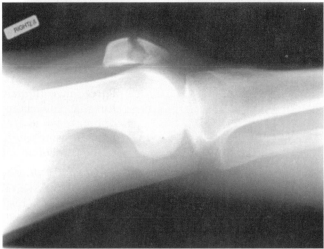

FIGURE 3–22 ■ Patella fracture. *Illustration continued on opposite page.*

mentous repair may or may not be necessary after early, emergent reduction and vascular management have been accomplished.

5. *Fracture of the tibial shaft.* This diaphyseal fracture presents a major problem from the standpoint of bony union. Because of the tenuous blood supply of the shaft of the tibia, fractures—particularly at the junction of the middle and distal third—are notorious for the high incidence of non-union. In adults, the preferred treatment has varied over the decades. It almost seems as though the pendulum from open to closed treatment of displaced tibial shaft fractures swings back every 10 years. Undisplaced

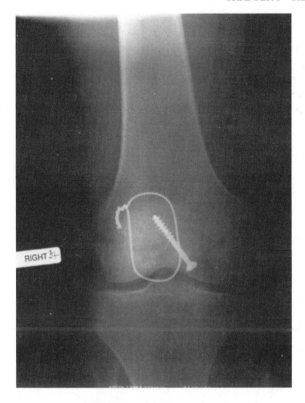

FIGURE 3-22 ■ *Continued*

or minimally displaced tibial fractures are generally treated by the application of a long leg cast. When some union has occurred, a shorter, so-called "patella tendon bearing" cast may be applied—ideally, within six to eight weeks. Some years ago the highly respected Swiss Association of Osteosynthesis recommended open reduction and plating of displaced tibial fractures to be its preferred method. In the years after World War II closed reduction and early weight-bearing gained favor. These methods resulted in a very high percent of solid union, but also in frequent shortening of the extremity. The present trend is toward intramedullary nailing of displaced and comminuted tibial fractures with locking screws above and below the fracture site. As has been mentioned in other locations, this allows relatively early function and healing while the patient temporarily depends on the intramedullary rod for stability. As in other bones, one might think in terms of a race occurring between the bone healing and the metal failing due to metal fatigue.

Ligamentous Injuries of the Knee

The knee is a relatively noncongruous joint that is stabilized through an elaborate symptom of ligaments, most noted are the medial and lateral collateral ligaments and anterior and posterior cruciate ligaments. Many sports related ligament injuries of the knee are seen on a regular basis and, generally speaking, are first treated conservatively by immobilization, then by physical therapy and muscle strengthening. After 6 weeks of rehabilitation, gaining quadriceps strength and a good range of motion, repair of the torn anterior cruciate ligament is frequently considered (see the chapter on sports medicine).

Fractures of the Ankle and Foot Region

Fractures of the lower end of the tibia, through the articular weight-bearing surface, may be quite serious. They are called "pilon" fractures, and unless early, excellent anatomic restoration and fixation is accomplished, traumatic arthritis of the ankle will follow. Fractures of the ankle itself—the distal end of the fibula (lateral malleolus), the medial malleolus, and the so-called "posterior malleolus" (a fragment of the posterior portion of the distal tibia)—are very common. While a nondisplaced fracture of the lateral malleolus may generally be treated by a simple below-the-knee immobilization cast, displaced ankle fractures are a different problem. If the student becomes familiar with any classification system, the Lauge-Hansen (Fig. 3–23) classification of ankle fractures would seem to be the recommended one. The first word in each heading of this classification system is the position the foot at the time the force was applied. The second word denotes the mechanism of load application. In any case, the importance of ankle fractures is the status of the mortise—that is, the joint in which the talar dome lies. Proximal is the distal tibia, medial is the medial malleolus, and lateral is the distal portion of the fibula or lateral malleolus. The ankle is very unforgiving. Perfect reduction is mandatory in order to produce an acceptable functional result. Just about all displaced ankle fractures, therefore, are treated surgically. Open reduction and internal fixation is performed, with the fibula being the critical segment; length and rotation must be corrected prior to fixation. Avoidance of any weight-bearing for six weeks is generally advised with or without the cast, depending on the reliability of the patient. Weight-bearing is then gradually advanced.

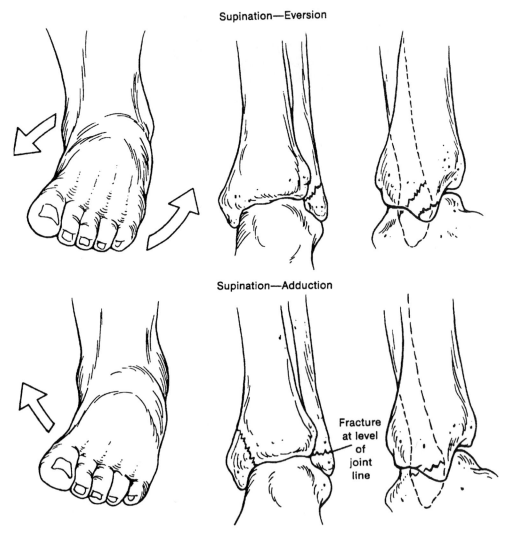

FIGURE 3–23 ■ Lauge-Hansen classification of ankle fractures. *Illustration continued on following page.*

Fractures and Soft Tissue Injuries of the Foot

1. *Fractures of the Os Calcis (Heel Bone).* This bone is unique in that it is essentially a cancellous bone (not unlike the vertebral body), yet it takes a great deal of load. If that load is applied vertically and quickly, crushing of the calcaneus can occur. This produces injury to the subtalar joint, and ultimately results in a certain degree of stiffness no matter what type of treatment is provided. Coincident fractures of the lumbar spine are not infrequent and should be sought out. Treatment of the os calcis fracture is often closed, but in expert hands open reduction and fixation may give a better result.

2. *Fractures of the Talar Neck.* Like the scaphoid bone in the wrist, the talus in the ankle is unusual among bones in that it has a retrograde blood flow. As such, fractures through the neck of the talus are frequently complicated by avascular necrosis of the dome of the proximal segment. Historically, this injury was called "aviator's astragalus." In an effort to minimize complications, open reduction and internal fixation with delayed weight-bearing are usually recommended, especially for displaced fractures.

3. *Ankle sprains.* Ankle sprains are common. The distal anterior tibiofibular ligament, the lateral ligament, and the medial deltoid ligament are the three important

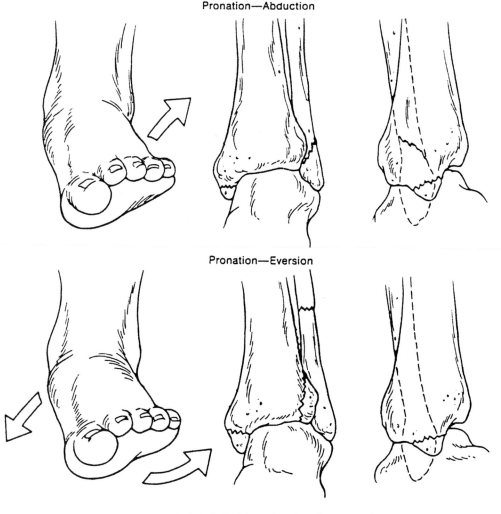

Pronation—Abduction

Pronation—Eversion

FIGURE 3–23 ■ *Continued*

ligament complexes. The biggest mistake in the treatment of ankle sprains is often found in the attitude of the first physician who sees such a patient and utters something to the effect of "This is only a sprain—you will be all right in a few days." Such a statement is, unfortunately, unrealistic and causes a great deal of patient dissatisfaction. Elevation and rest for a few days is generally helpful, but early motion and rehabilitation may also be recommended during this time. It appears that open suturing of torn ligaments at the ankle is very rarely necessary, but the use of a walking cast with the foot in slight dorsiflexion often allows patients to assume their normal activities much faster than otherwise might be the case. The cost of casting, however, is muscular atrophy of the calf and delayed rehabilitation. Various braces are commonly used, and these may then be continued for athletic activities in the subacute period. Pain, swelling, and/or disability lasting more than two months after a significant ankle sprain is a common outcome.

4. *Achilles Tendon Rupture.* Occurring in a sports-related injury in the middle-aged athlete, it may well be overlooked; but it should always be suspected, even though the patient may think that an ankle sprain has occurred. The Thompson test, which consists of squeezing the calf and noting the foot to plantar flex or, if positive, to fail to plantar flex, is most useful. These injuries may be treated by conservative means using a cast in plantar flexion or surgically by direct tendon repair. Occasionally, a sudden pain in the calf may be interpreted as a torn Achilles tendon, but more often only a few fibers of the gastrocnemius will tear. This is similar to the so-called "ruptured plantaris." Rest, elevation, and/or walking at first with an elevated heel amazingly relieves discomfort. Nonsteroidal anti-inflammatory drugs for prevention of deep venous thrombosis may be added to the treatment regimen.

5. *Lisfranc dislocation of the foot.* The Lisfranc joint, which is the joint between the tarsal bones and the metatarsals, may be injured in sport and other accidents. It is, unfortunately, frequently missed, and x-rays of the ankle are ordered which do not show this area. If the examiner is unsure and the pain and tenderness are in the midfoot rather than over the malleoli, a comparison foot x-ray may be useful. These injuries usually consist of lateral dislocation of one or more of the metatarsal bones, and if not treated (thus restoring perfect anatomical congruity of the joint), long-term disability will result.

6. *Distal Foot Fractures.* Most fractures of the metatarsals and toes are treated conservatively; although metatarsal fractures may be immobilized in a walking cast, this is often unnecessary. Fractured toes generally are treated by strapping the toe gently to its neighbor for support. The fracture of the base of the fifth metatarsal, which may be due to avulsion by the peroneus brevis tendon, is quite common and quite benign. This fracture is generally misinterpreted to be an ankle sprain by the patient. Walking cast, stiff sole shoes, and/or elastic stockings are all acceptable options. Excellent healing is the norm, with pain reduction occurring in about three weeks.

SUGGESTED READINGS

Rockwood Charles A Jr, Green David P, Bucholz Robert W, Heckman James D: Rockwood and Green's Fractures in Adults, ed 4. Philadelphia, Lippincott-Raven, 1996.

Rockwood Charles A Jr, Wilkins Kaye E, Beaty J: Fractures in Children. ed 4. Philadelphia, Lippincott-Raven, 1996.

Chapter 4

Orthopaedic Infections

Alan D. Aaron

INTRODUCTION

Musculoskeletal infections can prove to be extremely difficult to diagnose and treat. Unrecognized infections can be limb-threatening and potentially fatal if not recognized and treated. The most important aspect of caring for these patients is to recognize that an infection is present, with most problems occurring when treatment is delayed. Open fractures are discussed in detail, as appropriate intervention early on can often prevent the establishment of chronic osteomyelitis.

PATHOPHYSIOLOGY OF OSTEOMYELITIS

The pathogenesis of osteomyelitis, although conceptually similar in all cases, may vary depending upon the age of the host, duration of infection, etiology of infection, and type of host response to the infection. Osteomyelitis is often classified using these parameters, which can assist in defining the severity of infection, identify a mode of treatment, and assess the potential for recovery. Duration of infections is often divided into either acute or chronic osteomyelitis or septic arthritis. Although the distinction is somewhat arbitrary, acute osteomyelitis is usually considered to occur within the first 6 weeks following inoculation, with chronic osteomyelitis being greater than 6 weeks.

The development of bone and joint infections takes place via one of two basic mecha-

nisms, involving either exogenous or hematogenous pathways. Exogenous delivery involves direct inoculation of the bone from either trauma, surgery, or a contiguous focus of infection. Hematogenous spread is via the vascular tree into either osseous or synovial tissue producing a localized focus of infection. Local tissue compromise (i.e., in the case of fracture) or systemic tissue (i.e., diabetes) compromise is often associated with an increased risk of bone infection by either method.

Two patterns of response are noted and are often dependent on the infecting organism. Pyogenic organisms elicit a rapidly progressive course of pain, swelling, abscess formation, and aggressive bone destruction. A gram-positive staphylococci is a classic example of an organism that may produce a pyogenic response. In contrast, less aggressive nonpyogenic organisms invoke a more insidious granulomatous reaction, classically seen with acid-fast bacilli. Age of the host is important in that differences in bone vascular anatomy between adults and children slightly alter the mechanism of hematogenous delivery. In addition, children are susceptible to different organisms depending upon their age.

Exogenous osteomyelitis usually involves a clearly identified anatomic site, is usually inoculated with pyogenic organisms, and is often polymicrobial—frequently in association with foreign debris. The bacteria are inoculated into a compromised local environment, with bone and soft tissue disruption providing ample amounts of necrotic and devascularized material favorable for bacterial growth. In addition, tissue devascularization prevents host-response mechanisms from reaching bacterial colonies, thereby permitting unchecked proliferation.

Once a bone infection is recognized by the host, several steps are undertaken. Initial host responses to both the injury and infection include activation of inflammatory and immunological pathways. Inflammatory elements serve to destroy bacteria and remove nonviable material. Humoral and cellular immunologic mechanisms act to recognize specific bacteria and subsequently confer immunity to prevent further bacterial dissemination. The inflammatory response is initiated with increases in blood flow and vascular permeability, with the delivery of polymorphonuclear leukocytes. The leukocytes phagocytize and destroy bacteria and nonviable tissue. Mononuclear cells arrive within 24 to 48 hours and assist in eradication of bacteria and removal of necrotic bone. As a large number of these cells arrive and die, pus is formed, with an abscess often being clinically appreciable.

Eventually granulation tissue surrounds the infected area in an attempt to wall off the infection. Further isolation is achieved as chronic avascular fibrous tissue is produced around the infected area. Finally, reactive bone formation can occur to further sequester the infection from the host. Within the infected region, dead bone is often prominent, it is commonly termed the "sequestrum," while the reactive bone is known as the "involucrum." Unfortunately, this sequestrated area is isolated from host defense mechanisms due to the avascular fibrous tissue and can permit the continued proliferation of bacteria.

Pivotal to treatment of osteomyelitis is obtaining a better understanding of how bacteria achieve a foothold in either damaged tissues or surgical implants. Adhesion to the surface of tissue cells and implants depends on the physical characteristics of the bacteria, the fluid interface, and the substratum. Initially, bacteria arrive at random near a damaged tissue or implant surface by direct contamination, contiguous spreading, or hematogenous seeding. All surfaces, regardless of whether they are tissue- or implant-derived, acquire a glycoproteinaceous conditioning film when exposed to a biological environment. This surface is anionic and initially repels bacteria, whose surface is also anionic. However, attractive forces (Van der Waals), in conjunction with hydrophobic molecules on the exposed substrate and the bacteria, increase the duration of bacterial juxtaposition to permit the forma-

tion of irreversible cross-links between bacteria and host surfaces. Following anchorage of the bacteria, proliferation occurs with formation of a polysaccharide slime layer. The biofilm or slime layer is composed of bacterial extracapsular exopolysaccharides that bind to surfaces, thereby promoting cell-to-cell adhesion, micro colony formation, and layering of the microorganisms. Additional species of bacteria may attach to the surface of the biofilm, resulting in syntropic interactions between differing bacteria. Thriving bacterial colonies may be dispersed by shear force, enabling a localized colony to establish secondary sites of infection (Fig. 4–1).

Bacterial attachment and production of biofilms can lead to antibiotic resistance. Initially felt to be due to problems of antibiotic diffusion through the biofilm, more current theories center on decreased metabolic rates and phenotypic changes in surface adherent bacteria. Therefore, bacteria on surfaces or within micro colonies appear to be physiologically different from free-floating organisms, which may in part convey antibiotic resistance.

Treatment of osteomyelitis involves the disruption of these bacterial colonies. This is best achieved with aggressive debridement of nonviable tissues to remove an acceptable bacterial substrate and with the disruption of bacterial colonies and their associated biofilm. In the case of osteomyelitis involving removal of a prosthetic or fracture implant, it is often necessary to achieve eradication of the infection. Possible inhibition of infection may be achieved through modification of implant surfaces to enhance host tissue colonization in preference to bacterial colonization. By promoting tissue cell integration of these surfaces, inoculated bacteria are confronted with a living substrate capable of enacting a host defense mechanism.

PEDIATRIC INFECTIONS

Acute Hematogenous Osteomyelitis

The most common etiology for acute osteomyelitis is via hematogenous inoculation. The vascular anatomy of children's long bones can predispose them to hematogenous inoculation and proliferation of bacteria. The nutrient artery of long bones enters through the cortical bone to divide within the medullary canal, ending in small arterioles that ascend toward the physis (Fig. 4–2). Just beneath the

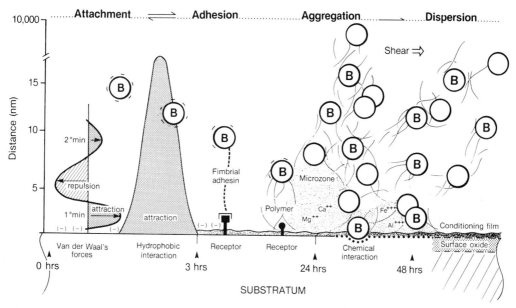

FIGURE 4–1 ■ Molecular sequence in bacterial (B) attachment, adhesion, aggregation, and dispersion at substratum surface. A number of possible interactions may occur depending on the specificities of the bacteria or substratum system (graphics, nutrients, contaminants, macromolecules, species, and materials).

From Gristina AG, Naylor PT, Myrvik QN: Mechanisms of musculoskeletal sepsis. Orth Clin North Am 22(3):363–371, 1991; reprinted by permission.

physis these arterioles bend away from the physis and empty into venous lakes within the medullary cavity. The acute bend in these arteriolar loops serve as points of diminished blood velocity promoting sludging of bacteria directly under the physis. In addition, phagocytic capability and reticuloendothelial function may be depressed in these vascular loops, promoting the establishment of bacterial colonies. Trauma, often associated with the emergence of osteomyelitis in children, may actually promote bacterial seeding and proliferation in metaphyseal sites (Fig. 4–3).

As previously discussed, an established infection will result in the delivery of inflammatory cells and, if the infection remains untreated, purulent material will be produced (Fig. 4–4). This pus can spread in one of three ways: through the physis, toward the diaphysis, or through the adjacent bony cortex (Fig. 4–5). This purulent material tends to seek the path of least resistance, through the metaphyseal cortex, to form a collection of subperiosteal pus. Though this is the most common route of egress, younger children (less than 1 year) with intact transphyseal vessels may demonstrate epiphyseal spread, with the development of epiphyseal abscesses.

In older children, the development of a subperiosteal abscess results in devascularization of the bone both from thrombosis of the endosteal blood supply and from the stripping away of the overlying periosteum. The periosteum, which is extremely thick and loosely

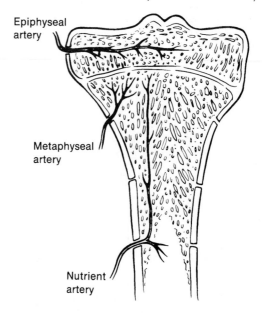

FIGURE 4–2 ■ Schematic representation of the blood supply to a long bone.

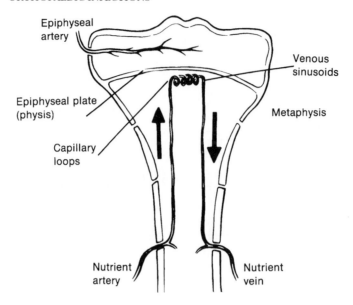

FIGURE 4–3 ■ Microcirculation of the metaphysis predisposes it to sludging and infection.

adherent in children, is not easily penetrated; in the devascularization process, it is lifted off of the bone, with the inner cambium layer producing a layer of new bone. In this case the devascularized bone is termed the "seques-trum," with the reactive periosteal bone being the "involucrum" (Fig. 4–6). A cellulitic phase precedes abscess formation, with medical management alone being successful to cure the infection. Once an abscess forms, surgical de-

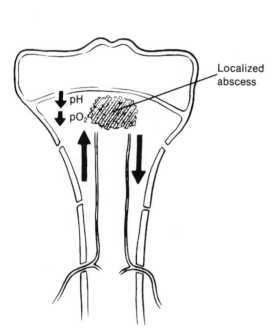

FIGURE 4–4 ■ A localized abscess develops, and the microenvironment is altered.

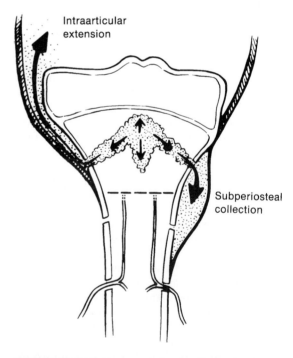

FIGURE 4–5 ■ Abscess perforates the metaphyseal cortex and spreads to the subperiosteal space and joint.

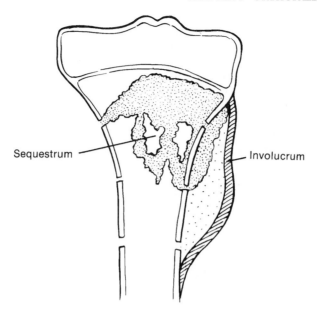

FIGURE 4–6 ■ Sequestered fragments of dead bone and periosteal new bone, or involucrum, may be seen on radiographs.

bridement is necessary to remove the nonviable bone, reduce the bacterial population, and provide for a vascularized tissue bed for antibiotic delivery. As the majority of pediatric infections emanate via hematogenous seeding from other sites, the specific organisms may differ depending upon the child's age. The vast majority of osteomyelitis in children is secondary to *staphylococcus aureus* (90%). In neonates the most common organisms include *staphylococcus aureus,* group B *streptococcus,* and gram-negative organisms.

Diagnosis and Treatment

A careful history and physical examination combined with a high index of suspicion is necessary to diagnose acute osteomyelitis. Invariably, patients present with pain for one to several days' duration, with onset of pain being fairly rapid. The pain is generally severe enough to limit or entirely restrict use of the involved extremity. Older patients may be able to assist in localization of the pain, with the clinician being cognizant of identifying potential sites of referred pain (knee pain for hip osteomyelitis). Children are usually irritable and febrile and often give a history of generalized malaise. Uncovering a potential site of a concomitant infection, such as a recent upper respiratory or ear infection, may provide the clinician with an etiology for hematogenous spread. Physical examination is extremely important, with localized swelling and tenderness often characterizing the physical presentation. Care must be taken to gain the child's confidence and to proceed in a slow, nonthreatening manner when examining the patient. Examination of an uncooperative child can be extremely frustrating for both the clinician and the patient, making interpretation of physical findings difficult.

Laboratory results are extremely important in diagnosing and treating osteomyelitis; however, they do not replace a complete history and physical examination. A complete blood count with differential and an erythrocyte sedimentation rate are imperative, with both being usually elevated. It must be emphasized that not all patients suffering from osteomyelitis present with a classic clinical history, physical findings, and laboratory values. Presentation at early onset may preclude a large amount of soft-tissue swelling and pain or an elevated sedimentation rate. In addition, diagnosis in neonates may be especially problematic due to the immaturity of their immune system, which may not be able to mount an identifiable host response.

Plain radiographs should be obtained of all involved areas and include adjacent joints to accommodate for referred pain. Unfortunately, initial radiographs may be negative, except for soft-tissue swelling, since the characteristic changes of osteomyelitis require 10 to 14 days to be appreciated. After 2 weeks, increasing radiolucency and a periosteal bone reaction are generally visible, with bone sclerosis, sequestra, and involucrum formation occurring much later (6 weeks).

Bone scanning, which has gained recent popularity, can serve as a valuable adjuvant in the identification of osteomyelitis. Technetium (^{99}Tc), coupled with methylene diphosphonate, is attracted to areas of rapid bone turnover. Though nonspecific, it exhibits a sensitivity for identifying areas of bone formation or destruction. Unfortunately it is <80% accurate when used to evaluate acute hematogenous osteomyelitis. This may be due in part to local thrombosis of vascular channels or devascularization of bone cortices thereby preventing delivery of the isotope to these surfaces. In fact a cold scan, in the face of an aggressive bone infection, is indicative of a high degree of bone necrosis and is a poor prognostic indicator for recovery. Bone scanning may be helpful in cases of multifocal infection found in neonates or when the exact site is not readily identifiable, such as seen in the pelvis. It must be remembered that bone scanning does not obviate a good clinical and physical examination. In addition, a bone aspiration should be performed in identifiable sites before embarking on a lengthy and possibly unproductive battery of radiographic examinations.

Bone aspiration is the best means of clinically identifying the presence of a bone or joint infection as well as any organisms associated with it. Aspiration should be performed immediately following acquisition of plain radiographs and directed toward the area of maximal swelling and tenderness. A large bore stiletted needle (18- or 16-gauge spinal needle) should be used to prevent plugging of soft tissue, bone, or thickened purulent material in the tip. Both subperiosteal and intramedullary sites must be aspirated. In addition, using a second needle, one should consider aspirating the adjacent joint if clinically indicated. Local anesthesia is given, with the needle being easily drilled through the soft metaphyseal cortex. If purulent material is obtained, the fluid is sent for immediate gram stain and culture. The presence of pus necessitates that the patient undergo an operative irrigation and debridement. However, antibiotics should be started immediately following aspiration, with these initial cultures serving as

possible later modifications in antibiotic coverage. The initial antibiotic choice is often based upon the "best guess" of the infecting organism. In patients, who are not allergic to penicillin, a semisynthetic penicillin that is beta-lactamase–resistant should be chosen. Good initial choices include oxacillin or nafcillin, with penicillin-allergic patients often being treated with cefazolin. The optimal length of therapy is still under debate, with a regimen of 3 weeks of intravenous (IV) antibiotics, followed by 3 weeks of oral therapy, being acceptable. In the event that purulent material is not aspirated, then sterile saline should be injected, aspirated, and sent for culture in the hopes of identifying an organism. Bacteriostatic saline should not be used as this may inhibit bacterial growth. In these cases, surgery is usually not indicated, as there is no pus to decompress or necrotic bone to debride; here, the administration of antibiotics is the mainstay of treatment. In the face of a negative aspirate, bone scans may provide more useful information in delineating the cause for bone pain.

Chronic infections are uncommon in children, as patients usually present early in the course of their disease. These patients almost invariably require surgical intervention to debride sequestrated tissues. Complications are high in this setting, from both the disease process and the surgical procedure, and include pathological fracture and physeal arrest.

Septic Arthritis

Acute septic arthritis may develop from hematogenous sources or more commonly from extension of an adjacent foci of osteomyelitis into the joint. Susceptible joints are those in which the metaphysis is intraarticular, such as seen in the hip and shoulder, where bacteria are afforded an avenue for dissemination (Fig. 4–7). Though uncommon, septic arthritis can be devastating and therefore requires complete exclusion by the clinician in the acute setting. Different organisms prevail, depending upon the age of the patient (see Table 4–1).

Diagnosis and Treatment

Clinical presentation and the physical finding are often similar to those seen with acute osteomyelitis (Fig. 4–8). However, patients tend to be sicker with higher temperatures, more pain, and an extremely high erythrocyte sedimentation rate (ESR). Patients are ex-

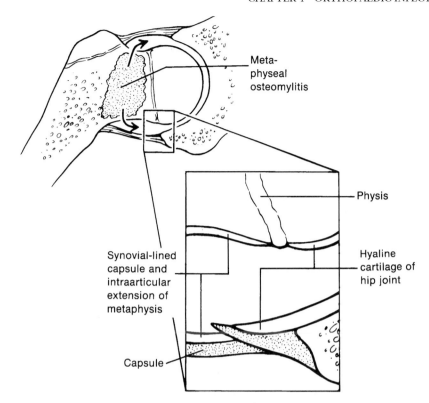

FIGURE 4–7 ■ Schematic representation of the immature hip. Metaphyseal osteomyelitis spreads by direct extension into the hip joint.

tremely reluctant to move the involved extremity or infected joint, often positioning the joint so as to maximally relax the surrounding joint capsule. For the hip this is usually flexion, abduction, and external rotation. Radiographs will demonstrate a joint effusion and associated soft-tissue swelling. Occasionally, adjacent bone involvement may be appreciable.

Joint aspiration is mandatory for diagnosis, with immediate gram stains and cultures being obtained of the joint fluid. The fluid should be analyzed for cell count and differential, protein and glucose levels, and pres-

ence of crystals. In addition, the adjacent metaphysis and subperiosteum should also undergo aspiration, as these are often sites of contiguous spread to the joint. In the majority of cases the white blood cell (WBC) count is >50,000 and often exceeds 100,000 in severe cases. The white cell population usually is comprised of polymorphonuclear lymphocytes, making up to 90 to 95 percent of the cells in fulminant cases. On occasion, circumstances may require the clinician to inform the laboratory of the possible organism as special techniques may need to be employed to obtain bacterial growth. *Haemophilus influenza* is diffi-

TABLE 4–1 ■ *Common Pathogens and Recommended Treatment for Septic Arthritis*

Age Group	Probable Organisms	Initial Antibiotic Choice
Neonate	Group B strep, *S. aureus,* Gram-negative coliforms	Penicillin, oxacillin, and gentamicin
Infants and children (4 wks to 4 yrs)	*S. aureus, H. influenzae,* Group B strep, Group A strep	Cefuroxime
Children (>4 yrs)	*S. aureus*	Oxacillin or Cefazolin
Adolescent	N. gonorrhoeae	

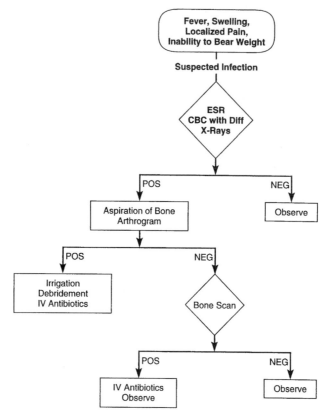

FIGURE 4–8 ■ Acute osteomyelitis and septic arthritis management algorithm.

cult to culture and must be incubated under a CO_2 environment. Because the percentage of organism retrieval has been reported by some series to be between 70 and 85 percent, blood cultures should also be obtained. Additional clues to possible infection include an elevated protein or a decreased glucose level.

Aspiration of accessible joints such as the knee and ankle can usually be performed at the bedside using appropriate analgesia and sterile techniques. However, inaccessible sites such as the hip may require that the patient undergo fluoroscopically directed aspiration. Requiring the patient to be sedated, this procedure is performed either in the radiology or operating room setting. If septic arthritis is suspected, the initial aspiration can be performed in the operating room under general anesthesia—to be followed by immediate open debridement and irrigation upon confirmation of the presence of pus or organisms. It is important to be assured that joint fluid has been sampled, with an arthrogram being necessary in the case of hip aspiration to confirm needle position. As with osteomyelitis, a nega-

tive aspiration should be followed by sterile saline flushing to obtain material for culture.

As a joint is considered a closed cavity and a joint infection an abscess, drainage of the joint is mandatory. Some controversy still persists as to whether septic arthritis can be adequately decompressed with serial aspirations and not surgery. Proponents of serial aspiration maintain the reduced risk of a local aspiration as compared to surgery. Disadvantages of serial joint aspiration include continual trauma to the joint and patient, higher risk for inadequate decompression, and repeated exposure to iatrogenic joint inoculation and infection. In addition, the joint must be readily accessible, which precludes the hip from being treated with aspiration. An infected hip joint is considered an operative emergency. The risk of avascular necrosis is especially high in the hip, as the blood supply is intracapsular and can be disrupted by intra-articular fluid secondary to a high intracapsular pressure. Reexamination of the joint is necessary following surgery or aspiration to be assured that purulent material has not reaccumulated. Arthroscopic debridement has become a popular modality for debriding affected joints. Regardless of the method employed the goals of treatment still hold true—namely, adequate decompression of purulent material, irrigation of both bacteria and host lysozymes from the joint, and debridement of nonviable tissues.

Intravenous antibiotics are initiated immediately following acquisition of joint fluid. Again antibiotic choice is based upon the suspected pathogens. Compared to treatment of osteomyelitis, the antibiotic course for septic arthritis is usually shorter (4 weeks), with 2 weeks of IV antibiotics followed by an additional 2 weeks of oral therapy.

ADULT OSTEOMYELITIS

Chronic Osteomyelitis

Management of chronic osteomyelitis involves consideration of several patient variables—physiologic, anatomic, and psychosocial. Utilizing these variables to assess and classify a patient's level of infection, goals of therapy can be determined. These include whether the infection is simple or complex, whether the goal of therapy is palliative or curative, and whether the patient would be better served by an amputation as opposed to a limb-sparing procedure. Host factors may adversely affect wound healing in cases of malnutrition, immune deficiency, malignancy, and diabetes just to name a few. Local factors, such as chronic lymphedema, venous stasis, major vessel disease, or extensive scarring, may also play a role. The Cierny-Mader classification has been developed to assist surgeons in classifying and selecting various modalities of treatment and to assist in predicting outcomes (Fig. 4–9). Local extent of disease is classified as medullary, superficial, localized, or diffuse osteomyelitis. Medullary involvement is entirely endosteal and does not require bone stabilization following debridement. Superficial osteomyelitis only involves the outer cortex and again does not require bone reconstruction following local excision of infected material. Localized osteomyelitis combines types I and II, thereby necessitating full-thickness cortical resection to effectively debride the bone. Though segmental instability is avoided, bone grafting techniques may need to be employed to reestablish bone continuity and subsequent stability. Type IV osteomyelitis results in widespread cortical and endosteal infection, with segmental resection being necessary to eradicate the osteomyelitis. Diffuse osteomyelitis is

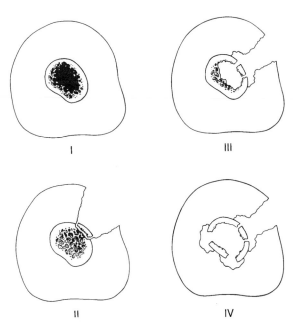

FIGURE 4–9 ■ The Cierny classification of chronic osteomyelitis: type I, medullary; type II, superficial; type III, localized full thickness; type IV, diffuse.

mechanically unstable both before and after debridement and requires bone reconstruction to attain stability.

Host variables are stratified with regard to physiologic capacity to withstand infection, treatment, and disease morbidity. A-hosts are normal, healthy patients. The B-host has a local (B^L), a systemic (B^S), or a combined local and systemic ($B^{L/S}$) compromise. The C-host, because of severe systemic problems, is not a treatment candidate. Treatment of C-hosts may potentially result in greater patient morbidity following treatment, then it would prior to intervention.

Surgical treatment of osteomyelitis involves three main facets: (1) extensive debridement, (2) vascular soft-tissue coverage, and (3) bone stabilization. An aggressive debridement is crucial to achieving successful eradication of osteomyelitis. All nonviable tissues must be removed to prevent residual bacteria from persistently reinfecting the bone. Removal of all adherent scar tissue and skin grafts should be undertaken. In addition, a high speed burr should be used to debride the cortical bone edges until punctate bleeding can be appreciated. Continuous irrigation is necessary to prevent bone necrosis with the burr. Multiple cultures of all debrided tissues should be obtained prior to the initiation of antibiotic therapy. The patient may require several debridements until the wound is considered to be clean enough to accept soft tissue coverage. Soft-tissue reconstitution may involve a simple skin graft, but often requires local transposition muscle flaps or vascularized free tissue transfers to effectively cover the debrided bone segment. These muscle flaps provide a fresh bed of vascularized tissue to assist in bone healing and antibiotic delivery. Finally, bone stability must be achieved with bone grafting being undertaken when necessary to bridge osseous gaps. Cancellous and cortical autografts are commonly used, with vascularized bone transfer (vascularized free fibular, iliac, and rib grafts) being occasionally necessary. Though technically demanding, vascularized bone grafts provide a fresh source of blood flow into previously devascularized areas of bone.

The recent advent of bone distraction has been used in lieu of bone grafting or complex soft-tissue procedures. Though technically demanding, application of a small-pin (Ilizarov) or half-pin (EBI-orthofix) external fixator with bone distraction following a cortical osteotomy can produce columns of bone to fill segmental defects. As distraction is carried out, the soft tissues regenerate along with the bone to cover the newly generated bone. Recent results appear to be encouraging, as these patients appear to achieve greater success rates for limb sparing as compared to patients undergoing more conventional bone replacement techniques.

Septic Arthritis

As with children, septic arthritis can develop from hematogenous sources, direct inoculation, contiguous soft-tissue infection, or periarticular osteomyelitis. Several factors have been implicated in predisposing to septic arthritis, with systemic corticosteroid use, preexisting arthritis, and joint aspiration being the three most common factors reported. As with children, *S. aureus* is the most common pathogen isolated from infected adult joints (44%). *Neisseria gonorrhoeae* is another common adult pathogen, with a reported incidence of 11 percent. The most commonly involved joints are the knee (40% to 50%), the hip (20% to 25%), and the shoulder and ankle (10% to 15%). In IV drug abusers, the sternoclavicular, sacroiliac, and manubriosternal joints are common sites with *Pseudomonas aeruginosa* often being isolated.

Adult patients present in a manner similar to children in that pain, swelling and a decreased range of motion are frequent complaints. Work-up involves routine laboratory tests, blood cultures, and joint aspiration. The appearance of the synovial fluid, as well as the white cell count and the percentage of polymorphonuclear cells, can assist in the diagnosis, with cultures of the fluid being mandatory (Table 4–2). Treatment, as with pediatric septic arthritis, requires aggressive irrigation and debridement utilizing either arthroscopy or an arthrotomy. Antibiotics are often delivered initially via parental routes, with patients being switched to oral therapy when demonstrating clinical improvement in conjunction with maintaining high bactericidal titers of at least 1:8.

OPEN FRACTURES

By definition an open fracture involves exposure of fractured bone to the extracorporeal environment, thus increasing the risk of bone contamination from foreign debris and bacteria. In addition, open fractures are often associated with severe soft-tissue damage,

TABLE 4–2 ■ *Synovial Fluid*

Examination	Normal	Noninflammatory	Inflammatory	Septic
Appearance	Transparent	Transparent	Opaque Translucent	Opaque Yellow to green
Viscosity	High	High	Low	Variable
White cells/mm^3	<200	<200	5000–75,000	>50,000
Polymorphonuclear cells (%)	<25%	<25%	>50%	>75%
Culture	---	---	---	Often positive
Associated conditions	---	Degenerative joint disease Trauma Neuropathic Pigmented villonodular synovitis Systemic lupus erythematosus Acute rheumatic fever	Rheumatoid arthritis Crystal-induced arthritis Seronegative arthritis Systemic lupus erythematosus Acute rheumatic fever	Bacterial infections Compromised immunity

Esterhai JL, Gelb I: Adult septic arthritis. Orthop Clin North Am 18:503–514, 1991; reprinted with permission.

devascularization, and devitalization of bone fragments, further increasing the susceptibility of the bone to infection. Open fractures are often graded on the degree of fracture comminution and the degree of soft-tissue disruption. Though not universally accepted, the Gustillo-Anderson classification is widely used due to ease of application and prognostic ability. It is divided into three grades based upon size of the soft-tissue wound, with grade III fractures being further subdivided based on bone devitalization. Other factors that place fractures into the grade III category include severe contamination, farm or barnyard injuries, or shotgun wounds. The three grades are defined as follows:

Grade I: less than a 1 cm of soft tissue laceration

Grade II: between a 1 cm and a 10 cm soft-tissue laceration.

Grade III: greater than 10 cm soft-tissue laceration and further subdivided into A) soft-tissue laceration with bone being covered by periosteum and muscle, B) severe periosteal stripping of the bone, and C) major arterial vascular laceration requiring repair.

Open fractures are considered operative emergencies and must be taken to the operating room as soon as the patient is considered medically stable enough to tolerate surgical intervention. With rare exception, patients should be taken to the operating room within 6 hours of injury. Wounds should not be explored in the emergency room, as further soft-tissue damage may be incurred. Active bleeding can almost always be controlled with local compression prior to surgical exploration. Cultures should be obtained in the operating room prior to irrigation and debridement. Wounds should be assessed, gently irrigated with sterile saline, and dressed with a sterile dressing in the emergency department. Reduction of severely contaminated fractures should be avoided in the emergency room to prevent the drawing in of foreign debris into the wound. In addition, IV antibiotics should be given immediately upon admittance to the emergency room. A good rule to observe is first-generation cephalosporins for grade I fractures, first-generation cephalosporins plus amino glycosides for grade II fractures, with grade III fractures requiring the addition of penicillin to the above regimen (Fig. 4–10).

Assessment of the injury extent and aggressive debridement should be undertaken in the operating room in an emergent manner. Wounds should be addressed sequentially with removal devitalized skin and subcutaneous fat followed by debridement of necrotic muscle

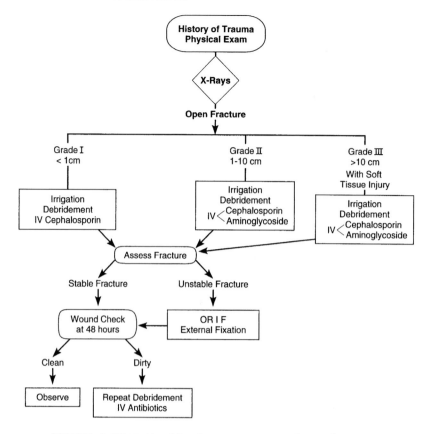

FIGURE 4–10 ■ Algorithm for management of open fractures.

and bone tissue. This prevents external contamination from being carried beyond the skin to the deeper tissues.

Another important concept is "the zone of injury." This refers to the area around the wound that has been traumatized but can recover with appropriate management of the soft tissues and bone. Though an initial debridement should aggressively remove necrotic or devitalized tissues, marginal tissue should be preserved to permit potential recovery. This is one of the reasons that a second assessment and debridement should be carried out 48 to 72 hours later. Tissues that have demonstrated local recovery can be preserved, while other tissues which have continued to remain ischemic should be excised. One cardinal rule is to never close the soft-tissue laceration of an open fracture. This is potentially disastrous in that an open drainage system is converted to a closed cavity, with gas gangrene possibly resulting. All open fractures should be covered with moist sterile dressings that prevent bone and soft-tissue desiccation. The principles of wound management are

undisputed when dealing with open fractures, with the majority of controversy surrounding when and what to use for bone stabilization. Suffice it to say that early bone stabilization via intramedullary nailing, plate-and-screw fixation, or external fixation optimizes soft-tissue healing and access to the extremity for examination and treatment. By preventing continued soft-tissue shearing forces, with the resultant further devascularization of soft tissue, further extension of the zone of injury can be minimized. Soft-tissue coverage of the fracture should be achieved within the first 5 to 7 days of injury. A delayed primary closure may be all that is required in grade I fractures, whereas skin grafting in grade II fractures and possible muscle transfers in grade III fractures may be required. Options for soft-tissue coverage should be individualized for the patient and the degree of injury.

Systemic factors may play a pivotal role in promoting wound healing. It has been estimated that 50 percent of metropolitan medical and surgical patients have overt or subclinical protein and caloric malnutrition. Multiple injuries or even isolated fractures result in a large increase in a patient's metabolic demand needed to assist in healing. Systemic parameters that have been shown to impede soft-tissue healing include a serum albumin <3.5 mg/dL or a total lymphocyte count <1500 cells/mL. Patients presenting with or developing malnutrition following multiple traumatic injuries are at increased risk of infection, delayed union, or nonunion of open fractures. Aggressive nutritional resuscitation is necessary with either oral or feeding tube supplementation or, in extreme cases, IV total parental nutrition via a central venous catheter.

If osteomyelitis develops following an open fracture, then the principles of treatment for adult osteomyelitis apply with one important exception—namely, the retention of implants for fixation of the fracture. In patients who present with an infection surrounding an intramedullary nail or plate, the wound should be aggressively debrided and the implant maintained if fracture stability is being achieved. Loose implants should be removed and either replaced or substituted for by another implant type (i.e., an external fixator replacing a loose plate and screws). Intravenous antibiotics should be administered and directed toward isolated organisms for at least six weeks. Once the fracture has healed, the implant can be removed and further debridement performed. This approach reduces the fracture complexity from an infected nonunion to an infected united bone, with a better prognosis for successful healing and eradication of the infection.

INFECTIONS ASSOCIATED WITH JOINT ARTHROPLASTY

As previously discussed, the presence of a foreign substrate (e.g., joint surface) can provide bacteria with an excellent opportunity for binding and colonization. Unfortunately, the diagnosis of an infected joint arthroplasty can be extremely difficult. Radiographs can demonstrate subtle or even profound bone resorption surrounding implants suspected of being infected. However, similar changes can be seen with aseptic loosening without an associated infection. Laboratory values, though often abnormal, are also not specific for infection. The WBC count is rarely elevated except in a fulminant infection. The ESR is generally elevated and has been estimated to be approximately 80

percent accurate in suggesting the presence of an infection. Aspiration still remains the best single test to identify a subclinical infection, with a sensitivity of 0 percent, specificity of 80 percent, and an accuracy of 78 percent. Fluoroscopy or ultrasound should be used to confirm needle localization within the joint. The use of radionuclide scanning has been utilized to diagnose joint arthroplasty infections. Studies have varied in reporting the accuracy of indium-labeled WBC and gallium scanning. At best the accuracy of either a indium labeled-WBC scan or a combined gallium-technetium scan is approximately 80 percent for identifying an infected arthroplasty. It has been recommended that all three methods—ESR, joint aspiration, and indium scanning—be used to determine whether an infection is present. If up to two of the three studies point toward an infection, appropriate treatment should be employed. Further evaluation may be necessary when only a single study is indicative for infection. Treatment of infected arthroplasties involves removal of the old implant, including all of the cement mantle, aggressive irrigation and debridement, and at least 6 weeks of antibiotics followed by reaspiration once the patient has been off of antibiotics for at least 2 weeks. A cement spacer impregnated with antibiotics is usually implanted at the time of initial debridement. Patients with cultures negative for bacteria may undergo reimplantation at a later date. Positive cultures necessitate redebridement and another course of antibiotics. In the case of gram-negative bacterial infections, reimplantation may be delayed for as long as 1 year. Antibiotics, specific for the infecting organism, are generally added to the bone cement at the time of reimplantation.

SUGGESTED READINGS

Cierny G: Chronic osteomyelitis: Results of treatment. Instr Course Lect 39:495–508, 1990.

Evarts CM (ed): Surgery of the Musculoskeletal System, ed 2. New York, Churchill Livingstone, 1990.

Esterhai JL Jr (ed): Orthopaedic infections. Orthop Clin North Am 22(3), 1991.

Green NE, Edwards K: Bone and joint infections in children. Orthop Clin North Am 18:555–576, 1987.

Gristina AG: Biomaterial-centered infection: Microbial adhesion versus tissue integration. Science 237:1588-1595, 1987.

Chapter 5

Tumors of the Musculoskeletal System

Alan D. Aaron and George P. Bogumill

INTRODUCTION

Tumors of the musculoskeletal system are uncommon when compared to tumors of the breast, uterus, lung, or skin. It is estimated that soft tissue sarcomas account for about 0.8 percent to 1.0 percent of all cancers and that about 5000 to 5500 new cases are diagnosed per year. Osteosarcoma, the most common primary malignant bone sarcoma afflicting children, is even less common, with only 900 newly diagnosed cases being reported annually. In contrast, 93,000 cases of lung carcinoma and 88,000 cases of breast cancer are newly diagnosed each year. It has been calculated that primary malignant lesions of the skeleton will be seen by a primary care practitioner only two or three times in a lifetime of practice. It is because of this that bone and soft tumors can often be underdiagnosed and neglected by both patient and physician. If a physician accepts that any mass is abnormal or significant, efforts can be made to ascertain the proper diagnosis. On occasion, the workup will prove to be more than necessary for an innocuous lesion, but a more serious lesion will seldom be neglected until it is too late for optimal treatment. Those lesions recognized as possibly being malignant should be referred to a surgical oncology specialist for appropriate

workup and treatment. Retrospective review of misdiagnosed malignant lesions often yields clues in both the clinical history and physical examination, which would have assisted in earlier recognition of these lesions. Therefore, the most important aspect of the initial evaluation of a patient with a musculoskeletal tumor is recognizing its presence. Musculoskeletal neoplasms should always be in the differential diagnosis of a patient with musculoskeletal symptoms or signs. A careful evaluation is necessary to prevent delays in diagnosis and treatment, which is often detrimental to patient outcome or survival.

HISTORY

Every patient with a soft-tissue mass, with or without associated symptoms, or radiographic evidence of a bone lesion, deserves a thorough and careful evaluation. Often patients seek out a physician because of pain, an unexplained soft tissue mass, or the presence of a suspicious radiographic finding. A good history and physical examination are mandatory. One should ascertain how and when the lesion was discovered and whether there has been any change in size (either increase or decrease). A rapidly increasing mass is more indicative of a malignant or inflammatory process, while slow growth is often characteristic of benign lesions. Associated symptoms such as pain or loss of function of the involved part are all important pieces of information. A dull aching type of pain, not relieved by rest and present at night are worrisome findings. In addition, children rarely complain of extremity or back pain. A complete evaluation is necessary in such cases to rule out the presence of an occult neoplasm.

Local or general symptoms, anorexia or weight loss, or any change in the function of other systems should be asked about and recorded since they may be indicators of a malignant process. A history of trauma is often recounted by patients, especially children, but it serves mainly to draw attention to the lesion in question. Pathologic fractures may serve as the initial presentation of a particular skeletal problem. A history of pain in the same region prior to fracture is concerning for either an aggressive benign tumor or possibly a malignant process. Adult patients with a history of a primary carcinoma occasionally sustain pathological fractures secondary to local bone destruction from metastatic bone disease. In both cases, a biopsy should be considered to establish the etiology of the lesion. Bone infections (osteomyelitis), which are considered to be the most common mimickers of malignant lesions, can often be established with a careful history. Recent infections, especially in children, may serve as sources for secondary seeding of skeletal sites.

The past medical history can provide vital information. A previous history of cancer should always be established, but may not be readily volunteered by the patient, especially for those considered to be in remission. In addition, chronic diseases (e.g., chronic renal failure) may secondarily involve the skeleton, with attendant radiographic changes. As there are no infallible features to distinguish a benign process from a malignancy by history or physical examination, it is imperative not to diagnose a malignancy without histological confirmation.

PHYSICAL EXAMINATION

The physical examination should include overall evaluation of the patient, as well as examination of the specific area of complaint. Metastatic tumors account for the most common malignancies of the skeleton, with common primary sites being lung, breast, prostate, kidney, thyroid, and gastrointestinal neoplasms. For example a destructive bone lesion in an elderly patient with a breast mass or a thyroid nodule is indicative of a metastatic carcinoma as opposed to a primary bone neoplasm. Other worrisome systemic manifestations can include recent weight loss, loss of appetite, cachexia, and malaise. Local examination should include careful palpation of the mass to determine size, extent of fixation to adjacent tissues, firmness or softness, local temperature change, and overlying skin changes (atrophy, telangiectasia, etc.). Although most malignant musculoskeletal tumors metastasize to the lung, some do go to the draining lymph nodes. Therefore, a careful physical examination of both regional and systemic lymph nodes for evidence of enlargement is required. In patients complaining of low back pain, a rectal examination can uncover an occult sacral lesion (e.g., chordoma), which may not be readily apparent with routine radiographs.

RADIOGRAPHIC AND LABORATORY EXAMINATION

Plain radiographs in two planes of the involved area are necessary and should be performed even on patients with only a soft-tissue mass. Radiographs should be of good quality, include the entire bone in question, with additional views being obtained of anatomic sites that potentially may refer pain to another location (e.g., hip lesion presenting as knee pain). It must be remembered that the best diagnostic radiographic examination of a bone lesion is the plain radiograph. Additional studies, such as a radionuclide scan, computerized axial tomography (CT scans), or a magnetic resonance imaging (MRI) study, only serve to confirm diagnostic impressions obtained from review of the plain radiographs.

A systematic approach to radiographic interpretation is needed with specific questions being asked. A good approach is to review the soft tissues before the bone, as this area is often forgotten and can provide valuable information. The initial radiographs may detect changes in soft-tissue densities, such as a calcification (Fig. 5–1) or ossification. Enneking has outlined four basic questions that should be asked when evaluating bone lesions on plain radiographs. These are important be-

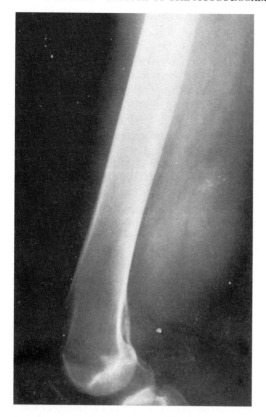

FIGURE 5–1 ■ Large soft-tissue sarcoma of posterior thigh containing scattered calcifications. The mass is ill-defined because it has the same water density as the surrounding muscle, although the fat densities provide some delineation.

cause particular tumors present in characteristic locations, interact with bone in a particular manner, and may produce a specific matrix that is apparent on a radiograph.

The first question is "Where is the lesion?" Is it in the appendicular (extremity) or axial (spine) skeleton, the hand or foot? Is it situated in the epiphysis, metaphysis, or diaphysis? Is it within the medullary canal, in the cortex, or outside of the bone?

The second question is "What is the lesion doing to the bone?" Is there bone destruction with a poor zone of transition or has bone formed around the lesion to sequester it (as in sclerosis)? Characteristic patterns of bone destruction typically include either geographic, motheaten, or permeative patterns (Fig. 5–2). Geographic bone destruction often presents with a clear zone of transition between the lesion and the surrounding normal bone. This type of pattern is usually indica-

tive of benign lesions (e.g., unicameral bone cysts, nonossifying fibroma, or giant cell tumors). A motheaten pattern presents with a poorly definable zone of transition and usually signals aggressive bone destruction characteristic of malignant tumors or infections (such as osteosarcomas or chronic osteomyelitis). Permeative patterns have no appreciable zone of transition and generally are associated with aggressive round cell tumors or acute infections (e.g., Ewing's sarcoma, lymphoma, or acute osteomyelitis).

The third question is "What is the bone doing to the lesion?" Is there an endosteal reaction, and if there is, how mature is it? Examples include sclerosis, usually seen with benign lesions, or endosteal scalloping, often a hallmark of aggressive behavior. Is there a periosteal reaction, and what type is it if present? Examples include aggressive patterns, such as sunburst or onion skinning, and benign patterns with a well-formed appearance (Fig. 5–3).

The fourth question is "Is there any characteristic within the lesion to suggest a specific diagnosis?" Is there calcification (mineralization of cartilage), ossification (bone formation), or a ground-glass appearance?

In addition to the initial radiographic interpretation, observation of a lesion over time can provide important information about rates of growth or any suspicious changes in radiographic appearance. Therefore, inquiries about previously obtained radiographs should be made and reviewed if available to evaluate bone lesions. If a bone lesion presents with a classic radiographic appearance of a benign lesion, such as an enchondroma or osteochondroma, treatment often can be performed without recourse to more elaborate and expensive studies. In addition one may choose observation rather than surgery for lesions which typically heal with time. This decision must be made by persons thoroughly familiar with musculoskeletal pathology and not by one who rarely sees such lesions.

Additional imaging modalities are often employed by physicians to gain more information, which can assist in surgical planning or systemic staging. These include bone scintigraphy, CT scans, MRIs, and angiograms. In addition, chest radiographs or CT scans of the chest, head, abdomen or pelvis may be indicated for staging purposes. When the bone changes are more ominous on plain radiographs, other imaging studies may be necessary.

Technetium-99m and gallium-67 scans are readily available, efficient, cost effective and can provide extremely useful information. These scans are used to determine the activity of the primary lesion, as well as the uncovering of occult metastatic sites. Though extremely sensitive, these modalities are not specific for neoplastic conditions and must be coupled with other modalities (plain radiographs) to be useful. Technetium-99 coupled with methylene diphosphonate is the most commonly utilized bone scintigraphy agent, largely because it is an avid bone-seeking agent and can be performed in a relatively short time (usually 6 hours). Lack of isotope uptake (cold scans) is usually indicative of a benign process. One noted exception is multiple myeloma, which characteristically demonstrates a normal or decreased pattern of uptake. Increased uptake can be seen in fractures including stress fractures, infection, metabolic disorders, trauma, and benign or malignant neoplasms. Bone scans with only a single region of uptake (monostotic) are more indicative of a primary bone condition, while multiple sites (polyostotic) patterns usually represent either metastatic disease or metabolic conditions. Gallium scans are less useful since the examination takes longer to perform (24 to 48 hours) and is more sensitive for the presence of inflammatory cells than bone activity.

Computed tomography scans, though recently supplanted by MRIs, are extremely useful in evaluating bone lesions. Better resolution of osseous structures and such features as calcification and ossification can be appreciated with CT scans. For example, osteoid osteomas, which are extremely small (<10 mm) benign bone tumors residing in the cortex, are better elucidated on CT scans as compared to MRIs. Intravenous (IV) contrast agents, which clearly define vascular structures and enhance soft-tissue masses, can be used in conjunction with CT scans in the place of MRIs in some circumstances.

Magnetic resonance imaging currently serves as the most utilized study, aside from plain radiographs, in the evaluation of bone neoplasms. The advantages of using MRI include the lack of radiation exposure for the patient, clear elucidation of soft-tissue masses, and the marrow extent of bone neoplasms. In addition, unlike CT, MRI is able to distinguish between histologically different tissues of identical densities. Utilization of IV contrast can readily distinguish between tumor margins and edematous normal tissues, thus enabling surgeons to better plan surgical procedures.

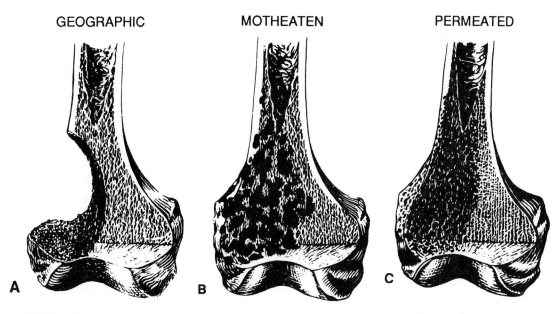

FIGURE 5–2 ■ Radiographic patterns of bone destruction. *A,* Geographic pattern implies slow rates of growth. *B,* Moth-eaten pattern implies intermediate rates of growth. *C,* Permeative pattern implies rapid rates of growth.

(Lodwick GS: Solitary malignant tumors of bone: The application of predictor variables and diagnosis. Semin Roentgenol 1:293, 1966; reprinted with permission.)

PERIOSTEAL REACTIONS

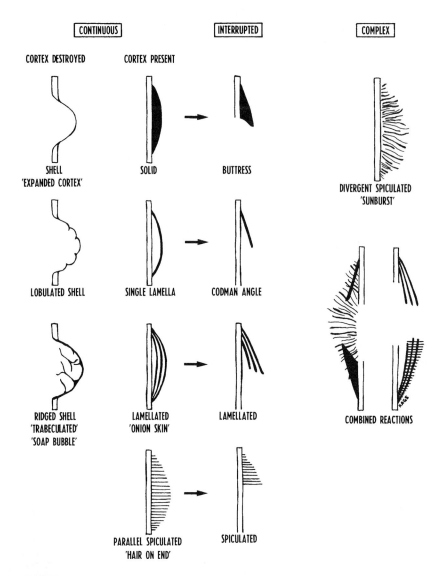

FIGURE 5–3 ■ Radiographic patterns of periosteal reaction. Continuous patterns tend to be less aggressive, with either onion skinning or sunburst patterns indicating rapid growth.

(Ragsdale BD, Madewell JE, Sweet DE: Radiologic and pathologic analysis of solitary bone lesions. Radiol Clin North Am 19(4):749–783, 1981; reprinted with permission.)

Disadvantages include high cost, long examination times, and poor tolerance for claustrophobic patients.

Whereas angiography was once the best modality available for judging the extent of bone or soft-tissue tumors, it has been largely replaced for this purpose by both CT scans and MRIs. Its primary applications include definition of vascular structures adjacent to or en-

cased by tumors or for the embolization of vascular lesions prior to a resection. In addition, chemotherapeutic drugs can be given intra-arterially utilizing angiographic techniques.

Laboratory studies of blood and urine often are not helpful in diagnosing primary musculoskeletal lesions. However, calcium, phosphorus, alkaline phosphatase, and other studies may provide clues to a proper diagnosis. An elevated white blood cell count and sedimentation rate can lead one to consider infection as the causative entity. Occasionally, an iliac-crest bone marrow biopsy may confirm a diagnosis of multiple myeloma without recourse to a biopsy of a major limb bone with its attendant risk of a post biopsy fracture.

BIOPSY

The biopsy should follow all radiographic imaging of the primary lesion. Proper planning of the biopsy is imperative to prevent complications that can lead to unnecessary amputations or death. Prebiopsy evaluation and planning improve the likelihood that adequate and representative tissue will be obtained with minimal normal tissue contamination. In addition, scans obtained after a surgical procedure may reflect a larger tumor image secondary to postsurgical edema and swelling. This may result in the unnecessary removal of normal tissue or adjacent structures. When performing a biopsy a specialized approach is necessary and is done with the anticipation that a more extensive surgical resection may need to be done later. Surgical guidelines for a biopsy include the use of longitudinal as opposed to horizontal incisions, contamination of only a single compartment, avoidance of neurovascular planes, and meticulous hemostasis to prevent tracking of tumor cells through a hematoma while avoiding the development of skin or muscle flaps.

Drains should be avoided, but if necessary should be brought out through the incision and not through a distant site. A tourniquet may be used, but must be released with adequate hemostasis being obtained prior to wound closure. In addition, if a tourniquet is used, exsanguination is contraindicated since tumor cells may be discharged into the local vascular system. Cultures should always be taken at the time of biopsy in lieu of an unsuspected osteomyelitis. A frozen section must be performed to be assured that adequate and representative tissue has been obtained. In addition, the clinical history and radiographs should be reviewed with the pathologist prior to the biopsy. Often review of these studies is necessary before the pathologist can properly interpret the histologic sections.

Types of biopsies include a needle biopsy, an open-incisional biopsy, and an excisional biopsy. Needle biopsies do not require a surgical procedure and are cost effective. However, a major disadvantage is the limited amount of material available for histologic review and processing. An open-incisional biopsy requires a surgical procedure, but provides a larger amount of lesional material for interpretation. Open-excisional biopsies are often reserved for small or benign lesions.

TUMORS OF THE SKELETON

Though relatively rare, bone and soft-tissue lesions vary widely in type, making assimilation of information about these lesions difficult to encompass. The simplest approach is to categorize tumors based upon tissue type or common attributes and then divide them into benign and malignant entities. This approach is helpful when evaluating radiographs, since a large differential diagnosis can often be trimmed to a few likely possibilities. For example, calcifications on a radiograph generally signify a cartilaginous tumor regardless of whether the tumor is benign or malignant. A strong emphasis can then be placed upon the cartilage subtype of tumors. These lesions can then be further categorized into benign or malignant lesions and intramedullary, cortical, or juxtacortical lesions based upon the radiographic appearance, permitting further identification.

Benign Cartilaginous Tumors

Osteochondroma is a cartilage-capped protuberance of bone growing outward from the surface of a normal bone (Fig. 5–4). Such tumors tend to grow until puberty, then mature with subsequent ossification of the cartilage cap. Some patients can present with multiple lesions, a tendency that is carried as an autosomal dominant gene (resulting, when expressed, in familial multiple osteochondromatosis). Continued growth beyond puberty is highly suggestive of malignant degeneration. This seldom occurs in isolated lesions but is fairly common with the familial generalized variety. Interference with normal growth of the parent bone is common in the generalized condition. Osteochondroma must be distinguished from parosteal osteosarcoma, an indolent but persistent malignancy. This distinction can often be made with CT or MRI or even

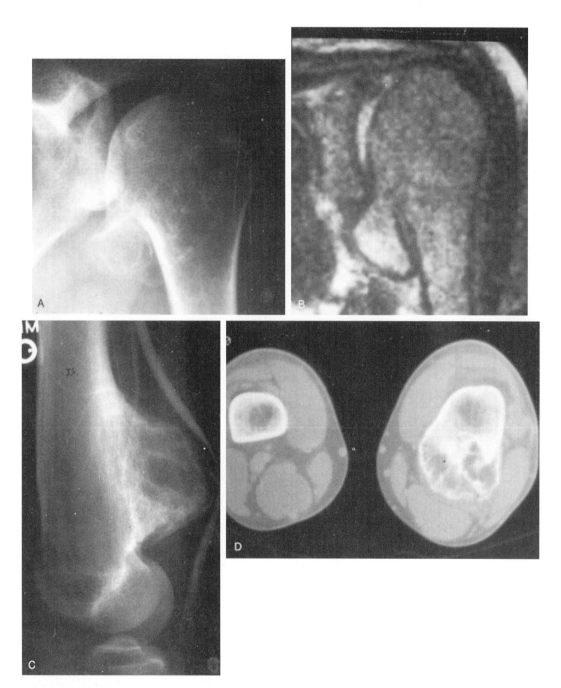

FIGURE 5–4 ■ Osteochondroma. *A* and *B,* radiographic and MRI studies of a shoulder joint with a bony excrescence from the head of the humerus. The cortical and cancellous bone of the osteochondroma are continuous with the same tissues of the parent bone (compare with Fig. 5–7). *C* and *D,* Osteochondroma arising from the posterior aspect of the femur. Again, the cortex of the protuberance is continuous with the cortex of the femur. Note the tenting of the femoral artery by the lesion.

a biopsy. Treatment is surgical excision if the patient is symptomatic.

Enchondroma refers to the accumulation of cartilage rests within the bone. They can be single (rarely symptomatic, often found incidentally) or multiple. Generalized enchondromatosis leads to growth disturbances, is often unilateral, and may be associated with malignant degeneration in later years, with lesions of proximal femur and pelvis being at particularly high-risk. Curettage is often done for diagnostic and treatment reasons. Radiographic changes may be diagnostic, with speckled calcifications apparent throughout the lesion on CT. Bone scans are positive and can lead to the discovery of additional lesions.

Chondroblastoma is a lesion of the epiphysis in adolescents. It is composed of uniform-appearing cartilage cells (or chondroblasts), occasional giant cells, and calcification in a lacy network ("chicken-wire" calcification) around the cells. It produces pain secondary to an associated joint synovitis and can progress to involve a fairly large area if untreated. Treatment is curettage.

Malignant Cartilaginous Tumors

Chondrosarcoma can occur in any bone preformed in cartilage. Patients with multiple benign cartilage lesions run the risk of eventually developing malignant change, particularly in the pelvis, proximal femur, or humerus. The patient population is thus in middle life or older for these secondary tumors. Primary chondrosarcoma may occur during the third or fourth decade of life. The tumors may grow to a very large size before the patient presents for treatment (Fig. 5–5), making surgical removal difficult without amputation. These tumors are not very responsive to adjuvant therapy, such as chemotherapy or radiation therapy. Death is by local invasion of vital structures or by pulmonary metastases.

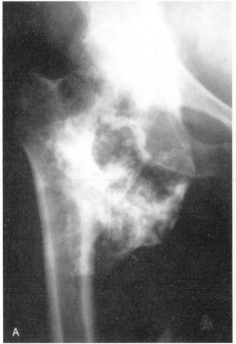
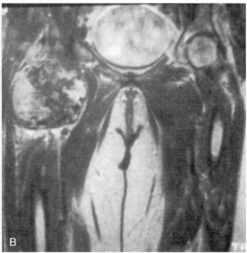

FIGURE 5–5 ■ Chondrosarcoma. *A,* A large lesion in a 74-year-old woman who had known of a mass in the groin for more than 20 years. Recent pain from a pathologic fracture led to treatment for the lesion. *B,* Coronal section of a MRI scan demonstrates nonhomogeneous nature of the large lesion. *C* and *D* is comparative axial view of MRI and CT scans. Although the CT scan illustrates the bony tissues more clearly than the MRI, the latter can give views in three planes and provides useful anatomical information to the surgeon. *Illustration continued on following page.*

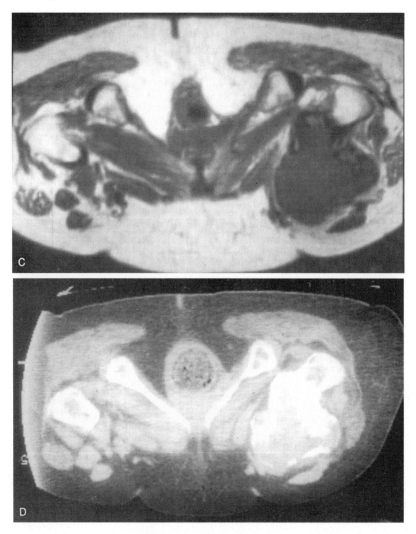

FIGURE 5–5 ■ *Continued*

Benign Osseous Tumors

Osteoid osteoma is a small (<10 mm), painful bone lesion that has many in the field questioning whether the lesion is neoplastic or inflammatory. It incites a fairly marked osteoblastic response in bone. The aching pain, worse at night, is often dramatically relieved with aspirin. Individuals of either sex or any age may be affected. Surgical removal of the small nidus is curative.

Osteoblastoma is uncommon and can occur in any bone. It is one of the more common benign osseous lesions afflicting the vertebral column. Histologically, it is composed of osteoblasts making osteoid, some of which calcifies. It is distinguished from osteoid osteoma by its larger size (>10 mm) and continued enlarge-

ment if left untreated. As with chondroblastoma, treatment is curettage.

Malignant Osseous Lesions

Osteosarcoma is a high-grade malignancy in which pleomorphic osteoblasts produce bone or osteoid of bizarre histological appearance. The calcification of the osteoid is usually prominent and leads to irregular sclerosis-mixed with radiolucent areas on radiographs (Fig. 5–6A–D). The patients are sometimes barely into adolescence, although most are in their late teens or early twenties. Disease in another group occurs in later life (usually the sixth or seventh decade) and is most often associated with Paget's disease of bone. Ag-

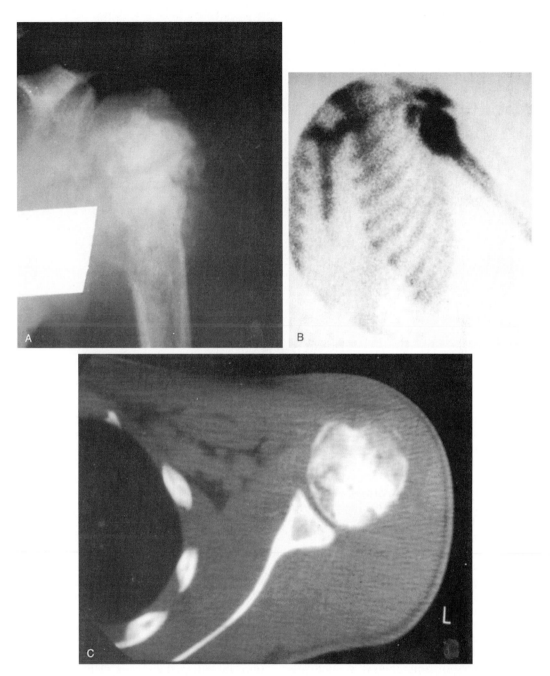

FIGURE 5–6 ■ Osteosarcoma. *A,* A radiograph of the shoulder shows the irregular destruction and production of bone with extension into the soft tissues. *B,* Bone scan shows marked uptake of the tracer in the tumor area, indicating intense bone production. *C,* The CT scan illustrates the extent of the osseous production by the tumor in the humeral head. *D,* A specimen radiograph can be useful to illustrate the extent of the tumor inside and outside the bone, as well as the repair attempts that occurred during the neoadjuvant chemotherapy. *E,* A large slice of the resected specimen gives a good gross picture of the tumor extent and repair attempts. The junction of an extraosseous tumor and cortical surface is called Codman's triangle and represents normal bone made by the periosteum elevated by tumor expansion. *Illustration continued on following page.*

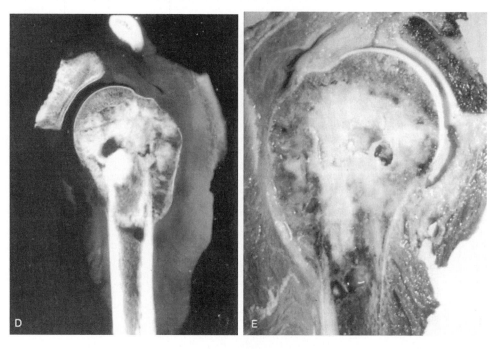

FIGURE 5–6 ■ *Continued*

gressive growth is recognized by a motheaten pattern of bony cortical destruction and spread of the tumor into the soft tissues, with characteristic ossification and periosteal reaction in a "sunburst" pattern and a "Codman's triangle" at the ends of the periosteal reaction (Fig. 5–6D,E). Patients have often experienced low-grade pain with steady progression for a number of months before diagnosis. Treatment must be aggressive, and amputation is often required, especially if there has been delay in diagnosis or inappropriate surgery. Limb-sparing surgery may be possible with either allograft or prosthetic reconstruction. Current methods of treatment involve neoadjuvant chemotherapy for several courses to "stun" or kill the tumor, followed by surgery and then completion of the course of chemotherapy. Older methods of treatment (mainly radical surgery or amputation) yielded less than 20 percent of patients surviving for at least 10 years. Newer methods are resulting in better cure rates, varying from 100 percent at 2 years to 75 percent at 10 years. Death is usually by pulmonary metastases.

Parosteal osteosarcoma is a bone-forming tumor arising from the outer surface of the cortex of any bone (Fig. 5–7). It is slow-growing, often underdiagnosed on a biopsy, particularly if the pathologist is not experienced at reading bone lesions. An incomplete resection invariably leads to recurrence. If the lesion is present long enough, it exhibits invasion into the medullary cavity of the parent bone and becomes more aggressive, with a prognosis similar to a conventional osteosarcoma. A distinction must be made with an osteochondroma, which is benign. Computed tomography scans or MRI will help make this distinction. In osteochondromas, the cortex and medullary cancellous bone are continuous from parent bone into the bony stalk (see Fig. 5–4). In a parosteal osteosarcoma, the lesion spreads along the cortical surface of the parent bone, but there is no continuity between the lesion and the host bone. On histology, the marrow one would expect to see is not normal fatty marrow but a low-grade fibrous sarcoma with innocuous-looking bone spicules. Recommended treatment is wide excision, including the cortex of the underlying bone.

Benign Fibrous Tumors

Nonossifying fibroma (fibroxanthoma) is one of the most common bone lesions, usually without symptoms unless it becomes large enough to fracture. It is seen on films as a radiolucent lesion with a sclerotic border, eccentrically situated in the long bones at the junction of

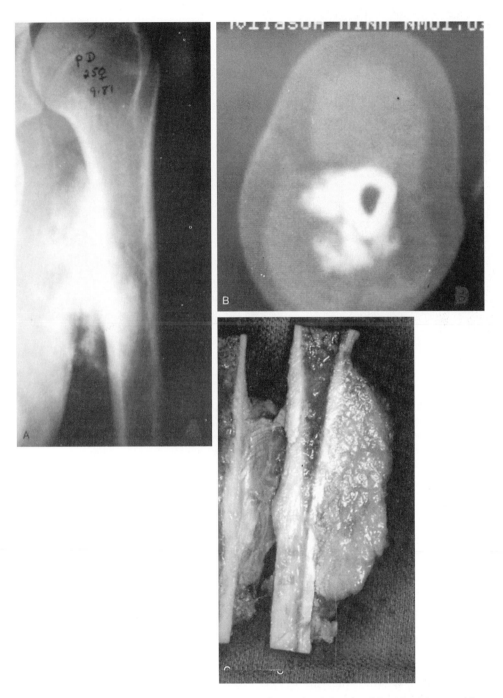

FIGURE 5–7 ■ Parosteal osteosarcoma. *A,* A radiograph of the shoulder of a 26-year-old woman shows a heavily ossified mass medial to the proximal humeral diaphysis. The tumor originates in a specific cortical location, and as it grows it extends around the bone, making the determination of intraosseous location difficult without CT scans or tomograms. *B,* CT scan of lesion shows clearly that the lesion is entirely on the outer surface of the bone, with no tumor in the medullary cavity. *C,* Longitudinal section of the resected specimen also shows that the cortex is abnormal on one side but that the medullary cavity is free of tumors.

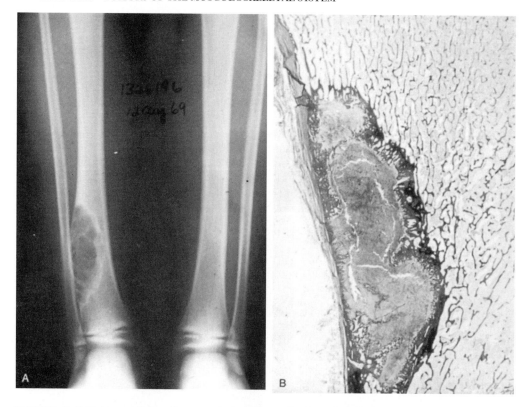

FIGURE 5–8 ■ Nonossifying fibroma. *A,* A radiograph of a typical lesion in the metaphyseal-diaphyseal location of a long bone. The eccentric position is classic, and the clearly defined inner border of sclerotic bone suggest an indolent process, most likely benign. *B,* A histologic macro-section of a fibroxanthoma illustrates the well-defined inner margin of bony rim as well as the lack of bone within the lesional tissue itself.

metaphysis and diaphysis (Fig. 5–8). These lesions present during adolescence and if they are small disappear over a period of several years. Larger ones may need curettage. Histology shows fibrous tissue, foam cells, and giant cells, with an internal border of sclerotic bone.

Fibrous dysplasia may involve one or many bones with a radiolucent appearance on radiograph. Expansion of the involved bone and thinning of the cortex, occasionally sufficient to lead to pathologic fracture, are seen. Histology shows abnormal fibrous tissue with curlicues of bone, giving it a "ground glass" appearance on radiographs. If multiple bones are involved, endocrine changes may be present along with pigmentation of the skin. This condition, known as Albright's syndrome, often presents with a triad of physical findings. They include polyostotic fibrous dysplasia, precocious puberty, and islands of skin pigmentation commonly termed "coast of Maine" lesions.

Malignant Fibrous Tumors

Fibrosarcoma and *malignant fibrous histiocytoma* are rare tumors that may arise within the medullary cavity or periosteal surface. These sarcomas can occur at any age from birth to the elderly but are more prominent in young adults. The most common sites include the long bones of the lower extremity or the humerus and are rare in the axial skeleton. As with most malignant lesions, patients often complain of pain and a mass, which is occasionally complicated by a pathological fracture. A motheaten appearance is characteristic, with regions of radiolucency representing localized bone destruction. Histologically, fibrosarcomas are characterized by interwoven bundles of spindled cells with narrow tapering nuclei and ill-defined cytoplasmic borders, accompanied by lower grade lesions often presenting with a "herringbone pattern." Malignant fibrous histiocytomas differ in that the cells show striking nuclear pleomorphism and abundant cytoplasm. The mononuclear cells are usually fibroblastic and show a cartwheel or storiform (derived from the Greek *storis,* meaning matted) growth pattern. Tumor necrosis is frequently present and mitoses are variable and sometimes common. Treatment for both sarcomas includes a wide surgical resection, with adjuvant radiation and chemotherapy not having any clear benefit.

Malignant Round Cell Tumors

Multiple myeloma is probably the most common primary malignancy in bone. Like Ewing's sarcoma, it arises in the diaphysis of long bones or other bones that contain marrow. Diagnosis occasionally can be made by needle biopsy, although bone lesions in general should be diagnosed by an adequate amount of tissue that can seldom be obtained by a fine needle. Blood or urine specimens may provide confirming evidence. A monoclonal globulin spike on serum electrophoresis or the presence of Bence-Jones proteins in the urine are intrinsic to the workup and evaluation of efficacy of treatment. Bone destruction is the rule, with severe osteoporosis occurring in later stages; surprisingly, bone response is minimal and bone scans are often negative. Treatment is radiation therapy and chemotherapy.

Ewing's sarcoma is a malignancy whose cell of origin is unproven. This sarcoma usually presents before the age of 30, arises in the diaphysis, grows rapidly, and spreads to the lungs early on. On radiographs we see radiolucency in the diaphysis with periosteal reaction in an "onion skin" pattern indicating the extent of the lesion in the bone and the intermittency of the growth pattern (Fig. 5–9). It is often confused with osteomyelitis. As is true of most rapidly growing tumors, Ewing's sarcoma is responsive to neoadjuvant chemotherapy and radiation therapy, and these treatment modalities are often used before surgery. Operations may be necessary later, particularly if growth disturbances from the tumor and/or its treatment occurs.

Other Commonly Seen Lesions

Unicameral bone cysts occur most commonly in the proximal humeral metaphysis (Fig. 5–10A), where they appear as a radiolucent expansion of bone. Other bones are commonly involved (Fig. 5–10B–D), including carpals

and tarsals. Pathological fracture is often the first indication of the lesion. Young children are principally involved. The lesion cavity is filled with a straw-colored fluid and has a lining containing numerous vascular channels, fibrous tissue, some giant cells, and foam cells. Treatment in recent years has consisted of transcutaneous injection of steroids; several injections may be needed. Surgical curettage may be required.

Giant cell tumors of bone usually are benign (90%) but behave in a locally aggressive fashion, and in 10% or more of cases it may metastasize to the lung. This controversial tumor is filled with giant cells that are thought to be osteoclasts, and thus it is not surprising that the major response in the bone is destruction, producing a lytic area in the end of long bones on a radiograph (Fig. 5–11A). Although the periosteum responds with new bone production (Fig. 5–11B), it is often unable to keep up with the destruction; when enough bone tissue is removed to weaken the bone, pathological fracture often occurs. Lesions originate in the metaphysis, particularly in the distal femur or proximal tibia, but extend into the epiphysis after growth plate closure (Fig. 5–11C–E). Curettage is the treatment of choice if the tumor is discovered early (Fig. 5–11E), but recurrences are disappointingly common. Larger lesions or recurrent ones may require *en bloc* excision with an allograft or prosthetic replacement. Amputation may be needed if the lesion leads to a nonfunctional limb, as determined by the extent of bone destruction or persisting infection after surgery. Radiation therapy has been used, especially for lesions that are surgically inaccessible, but it has a disturbing tendency to lead to malignant degeneration.

METASTATIC TUMORS

Metastatic bone disease is common and comprises the most frequent malignancy found in bone. The most common primaries originate from the breast, kidney, thyroid, prostate, or lungs. The radiographic appearance may mimic that of any of the primary tumors of bone. In 22 percent of cases, a biopsy of the bone lesion is the first indication that a patient has a primary tumor elsewhere. Often the patient is under the care of an oncologist who will refer the patient to an orthopaedist when symptoms of pain or a radiograph disclose a

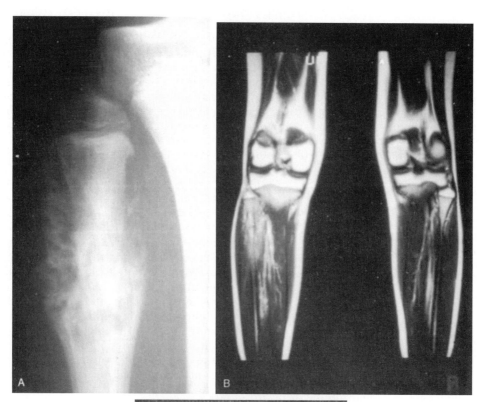

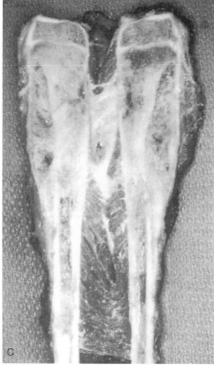

FIGURE 5–9 ■ Ewing's sarcoma. *A,* Anteroposterior radiograph of a proximal fibula in a 13-year-old boy shows irregular destruction of the bone with expansion and attempts at repair. *B,* A coronal view on MRI demonstrates extensive changes in the bone as well as surrounding soft tissues. *C,* The proximal fibula was resected after a course of x-ray and chemotherapy. The intraosseous and soft-tissue extensions of the tumor are well shown. *D–F,* Comparable CT and MRI views of the lesion demonstrate well how the differing techniques emphasize different aspects of the lesion.

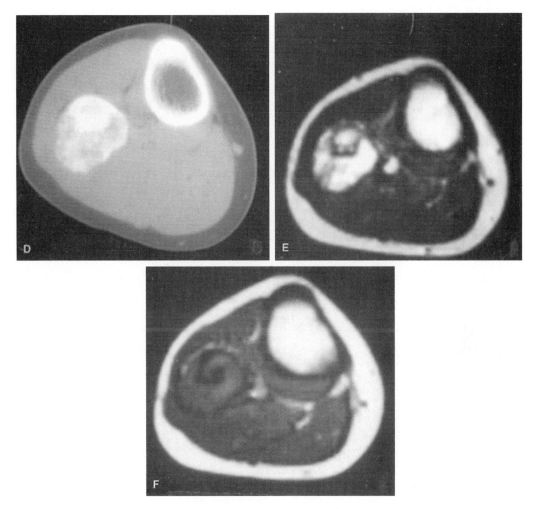

FIGURE 5–9 ■ *Continued*

pathologic fracture. In addition, there has been enough bone removal, stimulated by tumor growth in the bone, that an impending fracture may be imminent, or it may be a case of intolerable pain following radiation therapy. Treatment is directed toward providing support of the skeleton, usually by some form of internal fixation or prosthetic replacement of the involved area. Such treatment is used to provide comfort by stabilizing the skeleton during the patient's limited remaining life span. Lesions detected early may be treated with radiation therapy to decrease the chance of pathological fracture.

The Algorithm

The patient who presents with a lesion of bone requires careful evaluation by the clinician in order to make the appropriate diagnosis and provide the proper treatment (Fig. 5–12). The algorithm is designed to provide a series of steps to consider. If the lesion is on the cortical surface of the bone, steps must be taken to separate benign from malignant lesions. This distinction can be done on plain radiographs, although computerized axial tomography scans, MRI scans, or tomograms are helpful confirmatory studies. If the lesion is inside the bone, careful study of what the process is doing to the bone (destruction, bone production, or both), the bone's response to the lesion (whether it's a geographic, motheaten, permeative pattern, a periosteal reaction etc.), and the matrix of the lesion as seen on various studies all give critical preoperative information. Slower growing lesions with clear-cut borders and little periosteal reaction are usually benign. Lesions that are clearly growing too fast for the body to keep them walled off

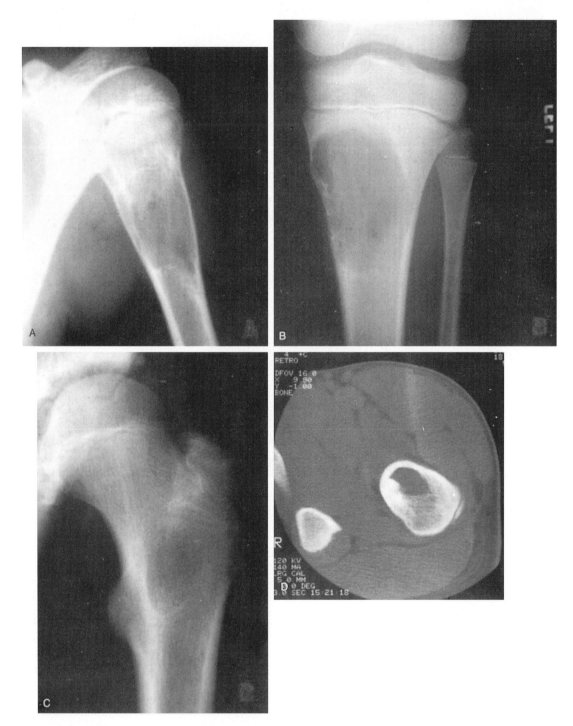

FIGURE 5–10 ■ Unicameral bone cyst. *A,* Typical location. The ill-defined proximal portion and the double cortical line medially suggest there has been a pathologic fracture that has healed. *B* and *C,* Typical cysts in other long bones. Note the metaphyseal location. *D,* The CT scan clearly demonstrates the lack of matrix. *Illustration continued on facing page.*

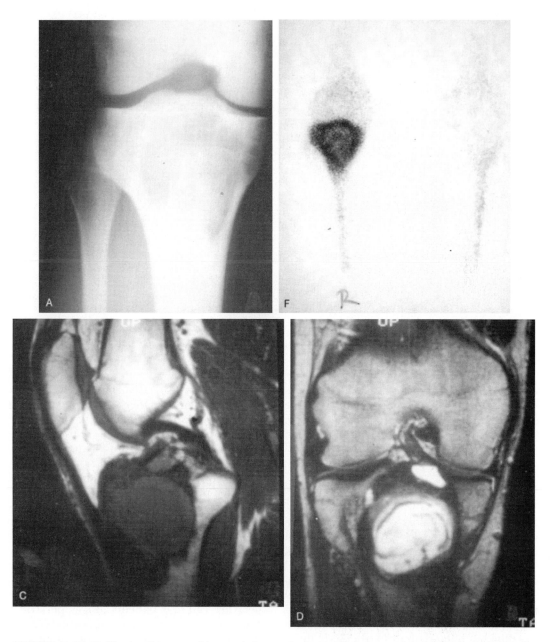

FIGURE 5–11 ■ Giant cell tumor of bone. *A*, Expansile, lytic defect in proximal tibial metaphysis of a young man, with slight extension into epiphysis. *B*, Bone scan is "hot" around periphery and "colder" in the center because the tracer is picked up where bone is being formed, which is at the periphery of the lesion as the result of a repair attempt. *Illustration continued on following page.*

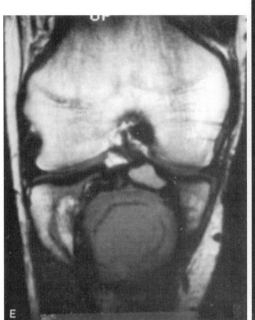

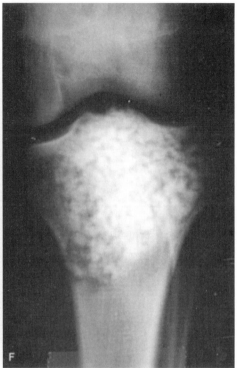

FIGURE 5–11 ■ *Continued C–E,* Three MRI views of the lesion illustrate its inhomogeneous nature. *F,* Curettage and packing the cavity with allograft cortical bone chips are a common form of treatment.

with bone production are much more worrisome and require a prompt search for the cause and plan for the cure. Many of these questions are best resolved at a tumor center.

TUMORS OF THE SOFT PARTS

Masses in the musculoskeletal soft tissues are more frequent than lesions in the skeleton itself. They can arise in any of the mesodermal tissues; thus we can see lesions of fat, blood vessels, fibrous tissue, synovium, and occasionally muscles. Plain radiographs are less helpful than they are when the lesions involve calcified tissues because the lesions are isodense with the muscles. Some lesions, particularly those with high fat content or vascular lesions that often contain calcifications, may be evident on plain films. Computed tomography scans can assist in delineation of the lesion, but MRI has been the most helpful diagnostic tool. Again, a thorough history and a careful examination—with particular attention to regional lymph nodes—are essential.

Malignant tumors of the soft tissues are approximately 3 to 4 times more common than malignant tumors of bone, although they com-

prise less than 2% of all malignancies. They are often discovered incidentally during a shower or when looking in a mirror; pain is seldom present to a major degree. Thus they may become quite large before a patient presents for treatment (Figs. 5–1, 5–13). They tend to grow outward by small extensions that are not detected by the naked eye. The tumors usually have an apparent capsule, which is deceptive because clusters of tumor cells extend beyond this pseudo capsule and can be left behind if the lesion is simply "shelled out." Radical surgery has been the mainstay of treatment in the past, but more recent regimens with radiotherapy and chemotherapy combined with surgery are offering patients longer periods of tumor-free survival and opportunities for limb-sparing surgery instead of amputation.

To accomplish optimal results, staging is necessary. Enneking and associates have proposed a staging system that can be applied to both bone and soft-tissue malignancies (see Table 5–1). Tumors are divided into low and high grade based on the histological appearance (Stages I and II). They are also separated into those that have escaped the anatomic compartment in which they arose (Stages IB and IIB) and those that have not (Stages IA and IIA). Stage III reflects a tumor that has

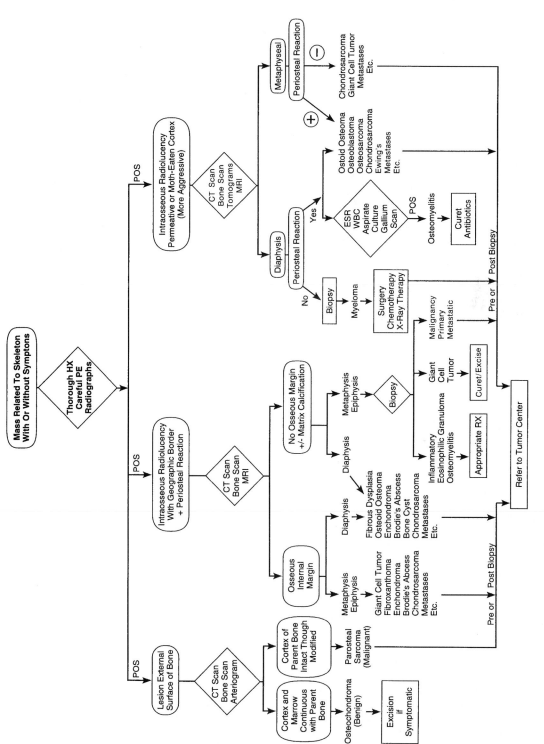

FIGURE 5–12 ■ Algorithm for management of skeletal tumors.

TABLE 5–1 ■ *Surgical Stages of Sarcomas*

Stages	Grade	Site
IA	Low (G1)	Intracompartmental (T1)
IB	Low (G1)	Extracompartmental (T2)
IIA	High (G2)	Intracompartmental (T1)
IIB	High (G2)	Extracompartmental (T2)
III	Any (G) Regional or distant metastasis	Any (T)

From Enneking WF, Spanier SS, Goodman MA: A system for the surgical staging of musculoskeletal sarcoma. Clin Orthop 153:106–120, 1980; reprinted with permission.

metastasized, either to local or distant sites. It can be seen that staging does not involve naming the tumor or detecting the presumed cell of origin, but rather is based upon the aggressiveness of the individual tumor, both on radiographic and histologic studies. The tumors usually arise in the deeper tissues and spread along tissue planes. Metastases are blood borne and tend to be seen first in the peripheral portions of the lung. Recurrence rates approach 15% with a combination of surgery and local radiation therapy. Recurrences usually present with 18 months of treatment.

Anatomic localization of any soft-tissue tumor is the most important factor to consider in surgical management. One must know the precise anatomic extent of tissue change in order to plan surgical removal through normal tissue. A small lesion in the thigh can be resected with minimal loss of function. The same-sized lesion in the foot often requires amputation to obtain adequate margins. A number of recent protocols utilize adjuvant preoperative radiotherapy to shrink the tumor, especially at the active margins, to allow for less extensive resection of normal tissue.

Tumors of Fatty Origin

Lipoma is a very common benign tumor in the extremities, usually near the proximal portions of the limbs or about the limb girdles (Fig. 5–13). They are painless, slow-growing lesions that are often neglected by the patient until they are quite large. Surgical excision is simple and curative with recurrences being rare.

Liposarcoma is the most common soft tissue sarcoma in the extremities. It ranges in type from the low-grade myxoid variant to the high-grade pleomorphic variety. It does not arise from the common lipoma. Eradication is very difficult, even with radical surgery. Adjuvant radiation therapy in conjunction with wide surgical resection is the treatment of choice.

Fibrous Tumors

Desmoid tumors are fibrous tissue tumors that have a disturbing tendency to behave in a locally aggressive manner with frequent recurrences even after wide excision. However, as opposed to malignant soft-tissue sarcomas, they do not metastasize to distant parts. Histologic appearance is one of dense collagen with low cellularity; some lesions may be more cellular with less collagen and a greater tendency to recur. Since they are composed of collagen, it is difficult at surgery to determine the margin of the lesion since it has an appearance similar to normal fibrous tissue. Treatment must be wide excision, with the role of radiation therapy not being fully elucidated.

Fibrosarcoma is diagnosed less commonly than some years ago. The presence of pleomorphic fibroblasts and collagen arranged in a herringbone pattern lead to this diagnosis. Histologic grading is useful in predicting the prognosis, with Grade I lesions growing slowly and metastasizing late.

Malignant fibrous histiocytoma is a popular diagnosis at present. Many cases that were originally diagnosed as fibrosarcoma in the past have been reclassified as malignant fibrous histiocytoma. It is characterized histologically by the whorled (storiform) arrangement of the pleomorphic spindle cells, which comprise the tumor. Wide surgical resection is necessary, in conjunction with radiation therapy, to effectively treat these sarcomas.

Vascular Tumors

Hemangiomas and *vascular malformations* are common. They may vary from a small raspberry hemangioma, easily removed, to extensive malformations involving half of the body and leading to gigantism or other growth disturbances. Surgical excision may be extremely difficult because of the extent of involvement of vital structures; recurrences are common with the larger lesions.

Angiosarcoma presents as a number of variants, but all tend to be quite aggressive, spread early, and recur often. There may even be multiple sites of origin. Chronic lymphedema, as seen with filariasis (elephantiasis), can predispose patients to angiosarcomas in the affected limb. Even with radical surgery combined with adjuvant therapy, eradication of the tumor is difficult to accomplish and survival is often quite limited.

Other Neoplasms

Neurofibromas and *neurilemomas* originate in peripheral nerves. Neurofibromas may be

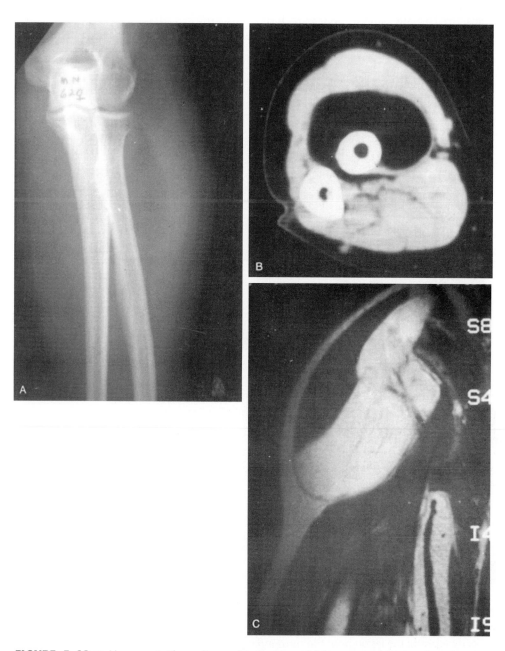

FIGURE 5–13 ■ Lipoma. *A,* The radiographic lucency of fat compared to muscle or bone makes the tumor clearly evident on plain film. *B,* The CT scan also clearly delineates the lesion from surrounding tissues. *C,* A large irregularly lobulated mass about the shoulder is well visualized on MRI.

single or multiple. They are very difficult to remove without removing the nerve, as they originate from the nerve itself. The multiple variety (i.e., neurofibromatosis) may be associated with overgrowth of a limb or digit or hormonal changes, with malignant degeneration being frequently reported. As opposed to neurofibromas, neurilemomas originate from the Schwann cell surrounding the nerve. Neurilemomas are usually single and can be "shelled-out" from around the nerve without loss of function.

Synovial sarcomas arise near, but seldom in, joints (Fig. 5–14). A biphasic histologic pattern of a fibroblastic component mixed with an epithelial component and slit-like space suggests the formation of primitive joints or bursae. These tumors often arise in the terminal portions of the limb and may show very little growth for a number of years, lulling

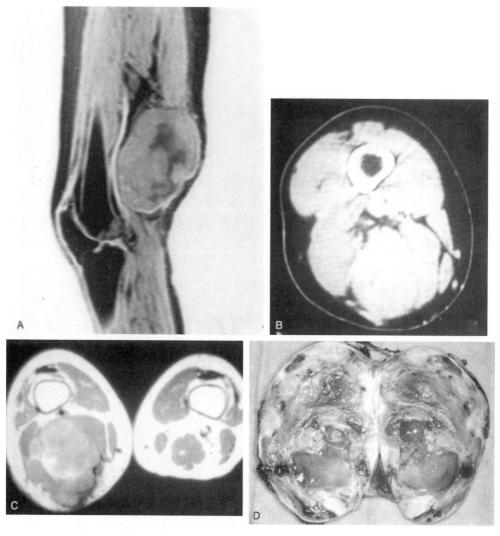

FIGURE 5–14 ■ Synovial sarcoma (compare with Fig. 5–1). *A,* A large mass is clearly visualized in the posterior thigh. *B,* The CT scan presents an axial view of the area but does not clearly separate the lesion from the surrounding muscle since they both have essentially the same water density on radiograph. *C,* The MRI scan of a comparable area shows more clearly the separation of the lesion from the muscle and even the underlying popliteal artery. *D,* Transection of the resected specimen illustrates the irregularity of the tissue components, with cystic areas representing zones of necrosis commonly seen in malignancies.

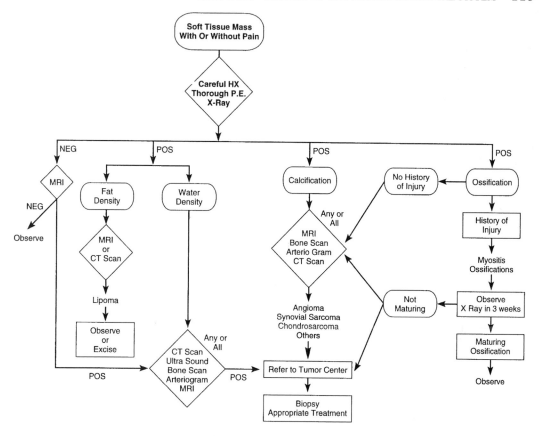

FIGURE 5–15 ■ Algorithm for management of soft tissue tumors.

the patient and physician into complacency. The onset of rapid growth requires prompt action for diagnosis and treatment. This is one of the few soft-tissue sarcomas that will spread to regional lymph nodes (in about 20% of cases).

Rhabdomyosarcoma is a malignant tumor of striated muscle and will show characteristic cross striations on microscopic exams. One third of the cases occur in children, often in the neck or urogenital tract. The two thirds that occur in adults appear in the soft tissues of the torso or extremities.

The Algorithm

Tumors of the soft tissues often present as a painless, progressively growing mass (Fig. 5–15). Separating the benign from the malignant is vital to proper treatment. Any such mass requires a careful history, physical examination, and plain radiographs. If the mass does not present obvious diagnostic features such as transillumination of a ganglion and the plain

radiograph is negative, an MRI should be considered. If this is also negative, observation would be in order. If positive, further workup is indicated, even including a biopsy. Plain radiographs that show the mass to be fat do not require further workup. If the mass is of water density, further workup is indicated, probably after referral to a tumor center. When the plain film shows ossification or calcification and there is no history of injury, workup for a potentially serious lesion is indicated. When to refer the patient to a tumor center depends on the individual situation of both patient and physician, but is often advisable to do early because of the potential for limb-sparing surgery and increased opportunity for a "cure" if delay or inappropriate surgery has not been done.

SUGGESTED READINGS

Bogumill GP, Schwamm, HA: Orthopaedic Pathology: A Synopsis with Clinical and Radiographic

Correlation. Philadelphia, WB Saunders Company, 1984.

Enneking WF, Spanier SS, Goodman MA: A system for the surgical staging of musculoskeletal sarcoma. Clin Orthop 153:106–120, 1980.

Lewis MM (ed): Musculoskeletal Oncology: A Multidisciplinary Approach. Philadelphia, WB Saunders Company, 1992.

Mankin HJ, Lange TA, Spanier SA: The hazards of biopsy in patients with malignant primary bone and soft tissue tumors. J Bone Joint Surg 64A: 1121–1127, 1982.

Mirra JM (ed): Bone Tumors: Clinical, Radiologic, and Pathologic Correlations. Philadelphia, Lea & Febiger, 1989.

Sim FH (ed): Diagnosis and Management of Metastatic Bone Disease: A Multidisciplinary Approach. New York, Raven Press, 1988.

Sugarbaker PH, Nicholson TH: Atlas of Extremity Sarcoma Surgery. Philadelphia, JB Lippincott, 1984.

Watt I: Magnetic resonance imaging in orthopaedics. J Bone Joint Surg 73-B: 539–550, 1991.

Chapter 6

Children's Orthopaedics

John N. Delahay

INTRODUCTION

Children are different! This statement has been presented in many different ways; but it is critically important that this one central fact be recognized, if one is to successfully diagnose and treat disease in this age group. Even within this rather broad range of ages there are dramatic differences among specific subsets: neonate, child, adolescent.

These differences are not only biological, but psychological, social, and emotional. It is likewise inappropriate to focus only on one aspect of these differences. For example, it would be unwise to ignore a young child's activity level when treating a fracture—inadequate immobilization or cast removal too early will have disastrous end results.

Recognition of this special group actually gave orthopaedics its name. The word means "straight child" and alludes to the interest and time spent correcting deformities in children. These deformities can result not only from injury but also from systemic and local disease states, both congenital and acquired. Because the child is *growing*, these diseases produce anatomic and physiologic effects not expected in the adult. Before discussing specific entities, it would therefore be appropriate to review some of the biological differences of the child's musculoskeletal system and the influences that act on the immature skeleton.

BIOLOGIC DIFFERENCES

Growth

As mentioned, the fact that the child's skeleton is growing, both longitudinally and latitudinally, positions it uniquely for damage due to the adverse effects of trauma and disease. The extent of this damage is a reflection of the rate of growth and the immaturity of the skeleton. Hence, an insult will have a greater impact, if applied at the time of more rapid growth (a growth spurt) or when the skeleton is very young (neonate).

Remodeling

The immature skeleton can remodel to a much greater degree than that of the adult. Due to the presence and activity of multiple cell populations, damage to the skeleton can be repaired more extensively than one should anticipate in the adult. The challenge for the physician is to be able to recognize the limitations of this remodeling process and work within the boundaries of this potential.

Specific Anatomic Structures

1. Bone: Although a child's bone is histologically lamellar in pattern, there remains enough flexibility in the skeleton

to permit what has been called "biologic plasticity," a phenomena not nearly as extensive in adult bone. Essentially, this allows a bone to "bend without breaking"; in point of fact, it is responsible for some of the unique types of fractures seen in the pediatric age groups—specifically, torus and greenstick fractures.

In addition, the mechanical properties of a child's bone vary from those of the adult. Such characteristics as modules of elasticity, ultimate tensile strength, and yield point, all reflect the elasticity and plasticity unique in this age group. However, the overall "strength" tends to be less than that of the adult in certain modes of loading, such as tension and shear.

2. Ligament: As a tissue, ligament is one of the most age-resistant tissues in the human body. The tensile strength in the child and older adult are virtually the same. Therefore, these structures remain as a constant in the musculoskeletal system. While the strength of bone, cartilage, and muscle tends to change, the ligamentous structures remain unchanged with growth and development.

3. Periosteum: The outer covering of the bone is a dense fibrous layer, which in the child is significantly thicker than that of the adult. The periosteum of the child actually has an outer fibrous layer and an inner cambial or osteogenic layer. Hence, the child's periosteum confers both mechanical strength as well as biologic activity. The effect of these biologic differences are far reaching when one discusses fractures in children. Due to this thickened periosteum, fractures do not tend to displace to the degree seen in adults, and the intact periosteum can be used as an aid in fracture reduction and maintenance. In addition, fractures will heal significantly faster than similar injuries in adults due to the fact that all the cellular precursors are already present. The osteogenic layer supplies active osteoblasts, ready to make bone for the fracture callus. The generation of these precursor elements in adults takes a period of time not required in the child.

4. Cartilage: As one will recall, the skeleton is developed embryologically within a cartilage model. At birth, large portions of any given bone remain largely cartilaginous. Unfortunately, cartilage is *not* seen on standard x-rays. The cartilage anlage are very labile and dramatically affected by external influences such as mechanical loading. It is important to realize that, in examining an x-ray, one should not be lulled into a false sense of security if all appears well; what you don't see (i.e., the cartilage) is more important than what you do! Aberrant cartilaginous growth will drastically affect the ultimate shape of bones and more importantly, joints. The best example is the proximal femur, where most of the upper end is cartilagenous. Adverse influences due to eccentric loading seen in developmental dysplasia of the hip can have far-reaching effects when applied to the immature cartilage of the neonatal hip.

5. The growth plate: By far and away, the most unique characteristic of the immature skeleton—indeed, what is the defining component of the immature skeleton—is the growth plate, or the "physis." The physis is a cartilage plate interposed between the epiphysis (the secondary ossification center) and the metaphysis (Fig. 6–1). It is essential for long-bone growth to occur. The down side is that this anatomic structure creates a "normal flaw" in the overall skeletal structure and thus a point of mechanical weakness. The physis histologically has four zones (Fig. 6–2), each with its own physiologic role:

   a. Resting zone: The top layer of flattened cells are germinal and metabolically store materials for later use, since they will ultimately "move their way" down the plate towards the metaphysis. The chondrocytes in this zone also are synthetic, as they fabricate the matrix within which they lie.

   b. Proliferating zone: The cells in this region are actively replicating and extending the plate. They have been described as looking like a "stack of plates." In this region, the cells are using the materials that they have previously stored for their "trip to the metaphysis."

   c. Hypertrophic zone: Having extended the plate in the former zone, the cells now tend to swell and switch over to a more catabolic state. They prepare

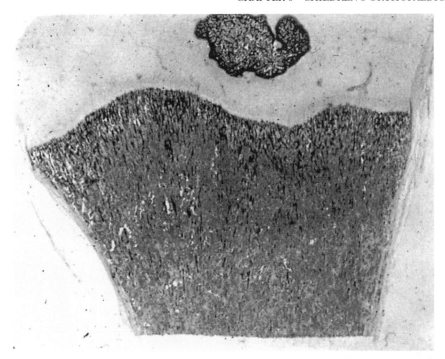

FIGURE 6–1 ■ Early secondary ossification center of mature fetus. The formation of the secondary ossification centers in the lower tibia and upper femur coincide with fetal maturity. The secondary center begins not in the center of the epiphysis, but nearer the growth plate. Expansion, therefore, is eccentric.
(From Bogumill GP: Orthopaedic Pathology: A Synopsis with Clinical and Radiographic Correlation. Philadelphia, WB Saunders Company, 1984, p 9; reprinted by permission.)

the matrix for calcification and ultimately for conversion to bone. Due to large swollen cells and the disorganized matrix, this zone has been cited as being the weakest mechanically; hence, it is here that failure tends to occur. Most, however, would agree that crack propagation can be seen throughout all zones in the case of trauma.

  d. Calcified zone: Metabolically, the matrix has been readied for the deposition of calcium salts, and the task of forming the osteoid is left for this lowest region of the plate. In the adjacent metaphysis, small vascular twigs can be seen arborizing toward the basal layers of the plate.

6. Peripheral structures of the plate: Two defined histologic regions have been identified with specific functional roles to play in skeletal development:

  a. Zone of ranvier: Around the circumference of the plate is an identifiable clustering of cells that are responsible for latitudinal growth of the plate.

  b. Perichondrial ring of lacroix: As the periosteum is continuous around the margins of the plate, this fibrous structure is apparent. Its function arguably has been to serve as a "girdle" for the plate and give mechanical support against translational movement.

Factors Affecting the Skeletal Growth

Numerous factors, both intrinsic and extrinsic, affect the way in which the skeleton develops. Some examples are noteworthy:

Genetic Impact: Inborn errors of metabolism (renal rickets) as well as chromosomal alterations (Down's syndrome) can cause phenotypic variations in the development of the skeleton. Abnormal histology, aberrational growth and variational development, all will affect the ultimate shape and behavior of the skeleton.

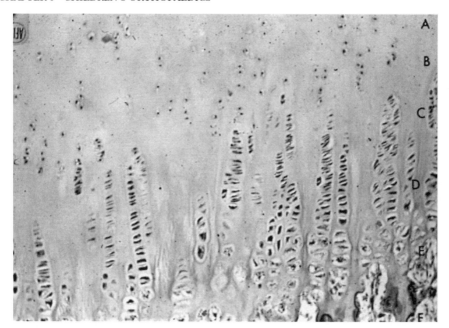

FIGURE 6–2 ■ Growth plate. Low-power view showing entire plate. At *(A)* resting zone has isolated cartilage cells in the upper portion together with empty lacunae. At *(B)* cell reproduction produces cloning of cells that "stack up" longitudinally. Successive generations occupy more space than each single progenitor cell and thus increase the length of the cartilage model. Secretion of new matrix at *(C)* is followed by dehydration with accompanying fibrillation of the territorial cartilage matrix between the "dinner plates" at *(D)*. Hypertrophy of cartilage cells at *(E)* is due to imbibition of water. Calcification of matrix is followed by vascular invasion at *(F)*.

(From Bogumill GP: Orthopaedic Pathology: A Synopsis with Clinical and Radiographic Correlation. Philadelphia, WB Saunders Company, 1984, p 12; reprinted by permission.)

Nutrition: Vitamins and proteins are required for normal skeletal development and without appropriate levels, abnormalities will be seen. Rickets, for example, will alter the shape of the metaphysis, in addition to disrupting normal physeal development.

Endocrine: Hormonal influences play a significant trophic or permissive role in the development of the skeleton. Shortages or excesses therefore will disrupt the way in which the skeleton matures. Thyroid hormone is a good example. Disrupted epiphyseal development is a hallmark of cretinism.

Environmental Factors: Mechanical effects as well as environmental toxins and drugs can adversely effect the development of the skeleton. Fetal alcohol syndrome and the use of illicit narcotics by the mother are just two examples of the growing compendium of skeletal aberrations due to externally applied toxins.

Coexistent Disease: Neuromuscular diseases of children, such as cerebral palsy, polio, and muscular dystrophy, provide good examples of the secondary effects seen in the skeleton due to extrinsic disease. In these examples, the final common pathway in the pathophysiology of the deformities is muscle imbalance, hence, eccentric and aberrational mechanical loading of the immature skeleton produce changes such as joint dislocations and deformities (e.g., scoliosis).

DEVELOPMENTAL VARIATIONS IN SKELETAL GROWTH

It seems axiomatic to say that children grow and develop at different rates and in different ways. Yet one of the most common reasons that children are brought to a physician is to evaluate the position of their lower extremities, and the way in which they stand and walk. Toeing in and toeing out, as well as knock knees and bow legs, are a major preoccupation of parents and especially grandparents—and a major source of orthopaedic referrals. The simple fact is that the vast majority of these children—well over 90%—are normal children who are simply reflecting variational growth and development. Dr. Mercer Rang, a preeminent pediatric orthopaedist, has tried to emphasize this important fact by referring to these conditions as "non-disease."

He further goes on to suggest that the appropriate management for "non-disease" is "non-treatment." It is important to recognize the difference between doing nothing and "non-treatment." As the physician seeing the child, one must be able to recognize the variational patterns and differentiate them from pathologic states. Once that has been accomplished, the physician may embark on a program of aggressive "non-treatment," which might include such things as:

■ Careful examination of the normal child
■ Reassurance of parents and grandparents
■ Supply educational information to

strengthen one's diagnosis and approach
■ Consider use of benign shoe adjustment (scaphoid pad) for the "terminally skeptical"
■ Offer the option of yearly follow-up "to be sure that the non-disease is getting better"

Torsional Variations

The newborn typically will reflect her intrauterine position and environment. Therefore, a certain amount of "molding" is to be anticipated. This usually, but not always, results in an internally rotated position of the lower extremities and the ultimate manifestation of this rotation is toeing-in when the child begins to walk. The two most typical variations leading to intoeing are:

1. Internal Tibial Torsion (Fig. 6–3): Axial rotation of the tibias can best be identified by examining the child supine with hips and knees flexed and evaluating the transmalleolar axis at the ankle for its relation to the knee axis. Normally, it

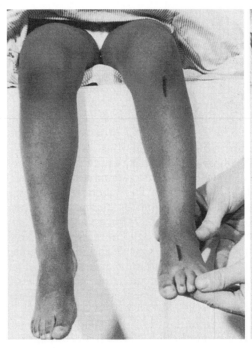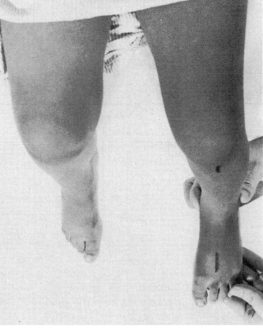

FIGURE 6–3 ■ Practical clinical method of measuring tibial torsion (see text for explanation). (From Tachdjian MO: Pediatric Orthopedics, ed 2, Vol 1. Philadelphia, WB Saunders Company, 1990, reprinted by permission.)

should lie 10 to 30 degrees externally rotated from that of the knee. Neonates typically have an internally rotated axis which causes intoeing with the initiation of walking and spontaneously corrects after about 1 year of walking. Tibial external rotation can occasionally be seen, but is far less common. Neither requires any specific treatment other than those recommended for "non-treatment."

2. Internal Femoral Torsion (Femoral Anteversion): The plane of the femoral head and neck in the normal adult lies 15 degrees externally rotated from that of the transcondylar plane of the distal femur. In the newborn, this relationship is more extreme: the head/neck plane is about 45 degrees external to that of the transcondylar plane, and it corrects spontaneously at a rate of about 2 degrees per year (Fig. 6–4). Persistence of this infantile pattern beyond the age of walking will cause intoeing as the leg internally rotates at the hip in order that the femoral head sits properly in the acetabulum. The rate of correction varies widely and "non-treatment" is usually all that is required. Additionally, two other recommendations might be made: first, the child should be discouraged from sitting in the so-called "W" or "TV position," since it seems to delay spontaneous correction; and second, lightweight footwear should be encouraged, since the child will toe-in less due to weight of shoes.

External femoral torsion is described, but most believe this actually represents the persistence of an infantile external rotational contracture of the soft tissues posterior to the hip; despite its etiology, spontaneous correction of this variation can similarly be anticipated.

When examining the child for femoral rotational patterns, it is best accomplished with the child prone, hips extended, and knees flexed 90 degrees (Fig. 6–5). Internal and external rotation of the hips can then be easily estimated using the leg as an angle guide.

Angular Variations

Knock knees (genu valgum) and bow legs (genu varum) are another common source of physician referrals. Recognition of the normal allows relatively easy determination of pathologic states.

Salenius examined thousands of "normal" children and has provided us with standard expectations for this group (Fig. 6–6). Newborns demonstrate 4 to 10 degrees of genu varus, which tends to spontaneously correct by 18 months of age. Thus, a child who presents with bow legs would be diagnosed as "physiologic genu varum." After 18 months of age, a child develops knock knees, which increases until about age 4 or 5 and then begins to improve. By age 7 or 8 most children have assumed more of an adult pattern: 5 to 7 degrees of valgus in males and 7 to 9 degrees of valgus in females.

It is best to record the degree of varus by measuring the number of finger breadths accommodated between the child's knees and the degree of valgus by recording the number of finger breadths accommodated between the medial malleoli.

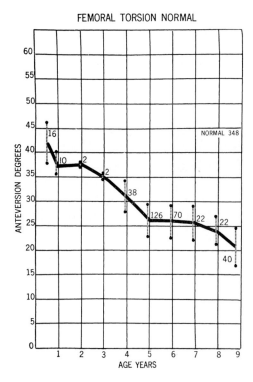

FIGURE 6–4 ■ The degree of normal femoral torsion in relation to age. The solid lines represent the mean; the vertical lines represent standard deviation.

(From Tachdjian MO: Pediatric Orthopedics, ed 2, Vol 1. Philadelphia, WB Saunders Company, 1990, reprinted by permission.)

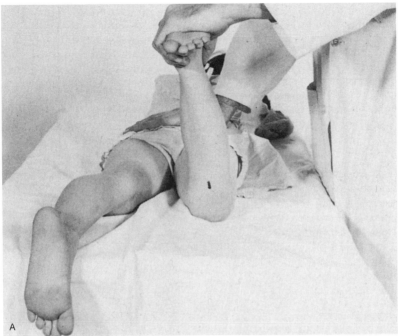

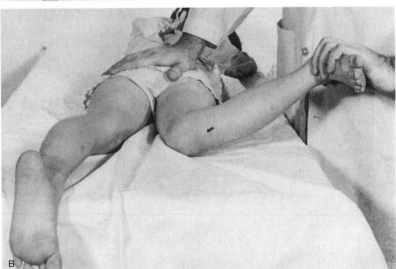

FIGURE 6–5 ■ Range of rotation of the hip in excessive femoral antetorsion. *A,* Lateral rotation of the hip in extension is exaggerated. *B,* Medial rotation of the hip in extension is limited to neutral.

(From Tachdjian MO: Pediatric Orthopedics, ed 2, Vol 1. Philadelphia, WB Saunders Company, 1990, reprinted by permission.)

Differential Diagnosis

Recognizing that the vast majority of children with angular patterns are normal and require "non-treatment," it is nonetheless important to realize that angular deformities can be a manifestation of pathologic states.

A. *Knock knees (genu valgum)* (Fig. 6–7)
   1. Physiologic
   2. Renal rickets
   3. Skeletal dysplasias
   4. Trauma
B. *Bow legs (genu varum)* (Fig. 6–8)

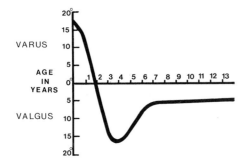

FIGURE 6–6 ■ Development of the tibiofemoral angle during growth.

(From Tachdjian MO: Pediatric Orthopedics, ed 2, Vol 1. Philadelphia, WB Saunders Company, 1990, reprinted by permission.)

1. Physiologic
2. Blounts' disease
3. Rickets (nutritional)
4. Skeletal dysplasias (achondroplasia)
5. Trauma

As one can appreciate from these lists, symmetry is important. Physiologic angular

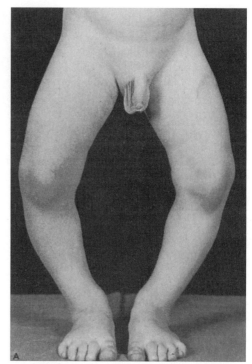

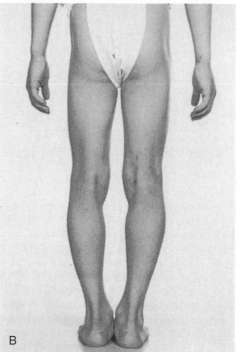

FIGURE 6–8 ■ Bilateral genu varum. *A,* At age one and one half years. *B,* At seven years, showing spontaneous correction without treatment.

(From Tachdjian MO: Pediatric Orthopedics, ed 2, Vol 1. Philadelphia, WB Saunders Company, 1990, reprinted by permission.)

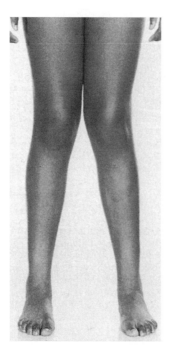

FIGURE 6–7 ■ Bilateral genu valgum in an adolescent.

(From Tachdjian MO: Pediatric Orthopedics, ed 2, Vol 1. Philadelphia, WB Saunders Company, 1990, reprinted by permission.)

deformity is virtually always symmetric; the finding of asymmetry should therefore suggest a pathologic state and trigger an appropriate work-up.

GENERAL AFFECTATIONS OF THE SKELETON

As mentioned earlier, many diseases will have skeletal manifestations; it is therefore impossible in one brief chapter to include every disease that affects the musculoskeletal system. Rather, by being introduced to several specific examples in each disease category, one can appreciate some of the general ways in which the skeleton can react to various insults. Since tumor and trauma are addressed elsewhere in the text, therefore this chapter can focus on the five disease categories—infection, arthritis, metabolic, vascular and hematologic, and congenital and neurodevelopmental.

Infection

Osteomyelitis

The pediatric skeleton is a prime location for bone and joint infections. In part, this is due to the many bacterial infections that small children seem to have—hence, providing organisms capable of hematogenously spreading from skin, ear, and nasopharynx. In addition, the unique metaphyseal blood supply (Fig. 6–9) in the child establishes the battlefield for the host–organism interaction. Since the physis creates a barrier to the vessels, they must double back on themselves, thereby forming end-loop capillaries and creating an area of stasis in the bony metaphysis. This area of stasis "catches" bacteria as they are showered hematogenously from distant sites. Once entrenched, the bacteria establish a focus of infection, and the classic case of osteomyelitis develops. It is important to recognize that the changes are not simply the result of the damage the bacteria do to the bone, but also the

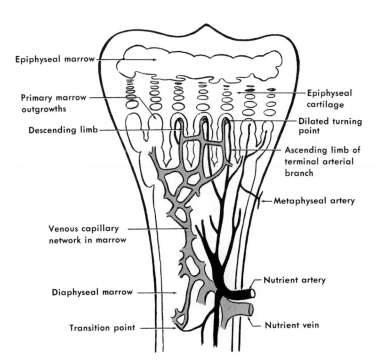

FIGURE 6–9 ■ Localization of osteomyelitis due to structure of metaphyseal sinusoids. Diagram of blood supply of long bones in children showing the structure of metaphyseal sinusoids to be the cause for localization of pathogenic bacteria in the metaphysis.

(From Tachdjian MO: Pediatric Orthopedics, ed 2, Vol 1. Philadelphia, WB Saunders Company, 1990, reprinted by permission.)

reparative changes initiated by the bone in an effort to localize the infection.

The result of this activity is a mixture of bony destruction by the organisms and new bone formed to wall off the infection and shore up the areas of damage. The dead and dying bony fragments are referred to as "sequestra," and the new viable bone being formed is called "involucrum" (Fig. 6–10; see also Chapter 4).

Clinical Features: One should inquire about a past history of trauma, as well as infections elsewhere, that may have provided a source for the organism. Occasionally, no such history will be available and one is evaluating a child who presents with pain in a limb and fever. The combination of these two findings—pain in an extremity and fever—should be presumed to be osteomyelitis until proven otherwise.

In children under 1 year of age, the findings may be more nonspecific and poorly localized—e.g., irritability, changes in feeding habits, and few signs of sepsis. Pseudoparalysis (failure to use the limb) may be the only localized finding.

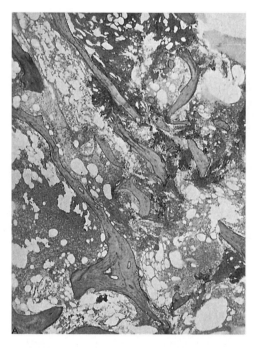

FIGURE 6–10 ■ Histologic findings in acute osteomyelitis. *A,* Necrotic trabeculae of bone surrounded by inflammatory cells (× 25).

(From Tachdjian MO: Pediatric Orthopedics, ed 2, Vol 1. Philadelphia, WB Saunders Company, 1990, reprinted by permission.)

Localized physical findings such as swelling, heat, localized tenderness, erythema, and signs of systemic sepsis are frequently seen in the older child.

Diagnosis: Standard laboratory studies will usually show an elevated white blood cell (WBC) count and sedimentation rate. X-rays initially may be negative since it takes 10 days for the pathology to become demonstrable radiographically. Bone resorption and new periosteal bone formation are the characteristic changes, but also may not be seen initially at presentation. A standard three-phase bone scan will assist in diagnosis from the standpoint of localization of pathology (Fig. 6–11).

Appropriate cultures are essential. Blood cultures will be positive about 50% of the time. Source cultures (throat, ear, skin, etc.) should also be obtained. Bony aspiration is essential. It is axiomatic that to diagnose a bone infection one must culture the bone. Using a large bore needle, one can aspirate the point of maximal tenderness in an effort to retrieve organisms. This is successful in 60 percent to 70 percent of cases. The organisms vary slightly with age, but generally the "big three" are staphylococcus, streptococcus, and hemophilus influenza. In neonates, one needs to consider Gram negatives.

Treatment: Diagnosis is critical prior to initiating antimicrobial treatment. All too often, broad-spectrum antibiotics are given before a bacteriologic diagnosis is made. The result is a "partially-treated osteo." These children present a challenging problem since the physical findings are damped or eradicated, but the organisms are not killed—they only await antibiotic withdrawal before initiating a new wave of bony destruction. The principles of management have been established for many years and are best summarized as follows:

1. Bacteriologic diagnosis
2. Appropriate antibiotic selection
3. Proper antibiotic delivery and duration
4. Immobilization
5. Surgical drainage of abscesses

For many years the tradition of intravenous (IV) antibiotic delivery has been accepted as essential. Although some would argue that the oral route is adequate, the IV route is still considered by most to be the standard mode of delivery, despite the inconvenience

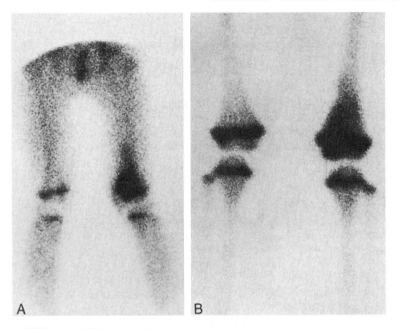

FIGURE 6–11 ■ Scintigraphic findings with technetium-99m in acute diphosphonate of the left distal femoral metaphysis. Note the increased localized uptake. *A,* Early vascular flush. *B,* Two hours later.

(From Tachdjian MO: Pediatric Orthopedics, ed 2, Vol 1. Philadelphia, WB Saunders Company, 1990, reprinted by permission.)

caused to child, family, and physician. The traditional duration of six weeks has been altered in some protocols to three weeks IV and three weeks oral, based on clinical response.

The indication for surgical drainage is the presence of loculated pus. Typically, this will be seen within the metaphyses or under the periosteum (Fig. 6–12). The subperiosteal abscess follows breakthrough of the metaphyseal cortical bone by aggressive organisms.

Septic Arthritis

Infection of a child's joint typically can result in one of three ways:

1. Hematogenous. Just as in osteomyelitis, organisms can localize in the joint, finding the highly vascular synovium a favorable location for replication.
2. Breakthrough. This occurs from an adjacent area of osteomyelitis. In certain specific joints, a portion of the metaphysis is intra-articular; thus, when the organism breaks through the metaphyseal bone, it enters the joint and creates a secondary septic arthritis. This phenomena is most typical in the hip (Fig. 6–13) but can also occur in the elbow, shoulder, and ankle.
3. Penetrating Trauma. This occurs with the subsequent injection of organisms directly into the joint.

Clinical Features: Although the most common organism to cause septic arthritis is gonococcus, this is clearly not an issue in younger children, where staphylococcus is the predominant organism. The clinical signs of sepsis are more obvious here than in osteomyelitis. The children tend to be toxic, exhibiting high fever, listlessness, and poor feeding. They will resist any attempts to move the involved joint.

Diagnosis: A work-up similar to that for osteomyelitis should be carried out and, at the risk of appearing repetitious, one cannot seriously consider this diagnosis without having made an attempt to retrieve organisms from the joint. It is important to be sure that the joint was aspirated, and frequently this mandates a fluoroscopically controlled arthrogram to document this fact. This is especially true of the pediatric hip, which is difficult to enter under the best of circumstances.

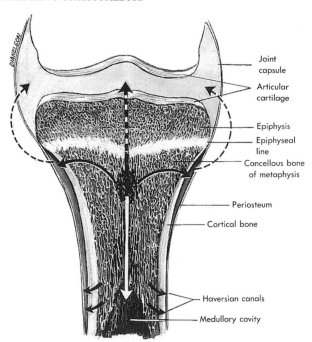

Joint capsule

Articular cartilage

Epiphysis

Epiphyseal line

Cancellous bone of metaphysis

Periosteum

Cortical bone

Haversian canals

Medullary cavity

FIGURE 6–12 ■ Diagram showing spread of acute hematogenous osteomyelitis. The interrupted lines are rare routes.

(From Tachdjian MO: Pediatric Orthopedics, ed 2, Vol 1. Philadelphia, WB Saunders Company, 1990, reprinted by permission.)

Treatment: Septic arthritis, unlike acute hematogenous osteomyelitis, is a surgical emergency. It is imperative that the pus be removed from the joint as soon as possible. The cartilage is extremely vulnerable and easily damaged by enzymes—those of the organisms, as well as those of the WBCs. It is therefore, *NOT* enough to simply kill the organisms in the joint; the joint must be rid of all WBCs, bacterial by-products, and enzymes. In most young

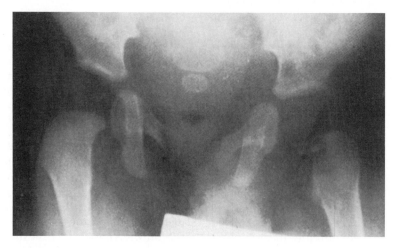

FIGURE 6–13 ■ Septic arthritis of left hip. Lateral subluxation and area of rarefaction in the femoral neck are evident.

(From Tachdjian MO: Pediatric Orthopedics, ed 2, Vol 1. Philadelphia, WB Saunders Company, 1990, reprinted by permission.)

children this requires an arthrotomy. Occasionally, arthroscopy is adequate for the knee in an older child; but repeated needle aspirations are rarely adequate to clean the inflamed joint and serve as yet another example of "man's inhumanity to man."

Antimicrobial management—choice, delivery, and duration—is similar to that for osteomyelitis, and one can anticipate that the usual organisms are also likely to be similar.

Complications of Bone and Joint Infections

Long-term sequelae can result from bacterial damage to these relatively vulnerable tissues (see Figure 6–14). In addition to the bone and articular cartilage, the child has a physis, which is likewise exposed to the insult.

Septic Joint Destruction: Loss of articular cartilage and arthrofibrosis ultimately result in joint contracture, deformity, and occasionally bony ankylosis (fusion). Salvage of the irreparably damaged articulations is difficult at best and frequently impossible.

Physeal Damage: Injury to the plate can have long-term effects, especially when it occurs in a very young child with significant growth remaining. Complete arrest and subsequent limit-length inequality or partial arrest and the resultant angular deformity are the two standard patterns of post-injury development.

Pathologic Fracture: Although infected bone will frequently look more dense (i.e., sclerotic) on x-ray, it should not be assumed that is mechanically stronger. In point of fact, the dense bone is disorganized, its lamellar pattern disrupted, and therefore it is mechanically less sound. Pathologic fracture can occur even in the immobilized limb, although the risk is less.

Chronic Infection: Despite aggressive treatment, some infections are not completely eradicated, and a "stalemate" is established between the host and the organism. Occasionally, at times of psychological or environmental stress, the infection will reactivate and produce additional damage (see Chapter 4).

Arthritis in Childhood

Juvenile Rheumatoid Disease

Frequently referred to as Still's disease, juvenile rheumatoid disease (JRA) is the most common connective tissue disease in children. In fact, George Still specifically described the systemic form of the illness. Children have systemic symptoms—fever, rash, hepatosplenomegaly—and develop a polyarticular arthritis. This is the most destructive form of the disease and leaves multiple destroyed joints in its wake.

The other two forms of the disease are definitely less virulent. Polyarticular disease, as the name implies, takes its toll on the joints but is not associated with systemic findings. Pauciarticular JRA is the most common and the most benign form of the disease. Typically, it is a monarticular arthritis, with the knee, elbow, and ankle being the joints most commonly involved. Frequently, children suffering from the pauciarticular form of the disease present with an isolated chronically swollen joint. This finding should trigger a diagnostic work-up. Diagnostic blood studies are usually negative (rheumatoid factor is positive in only 10% of cases). X-rays usually only show juxtaarticular osteopenia, and frequently a synovial biopsy may be needed (Fig. 6–15). The histology of the synovium is similar to that of the adult disease—namely, hyperplasia and villous hypertrophy of the synovium. It is imperative to recognize that JRA is the leading cause of blindness in children due to the destructive iridocyclitis that can accompany the joint disease. All children with JRA should be under the care of an ophthalmologist since eye involvement does NOT parallel the degree of joint involvement; those with minimal joint disease can have the most severe eye changes.

Treatment should be directed toward control of the synovitis with medications, physical therapy to maintain joint motion, psychologic support for those chronically impaired children, and ultimately arthroplasties or fusions for those joints most severely involved.

Hemophilia: Children with bleeding dyscrasias frequently have repeated hemarthroses. Initially, the blood in the joint simply distends the capsular structures and causes a mild synovitis. With repeated bleeds, the synovium becomes hyperplastic and ultimately pannus formation is seen. At this point, the joint changes appear very similar to those seen in rheumatoid disease—e.g., osteopenia, enzymatic cartilage degradation, bony erosions and lysis (Fig. 6–16).

Lyme Disease: In the endemic regions of the Northeast and Middle Atlantic states, the child

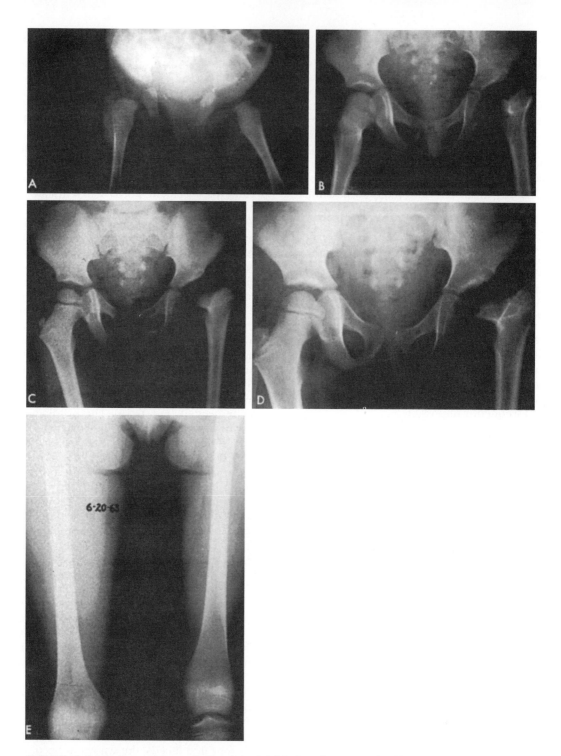

FIGURE 6–14 ■ Suppurative arthritis of the left hip in a three-month-old infant. Onset was at four weeks of age. Erroneous diagnosis of fibrocystic disease and thrombophlebitis resulted in a two-month delay in diagnosis. *A,* Radiograms of hips show marked effusion of left hip with lateral subluxation. *B to D,* Serial radiograms of hips show failure of ossification of the femoral head (due to avascular necrosis) and the development of coxa vara. *E,* Teleoradiograms taken nine and one half years after onset of sepsis in left hip. There is a 3.9-cm. shortening of left femur. A subtrochanteric abduction osteotomy was performed four years earlier. The left hip has functional range of motion. Skeletal growth of lower limbs is being followed, and the plan is to perform distal femoral epiphyseodesis on the right at the appropriate age.

(From Tachdjian MO: Pediatric Orthopedics, ed 2, Vol 1. Philadelphia, WB Saunders Company, 1990, reprinted by permission.)

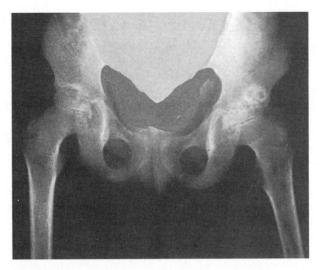

FIGURE 6–15 ■ Rheumatoid arthritis of both hips. Radiogram of hips taken three years later. The child was allowed to be ambulatory without protection of the hips. Note the destructive changes with fibrous ankylosis on the right and bony ankylosis on the left.

(From Tachdjian MO: Pediatric Orthopedics, ed 2, Vol 1. Philadelphia, WB Saunders Company, 1990, reprinted by permission.)

who presents with a swollen knee needs to be considered as a potential victim of Lyme disease. This infectious arthritis is due to a specific spirochete, *Borrelia burgdorferi*. The organism is

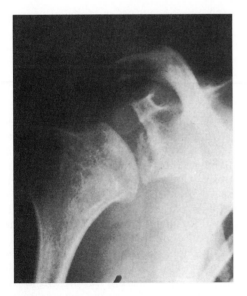

FIGURE 6–16 ■ Hemophilic arthropathy of shoulder.

(From Tachdjian MO: Pediatric Orthopedics, ed 2, Vol 1, Philadelphia, WB Saunders Company, 1990, reprinted by permission.)

transmitted to the human host by the bite of a deer tick. These ticks are significantly smaller than the common wood tick, and they are barely visible with the naked eye. Unfortunately, a history of a bite is rare and usually the diagnosis is reached by a high index of suspicion in a susceptible host. The combination of endemic region, erythematous annular skin lesions, and monarticular arthritis should lead the physician to order a Lyme titre.

Treatment is generally successful if begun early. Penicillin is adequate in the young child, and tetracyclines are used in the older age group. Occasionally, despite adequate treatment, the arthritis can progress to chronic joint destruction mandating further care.

Metabolic Disease

Perhaps the classic metabolic disease to affect the pediatric skeleton is rickets. The etiologies of rickets are multiple (Table 6–1), but the important pathophysiologic step is a relative paucity of vitamin D. It will be remembered that vitamin D is essential for normal progression of physeal bone development, and without it provisional calcification will not occur in the deepest layer of the growth plate.

As a result, physeal disorganization (Fig.

TABLE 6–1 ■ *Etiologies of Rickets*

1. Vitamin D dietary deficiency
2. Malabsorption states
3. Renal rickets
   a. Tubular defects (generally congenital)
   b. Glomerular disease (generally acquired)
4. Miscellaneous causes
   a. Associated with neurofibromatosis
   b. Complication of dilantin therapy

6–17) can be anticipated with subsequent physeal widening, trumpeting of the metaphysis, and aberrant enchondral bone growth. The clinically apparent changes of knobby joints, beading of the costochondral joints, and genu varum are all phenotypic reflections of the underlying histologic disruption of bone formation (Fig. 6–18).

Depending on the etiology of the rickets the histologic pattern will vary slightly, but the overall skeletal changes remain relatively constant.

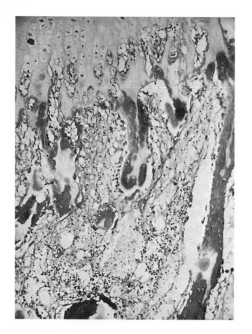

FIGURE 6–17 ■ Histologic appearance of rickets. Photomicrograph through the epiphyseal-metaphyseal junction. Note the uncalcified osteoid tissue, failure of deposition of calcium along the mature cartilage cell columns, and disorderly invasion of cartilage by blood vessels (× 25).
(From Tachdjian MO: Pediatric Orthopedics, 2 ed, Vol 1. Philadephia, WB Saunders Company, 1990, reprinted by permission.)

Vascular and Hematologic Disease

Vascular diseases of the pediatric skeleton are typified by osteochondroses such as Perthes disease of the hip and Osgood-Schlatter's disease of the knee. These will be considered regionally, leaving the hematologic diseases to be discussed here.

Sickle Cell Disease

The red cell deformation that occurs in sickle cell patients due to the abnormal hemoglobin is responsible for the skeletal changes. The abnormally shaped cells cause stasis and sludging in small arterioles and capillaries. The effect as expected is disrupted flow and bony necrosis. The bony infarcts seen in sickle cell disease can occur anywhere in the bone, but are more typical in the metaphysis (Fig. 6–19).

These children are also predisposed to osteomyelitis, probably due to the already sludged vessels in the metaphysis, making bacterial trapping even easier. Even though *staphylococcus* is the most common organism retrieved, this patient population is also susceptible to infection with salmonella. This organism gains access to the circulatory system through small infarcts in the intestinal wall and then enters the bone hematogenously. The incidence of salmonella osteomyelitis is approaching that of *stapylococcus* in this population.

The treatment for the infarcts is appropriate hematologic care—hydration, analgesics, etc. Antibiotic selection for osteomyelitis should take into consideration the incidence of salmonella.

Leukemia

This is the most common malignancy of childhood, and the skeleton is not spared its ravages. The bones by x-ray will show nondescript lytic changes most characteristically seen in the metaphyseal region and referred to as "metaphyseal banding" (Fig. 6–20). The areas of osteopenia parallel and are adjacent to the physis; although suggestive of leukemia, they are NOT pathogneumonic of it.

Although usually the diagnosis has been made well before skeletal complications develop, occasionally a child will present for the evaluation of "growing pains" only to have a work-up reveal this disease. Ordinarily "growing pains" occur in children 2 to 7 years of age, affect primarily the legs, are symmetric (although not simultaneous), occur in early evening or just after going to bed, and are NOT

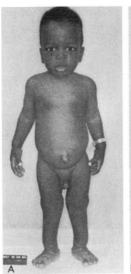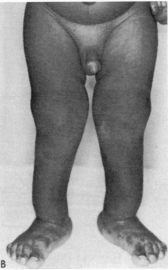

FIGURE 6–18 ■ Simple vitamin D deficiency rickets. *A* and *B,* Clinical appearance of patient. The legs are bowed anterolaterally. Note the protuberant abdomen with the umbilical hernia.

(From Tachdjian MO: Pediatric Orthopedics, ed 2, Vol 1. Philadelphia, WB Saunders Company, 1990, reprinted by permission.)

associated with any systemic complaints. Any variation from the usual pattern should suggest a basic work-up to include x-rays and a white count with differential.

Congenital and Neurodevelopmental

This is the largest and most nondescript "waste basket" of pathologic states, many of which

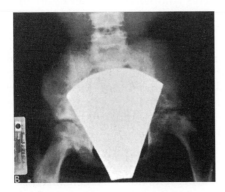

FIGURE 6–19 ■ Sickle cell disease in an 11-year-old girl. Anteroposterior radiogram of the hips. Note the avascular changes in the left femoral head.

(From Tachdjian MO: Pediatric Orthopedics, ed 2, Vol 1. Philadelphia, WB Saunders Company, 1990, reprinted by permission.)

have severe impact on the pediatric skeleton. Included here are congenital birth defects of no known etiology, such as proximal femoral focal deficiency, as well as genetic diseases transmitted in classic Mendelian fashion (e.g., hemophilia) or due to chromosomal defects (e.g., Down's syndrome).

In addition, the neuromuscular diseases frequently have an immense impact on the skeleton, as aberrant and eccentric muscular forces are created. Unfortunately, it is difficult to find many common themes that make an appreciation of the skeletal impact easier to understand.

Osteogenesis Imperfecta

This disease is transmitted in a classic autosomal dominant pattern with only rare exception. The basic defect is one of abnormal collagen synthesis due to impotent osteoblasts. For this reason it has been grouped with other "sick" cell syndromes. Certainly the osteoblasts are normal in number, but incapable of normal synthetic activity. The collageous product of their incompetence is poorly formed and poorly cross-linked, making it weak. The subsequent bone that is made is similarly architecturally thin and mechanically weak.

The severity of the disease is as expected, a function of the dose of abnormal genetic material. Some of the severe homozygotes are stillborn due to intracranial bleeds occurring in the perinatal period. As with most genetic diseases, phenotype penetrance varies such that some children have multiple fractures and severe shortening and others less involved have only the occasional fracture.

Typically, the bones are osteopenic (Fig. 6–21) with thinned cortices and decreased diameter. Multiple fractures with resulting deformities are the norm. These fractures respond to appropriate treatment, and healing is only slightly prolonged. Occasionally, it is necessary to correct long-bone deformities, and this is best accomplished operatively by performing multiple osteotomies in a single bone (Fig. 6–22) and lining the resultant fragments up on an intramedullary rod (Sofield "shish kabob").

Scoliosis can also complicate this disease, and its management can be very challenging,

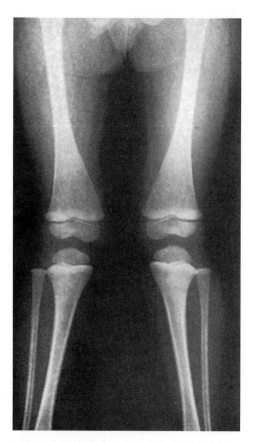

FIGURE 6–20 ■ Bone manifestations of acute leukemia

(From Tachdjian MO: Pediatric Orthopedics, ed 2, Vol 1. Philadephia, WB Saunders Company, 1990, reprinted by permission.)

especially if surgical management is required to correct the deformity. It is very difficult to use spinal instrumentation in the face of this osteopenic, softened bone.

Down's Syndrome

First described in England in the 1800s, Down's syndrome is now understood as involving a chromosomal abnormality on Trisomy 21. It is the most common chromosomal abnormality that we see today and occurs in about 1 in 500 live births. Because of its frequency, it is a prototype for the other chromosomal aberrations, and the orthopaedic manifestations tend to be somewhat common to all.

Hypotonia and ligamentous laxity typify the group. The ligamentous laxity probably results from an inordinate number of elastic fibers relative to the number of collagen fibers in ligament and joint capsule. In any event, the joint changes typical of the disease can be directly related to this laxity:

1. C_1 to C_2 instability (Fig. 6–23): Due to laxity of the transverse ligament of the dens, anterior translation of C_1 on C_2 occurs, frequently to alarming degrees. Routine lateral cervical spine radiographs in flexion and extension should be obtained to evaluate the child for this problem.
2. Hip subluxation and dislocation
3. Patellar subluxation: This phenomena frequently causes the child with Down's syndrome to walk with a stiff-legged gait. This compensation is an effort to keep the patellae from dislocating.
4. Hypermobile flat feet and bunions.

The management of these problems is primarily directed at controlling the deformity, if possible, and minimizing the pain, which is rarely a problem. Despite fixed deformities, it is frequently surprising how well these children do.

Skeletal Dysplasias

There are several hundred recognized skeletal dysplasias each with its own unique clinical characteristics and specific skeletal abnormalities. It is impossible to recall all of the features, which define a given dysplastic condition, especially in light of the fact that each is usually quite rare. At best, generalizations can be employed to assist in the diagnosis of a specific patient and thereby guide the appropriate

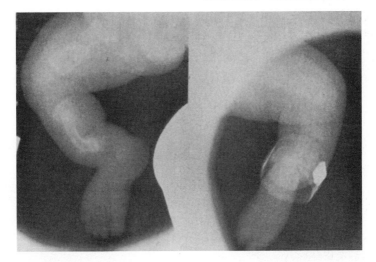

FIGURE 6–21 ■ Osteogenesis imperfecta congenita in a
newborn. Radiogram of lower limbs, showing multiple fractures.
(From Tachdjian MO: Pediatric Orthopedics, ed 2, Vol 1. Philadelphia,
WB Saunders Company, 1990, reprinted by permission.)

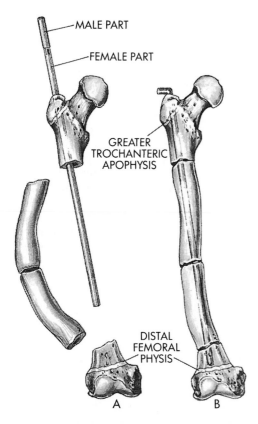

MALE PART

FEMALE PART

GREATER
TROCHANTERIC
APOPHYSIS

DISTAL
FEMORAL
PHYSIS

A   B

FIGURE 6–22 ■ Williams modification of
Sofield-Millar intramedullary rod fixation.
(From Tachdjian MO: Pediatric Orthopedics, ed 2,
Vol 1. Philadelphia, WB Saunders Company, 1990,
reprinted by permission.)

work-up and referral to an individual skilled in definitive diagnosis. The anticipated orthopaedic problems, treatment, and prognosis will hinge on the diagnosis.

When presented with an individual displaying dysplastic findings, especially short stature, chromosomal evaluation and standard x-rays are good starting points once appropriate history (especially family history) and a careful physical examination have been carried out. The x-rays should include a lateral of the cervical and thoracolumbar spine, an anteroposterior view of the pelvis and anteroposterior views of the wrists and the knees. These views will allow one to evaluate epiphyseal, physeal, metaphyseal, and diaphyseal growth and their aberrations.

Most of the dysplasias tend to affect a specific region of the bone; by assessing each region, clues can be gotten regarding the specific type of dysplasia. For example, spondyloepiphyseal dysplasia affects primarily epiphyseal growth as the name implies. One should expect to see deformities of the epiphyseal nuclei and disordered apophyseal growth. On the other hand, achondroplasia is a defect in physeal growth and will therefore produce significant dwarfing; in fact, it is the most common cause of pathologic short stature.

Most of the skeletal dysplasias are genetically transmitted, and a careful family history will define the pattern. Many, however, are spontaneous mutations or without a defined

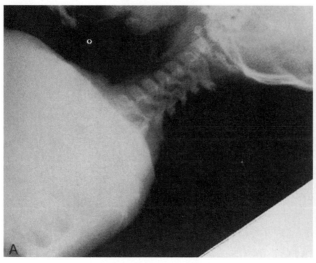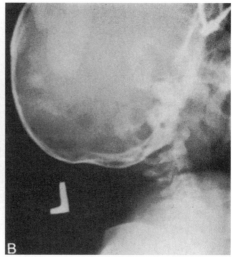

FIGURE 6–23 ■ Atlantoaxial instability in Down's syndrome.

(From Tachdjian MO: Pediatric Orthopedics, ed 2, Vol 1. Philadelphia, WB Saunders Company, 1990, reprinted by permission.)

etiology. It is important to keep in mind that by definition a skeletal dysplasia is a GENERALIZED affectation of the skeleton with all bones showing some changes. Obviously, the end of the bone growing more rapidly will demonstrate the defect to a greater degree; thus, the knee and wrist films are more likely to show changes than the hip or elbow views.

Achondroplasia

As an example of how a dysplasia affects the skeleton, one should consider the most common, achondroplasia. Transmitted as an autosomal dominant in most cases, it is usually apparent at birth. The infant will be rhizomelically shortened; that is to say the proximal segment of the limbs is relatively shorter, than the middle or distal segments (Fig. 6–24). In addition, the child is disproportionately built since the limbs are preferentially involved, and therefore very short relative to the spine and trunk.

These children follow the growth curve, but several standard deviations below normal, achieving a mature height between 3 to 4 feet. As with all of the true dysplasias, intelligence is not impaired and life expectancy is virtually normal.

Clinical Features: The child's head shows flattening of the nasal bridge and prominent frontal bones. Both findings are due to the disparity between the normal intramembranous calvarial growth and the retarded en-

chondral growth of the basilar portions of the skull.

The extremities are short, with each of the bones being short in length but relatively normal in girth, since periosteal bone formation remains relatively unaffected.

The spine and pelvis also show some decrease in height, but of greater significance is the decrease in the interpedicular distance, which effectively creates a spinal stenotic syndrome. This coupled with a hyperlordotic lumbar spine causes many achondroplasts to develop disc symptoms at an early age.

The major problem of the older adolescent is obesity, which complicates many of their other abnormalities. As adults, problems with multiple tendonitises and bursitises are commonplace.

Neuromuscular Disease

Unlike the skeletal dysplasias which are intrinsic abnormalities of the skeleton, this group of diseases are extrinsic, but drastically alter the normal skeleton due primarily to the muscle imbalance they create.

Common themes can be seen that emphasize the fact that the problem is disparity in the agonist-antagonist relationship. Major joints tend to dislocate with the hip being a prime example. The flexor pattern tends to become dominant, causing the femoral head to dislocate posteriorly. Scoliosis should be expected as asymmetry of spinal muscle action alters normal balance. If the neurologic defect is asymmetric, as in polio, then the growth plates in one leg will "feel" a different muscle pull than those of the other and a leg-length discrepancy can be anticipated.

Cerebral Palsy

This is a static neurologic disease of children due to an insult to the immature brain during

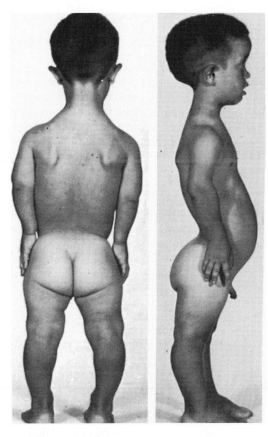

FIGURE 6–24 ■ *A,* Posterior photograph of achondroplastic dwarf showing distorted growth of long bones. The proximal limb segments are proportionately shorter than the distal, with the hands reaching only to the hip region. The legs are bowed, and the scapulae and pelvis are smaller than normal. Scoliosis is uncommon. *B,* Lateral photograph of child with achondroplasia. Note marked lumbar lordosis with prominent buttocks as a result of pelvic tilt. The lordosis is due in part to differential growth of vertebral body versus posterior elements.

(From Bogumill GP: Orthopaedic Pathology: A Synopsis with Clinical and Radiographic Correlation. Philadelphia, WB Saunders Company, 1984, p 48; reprinted by permission.)

the perinatal period. The defect is therefore central, damaging the normal inhibitory influences on the peripheral gamma efferent system. Without central damping, the peripheral reflex arc functions autonomously, and the result is increased tone or spasticity.

Cerebral palsy is classified in one of two ways:

1. Physiologic classification
   a. Spastic: Hypertonia, hyperflexia, and contractures are seen. This is the most common form of the syndrome.
   b. Athetoid: This is far less common today than it was in years past. Rh incompatibility and erythroblastosis fetalis was a common etiology of this form.
   c. Rigid
   d. Ballismic
   e. Mixed
2. Geographic Classification
   a. Hemiplegia: The most common form, it is frequently associated with seizures
   b. Diplegia: Both lower extremities predominate the pattern.
   c. Quadriplegia: The most severe cases involve children, many of whom are retarded and few of whom will ever walk.

Cerebral palsy is really a syndrome rather than a disease (Fig. 6–25), and no two children are really the same. This makes comparison of procedures and other treatments extremely difficult, if not impossible. The muscles all tend to be spastic, however; the muscle imbalance is created between spastic and more spastic muscles. Contractures, joint dislocations, limb deformities, and scoliosis should all be anticipated.

Polio

With the introduction of the Salk vaccine in 1954, this disease has become rare in the United States; however, it is certainly not eradicated in the Third World. Since immigrants are seen in our larger cities on an increasingly frequent basis with the sequelae of this disease, some familiarity with it seems appropriate.

The polio virus has unique predilection for the anterior horn cells of the cord and the bulbar portion of the brain. In most cases the involvement is spotty and the degree of paralysis is variable. The victim is left with a mix of normal muscle, weak muscle, and absent muscle—hence, creating a broad spectrum of muscle imbalance, but in an asymmetric distribution. It is important to remember that the sensory fibers are NOT affected, which gives these children a clear and distinct benefit over the children with spina bifida.

Spina Bifida

Despite the improvement in antenatal testing, many children with myelodysplasia are still born in the United States each year. Due to open cord defects at a certain level (Fig. 6–26), these children are essentially congenital paraplegics. They are without motor and sensory modalities below the level of the defect. Needless to say, the higher their level of defect, the poorer their function and, hence, the prognosis (Fig. 6–27). For example, a child with a T_{12} level (the spinal roots that are the last to function are T_{12}) has no motor power and no

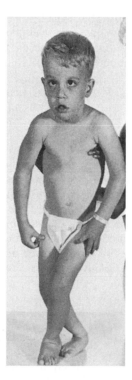

FIGURE 6–25 ■ Spastic quadriplegia with total body involvement. At four years of age. The marked scissoring of the hips and equinus deformity of the ankles provide a poor base upon which balance can develop. Note the pes valgus.

(From Tachdjian MO: Pediatric Orthopedics, ed 2, Vol 1. Philadelphia, WB Saunders Company, 1990, reprinted by permission.)

sensation below the waist. They will be wheelchair-confined and have bowel and bladder compromise. On the other hand, children with an S_1 level (the last functioning spinal level is S_1) will have only minimal motor involvement and will usually walk without braces. Their major problems are the bowel and bladder malfunction.

The absence of sensation below the level of the lesion creates many additional problems for these children. Not unlike a diabetic patient with severe neuropathy, children with spina bifida are prone to foot ulceration, infection, and the development of neuropathic joints.

One recently identified problem in this group is latex allergy. Perhaps due to repeated catheterization with latex rubber catheters, these patients can become severely sensitized to all latex contact, to the point of anaphylaxis. Specific protocols are now used at the time of surgical procedures to avoid contact with any latex products, including gloves, catheters, and IV tubing.

Lastly, it is important to realize that these children, as well as many of those with cerebral palsy, are multiply handicapped. They have learning difficulties, perceptual problems, hearing and visual impairments, not to mention emotional issues—all of which require a coordinated effort by multiple specialists to provide optimal care.

REGIONAL ORTHOPAEDIC PROBLEMS

The Pediatric Hip

Most of the showcase pediatric orthopaedic maladies affect the hip. Developmental dysplasia, Perthes' disease, and slipped capital epiphysis have established the hip as the preeminent joint of a child's musculoskeletal system. Several unique anatomic features predispose this joint to long-term problems following septic, vascular, developmental, and traumatic insults.

In the newborn, the upper end of the femur (Fig. 6–28) is entirely cartilaginous, representing the secondary ossification centers of both the greater trochanter and the femoral head (capital femoral epiphysis) as a composite chondroepiphysis. The two bony ossification centers will develop within this one cartilage mass and grow differentially to their ultimate adult size and shape. Implicit in this

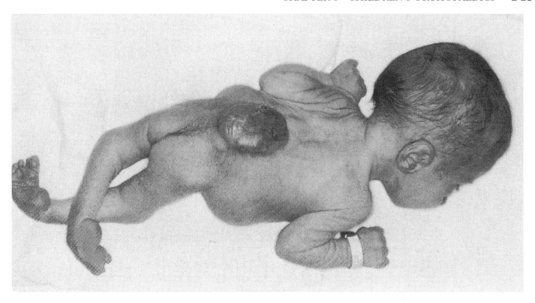

FIGURE 6–26 ■ Newborn infant with lumbosacral myelomeningocele. Note the severe equinovarus deformity of both feet.

(From Tachdjian MO: Pediatric Orthopedics, ed 2, Vol 1. Philadelphia, 1990, reprinted by permission.)

fact is that the growth of one is in part dependent on the growth of the other. Normally the bony centrum of the capital femoral epiphysis should be radiographically visible by 3 to 6 months of age.

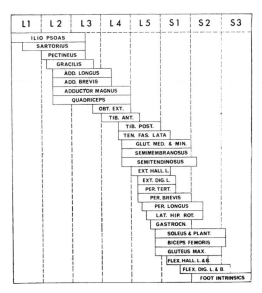

FIGURE 6–27 ■ Neurosegmental innervation of muscles of lower limb.

(From Tachdjian MO: Pediatric Orthopedics, ed 2, Vol 1. Philadelphia, WB Saunders Company, 1990, reprinted by permission.)

The growth of this epiphysis is dependent primarily on the blood supply of the upper end of the femur (Fig. 6–29). It is essential to recognize that up until 1 year of age there is communication between the metaphyseal and epiphyseal circulations. This protects the capital femoral epiphysis from isolation in the event of an insult to the epiphyseal side. Unfortunately, as the physis thickens and matures by 18 months of age, it becomes an impenetrable barrier between the two circulations, leaving the epiphysis of the head totally dependent on the epiphyseal vessels for its viability. Less than 10 percent of the femoral head is supplied by the branch of the obturator artery through the ligamentum teres. The epiphyseal vessels are supplied by the medial and lateral circumflex branches of the femoral artery. This vascular isolation of the upper end of the femur is largely responsible for the disastrous complications of developmental dislocation of the hip (DDH), Perthes' disease, and slipped capital femoral epiphysis (SCFE).

The acetabulum develops from two cartilage segments. The first is the triradiate cartilage, which a bilaminar physis formed at the junction of the ilium, ischium, and pubis. Integrity of this growth plate is essential for acetabular *height* to be normal. The *depth* of the acetabulum is a function of the cartilaginous labrum that circumferentially surrounds the developing acetabulum.

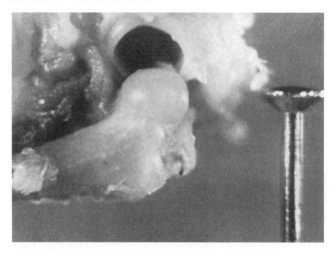

FIGURE 6–28 ■ Embryology of the hip joint. Note the spherical configuration of the femoral head and acetabulum. The limbus and transverse acetabular ligament are well-formed structures.

(From Tachdjian MO: Pediatric Orthopedics, ed 2, Vol 1. Philadelphia, WB Saunders Company, 1990, reprinted by permission.)

Developmental Dislocation of the Hip

The previous nomenclature, "congenital dislocation," was recently changed to "developmental dislocation" in recognition of the fact that some of these hips are located at birth and go on to dislocate in the postnatal period. The incidence of this condition is about 1 per 1000 live births and is more common in females. Although it is fair to say that the etiology is unknown, it is important to recognize that there are both genetic and environmental factors; hence, it is considered a multifactorial trait. It is also critical to recognize that this is a

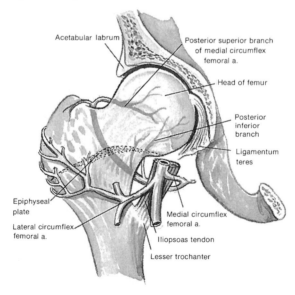

Acetabular labrum

Posterior superior branch of medial circumflex femoral a.

Head of femur

Posterior inferior branch

Ligamentum teres

Epiphyseal plate

Lateral circumflex femoral a.

Medial circumflex femoral a.

Iliopsoas tendon

Lesser trochanter

FIGURE 6–29 ■ Posterior view of the normal blood supply of the upper end of the femur in an infant.

(From Tachdjian MO: Pediatric Orthopedics, ed 2, Vol 1. Philadelphia, WB Saunders Company, 1990, reprinted by permission.)

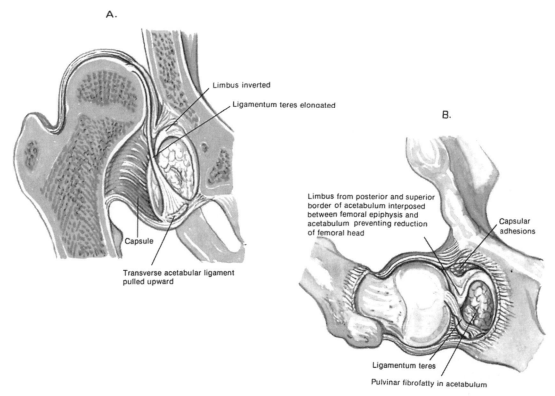

A.

Limbus inverted

Ligamentum teres elongated

Capsule

Transverse acetabular ligament
pulled upward

B.

Limbus from posterior and superior
border of acetabulum interposed
between femoral epiphysis and
acetabulum preventing reduction
of femoral head

Capsular
adhesions

Ligamentum teres

Pulvinar fibrofatty in acetabulum

FIGURE 6–30 ■ Pathology of the dislocated hip that is irreducible owing to intra-articular obstacles. *A,* The hip is dislocated. *B,* It cannot be reduced on flexion, abduction, or lateral rotation. Obstacles to reduction are inverted limbus, ligamentum teres, and fibrofatty pulvinar in the acetabulum. The transverse acetabular ligament is pulled upward with the ligamentum teres.

(From Tachdjian MO: Pediatric Orthopedics, ed 2. Vol 1. Philadelphia, WB Saunders Company, 1990, p 308; reprinted by permission.)

true dysplasia (i.e., aberrant growth), and NOT simply a femoral head that is not located in the acetabulum (Fig. 6–30). It is important to stress this fact to the parents in an effort to assist them in understanding the pathology.

Early diagnosis is the key to optimal treatment and the best prognosis. First, consider the risk factors:

1. First-born female
2. Breech presentation
3. Positive family history
4. Hip "click"
5. Presence of a muscular torticollis

With these in mind, a careful physical examination of the hips is the logical next step. In the newborn, one should attempt to demonstrate laxity and instability (Fig. 6–31). The Barlow test is performed with the infant supine and the hips flexed. As the hips are brought from the abducted to adducted position, a positive test is noted as the femoral head subluxes posteriorly over the posterior rim of the acetabulum. This would indicate instability. The Barlow is a provocative test: the hip is located and the maneuver dislocates it. Conversely, the Ortolani test is a reduction maneuver: the hip is dislocated and the test reduces it. This is accomplished by abducting the adducted hip and noting a palpable (but rarely audible) "clunk" as the femoral head reduces over the posterior acetabular rim.

As the child gets older (by 3 months old), the dislocated hip tends to become fixed in that position, and the classic signs of instability disappear in favor of those indicating a fixed dislocation deformity. Limited abduction is perhaps the most important finding to note. Examining the child on a firm surface, subtle differences in the degrees of hip abduction may herald a dislocated hip on the restricted side. Similarly, viewing knee height with the child supine and the hips and knees flexed may

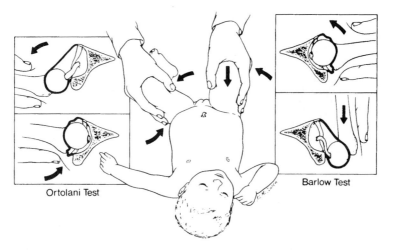

Ortolani Test   Barlow Test

FIGURE 6–31 ■ On the left, the Ortolani (reduction) test is demonstrated. The Barlow (provocation dislocation) test is shown on the right. These tests must be performed on a relaxed infant.

(From Sabiston DC Jr: Essentials of Surgery. Philadelphia, WB Saunders Company, 1987, p 776; reprinted by permission.)

reveal a positive Allis sign (Fig. 6–32): one knee higher than the other, again indicating a dislocation on the low side.

Imaging studies are important in both diagnosis and treatment. The current popularity of ultrasound is based on the fact that under 3 months of age much of the proximal femur is cartilaginous. Ultrasound has been helpful in the diagnosis of DDH (Fig. 6–33), as well as in defining relatively subtle degrees of acetabular dysplasia. The value of ultrasound after the child is 3 months old decreases, and standard x-rays assume a more central role. Many still feel that a standard AP of the pelvis with the

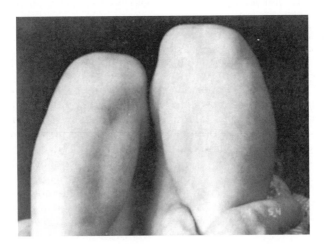

FIGURE 6–32 ■ The Galeazzi test is performed by comparison of the relative height of the femoral condyles by holding the hips in flexion. The right femur appears shorter because of a right hip dislocation. This test is usually not helpful in the case of bilateral hip dislocations.

(From Sabiston DC Jr: Essentials of Surgery. Philadelphia, WB Saunders Company, 1987, p 777; reprinted by permission.)

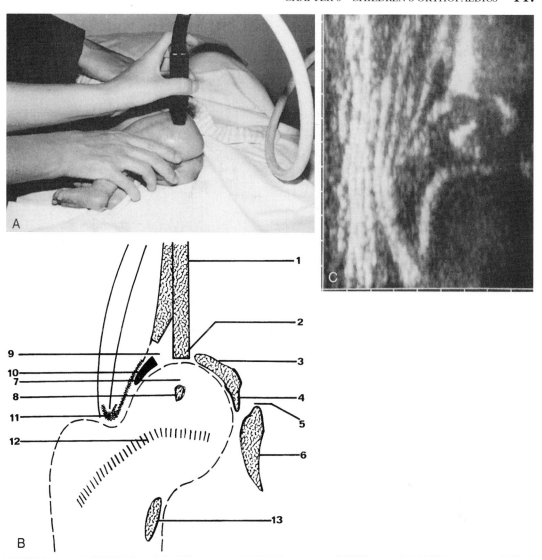

FIGURE 6–33 ■ Ultrasonography of the hip in congenital hip dislocation. *A,* Lateral decubitus position of the infant for ultrasonographic examination of the hip.*B,* Diagram of structures identified during static non-stress ultrasonography of the hip: (1) Iliac bone. (2) The most distal point of the ilium in the roof of the acetabulum. (3) Ossified medial wall of the acetabulum. (4) The inferior end of the iliac bone at the triradiate cartilage. (5) Triradiate cartilage. (6) Ossified ischium. (7) The cartilagtinous femoral head. (8) Ossific nucleus of the femoral head. (9)Cartilaginous roof of the acetabulum. (10) Labrum. (11) Intertrochanteric fossa. (12) Cartilaginous growth plate of the femoral head. (13) Ossified metaphysis of the femoral neck. *C,* Ultrasonogram showing structures.

(From Tachdjian MO: Pediatric Orthopedics, ed 2, Vol 1. Philadelphia, WB Saunders Company, 1990, reprinted by permission.)

hips in neutral is the "gold standard" to which all other studies need to be compared (Fig. 6–34). Historically, many classic measurements are made on this x-ray that allow one to determine the location of the femoral head as well as the degree of acetabular dysplasia. In addition, subsequent x-rays are important to monitor the progress of treatment, despite the enthusiasm in some centers to use ultrasound for therapeutic monitoring.

Treatment: Simply stated, the goals are:

1. Reduce the femoral head concentrically into the acetabulum.

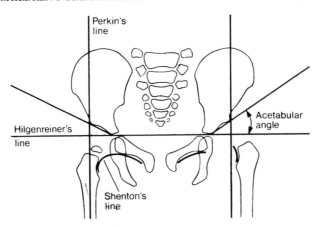

FIGURE 6–34 ■ Radiographic features of congenital dislocation of the hip (left hip dislocated, right hip normal). There is a delay in ossification of the capital femoral epiphysis. Shenton's line, a smooth continuation of an imaginary line drawn along the femoral neck and superior margin of the obturator foramen, is disrupted. The acetabular angle is increased usually greater than 30 degrees. The proximal media l margin of the femoral metaphysis is displaced lateral to Perkin's line, a line drawn from the lateral margin of the acetabulum perpendicular to Hilgenreiner's line.

(From Sabiston DC Jr: Essentials of Surgery. Philadelphia, WB Saunders Company, 1987, p 777; reprinted by permission.)

2. Maintain this reduction.

3. Avoid the complications of doing both.

There is probably no other pediatric orthopaedic malady in which there is a greater understatement of treatment. The pitfalls in accomplishing these apparently simple goals qualify more as "land mines." The adage, "The first physician to treat DDH is the last physician with the opportunity to achieve a normal hip," emphasizes the difficulties frequently encountered in the management of this problem. Also implied is the fact that the younger the child is when treatment is initiated, the better the prognosis will be. Indeed, it is generally believed that if treatment is delayed until after the age of walking, it will not be possible to produce a normal hip.

The use of a Pavlik harness (Fig. 6–35) as initial treatment in the infant has become the international standard. For the child under 3 months of age with a frank dislocation or with persistent instability (as documented, for example, by a positive Barlow test in a 3-week-old), appropriate application and use of a Pavlik harness will assure a normal hip in about 80 percent of cases. The device, how-

ever, is not foolproof, with avascular necrosis, inferior dislocation, and femoral nerve palsies reported as complications, not to mention failure to achieve a reduction. One should be familiar with the appropriate use of this device and NOT randomly apply it as a panacea in all children with hip clicks.

If diagnosis for some reason is delayed and the child presents after 6 months for treatment, more aggressive modalities are generally required to achieve a reduction. Closed reduction under anesthesia, adductor tenotomy, and occasionally prereduction traction are generally employed at this point, with open reduction indicated for those who cannot undergo closed reduction. Immobilization in a spica cast is essential to maintain the reduction.

After 18 months of age, operative approaches are required to reduce the hip and also to reconform the acetabulum. Pelvic osteotomies and proximal femoral osteotomies are utilized in the older age groups. Keep in mind that it is rarely possible to produce a normal hip when treatment is initiated after the age of walking.

The prognosis for DDH is generally very

good, when the diagnosis is made early and treatment initiated in infancy. With delay in diagnosis and therefore in treatment, the prognosis worsens. The complication most dreaded, avascular necrosis, can occur at many points in the treatment algorithm. Despite earlier diagnosis and advances in treatment, many reported series still record about a 10 percent incidence of avascular necrosis. If it occurs, the prognosis is fair at best.

Perthes' Disease

Idiopathic avascular necrosis of the femoral head in the child was originally described in 1909 by multiple authors—Legg in Boston, Calvé in France, and Perthes in Germany. Unfortunately, all authors interpreted that the observed changes were due to nontuberculous sepsis. Slowly it was recognized that the cause was, in fact, an avascular event. It has more recently been shown that the changes cannot be produced by a single period of avascularity. Rather, multiple episodes are needed to cause the characteristic pathologic changes. The exact trigger for this vascular disruption has remained elusive.

The affected children are typically males,

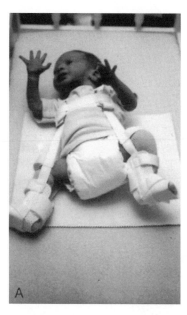

FIGURE 6–35 ■ The Pavlik harness.

(From Tachdjian MO: Pediatric Orthopedics, ed 2, Vol 1. Philadelphia, WB Saunders Company, 1990, p 331; reprinted by permission.)

from a lower socioeconomic status, aged 4 to 9 years, and slightly delayed in skeletal growth. Generally, the child presents with a limp and the absence of any systemic symptoms. Clinically, the child will usually have restricted hip motion, especially rotational, and some adductor muscle spasm. Local findings of tenderness and erythema are not seen. Since standard laboratory studies are usually normal, imaging studies are paramount in the diagnosis and treatment of the disease.

Pathologically, the disease progresses through four stages (Fig. 6–36), and these are reflected by the x-rays and MRI scans. Initially, the stage of synovitis, which lasts 2 to 3 weeks, produces an irritable hip syndrome easily confused with toxic synovitis. The x-rays are negative at this time. Subsequently, the stage of avascularity onsets, lasting 2 to 3 months, during which time the femoral head necrosis occurs. Fragmentation changes of the capital femoral epiphysis herald this stage. Once the avascular event has occurred, the femoral head will revascularize and the process will "heal"—resulting in the stage of revascularization. The critical issue is the degree of deformation of the normally spherical femoral head before complete healing occurs. Eccentric mechanical loads applied to the softened, diseased head frequently alter its sphericity. Ultimately, the process burns itself out, leaving the hip in the stage of residua. The healing phase lasts approximately two years, at which time only the residual deformity remains as the permanent marker of the disease.

The treatment principles for this disease are really no more advanced than they were 30 years ago. Nevertheless, certain facts seem generally accepted. The prognosis seems to hinge on two basic features. First is the patient's age at onset of the disease. Children under age 5 will do well left untreated, which is the current recommendation. Those over age 8 do poorly despite treatment. The other factor is the extent of head involvement. Obviously, a head that is completely necrotic is more likely to sustain permanent deformation than a head only partially involved. For children of intermediate age, 5 to 8 years, the principle of "containment" continues to be accepted. Conceptually, the thought is to place the softened femoral head concentrically into the acetabulum, which will in turn act as a mold or template as the head revascularizes. This can be accomplished in the smaller child by using an abduction orthosis (Fig. 6–37) and in the larger child by using either a femoral or

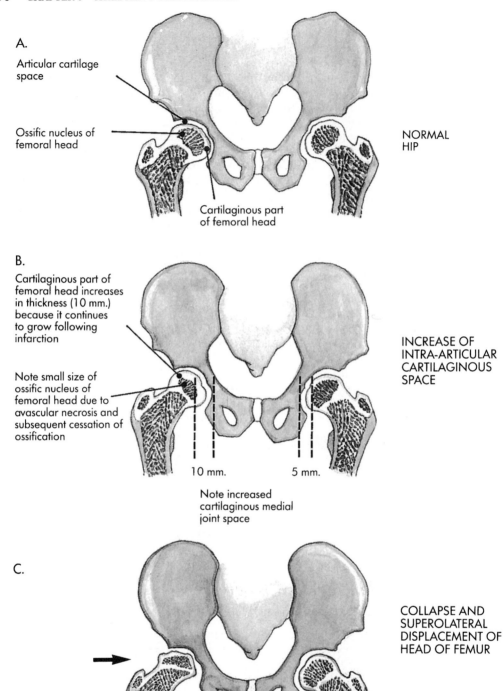

A.

Articular cartilage
space

Ossific nucleus of
femoral head

Cartilaginous part
of femoral head

NORMAL
HIP

B.

Cartilaginous part of
femoral head increases
in thickness (10 mm.)
because it continues
to grow following
infarction

Note small size of
ossific nucleus of
femoral head due to
avascular necrosis and
subsequent cessation of
ossification

10 mm.   5 mm.

Note increased
cartilaginous medial
joint space

INCREASE OF
INTRA-ARTICULAR
CARTILAGINOUS
SPACE

C.

COLLAPSE AND
SUPEROLATERAL
DISPLACEMENT OF
HEAD OF FEMUR

FIGURE 6–36 ■ Pathogenesis of deformity of the femoral head in Legg-Calvé-Perthes'
disease. *A,* Normal hips. *B,* Widening of the medial cartilaginous joint space due to
hypertrophy of the cartilage covering of the femoral head. Note the smaller ossific nucleus due
to cessation of bone growth as a result of avascular necrosis. *C,* Collapse of the femoral head
with superolateral displacement.

(Continued)

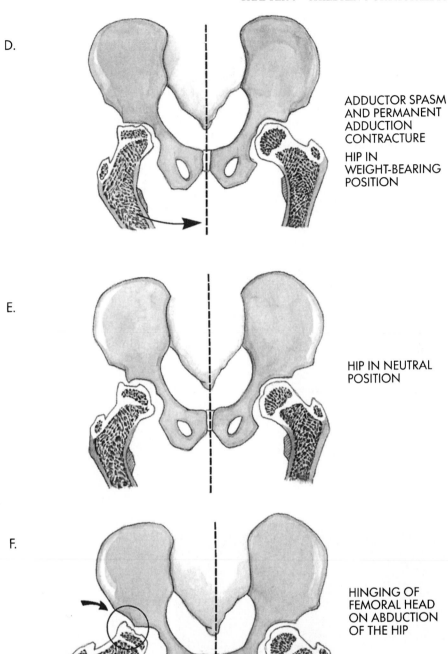

D.

ADDUCTOR SPASM
AND PERMANENT
ADDUCTION
CONTRACTURE

HIP IN
WEIGHT-BEARING
POSITION

E.

HIP IN NEUTRAL
POSITION

F.

HINGING OF
FEMORAL HEAD
ON ABDUCTION
OF THE HIP

FIGURE 6–36 ■ (continued). Pathogenesis of deformity of the femoral head in Legg-Calvé-Perthes' disease. *D,* The hip is adducted in weight-bearing position. Note in *(E)* the dent in the lateral part of the femoral head blocking concentric reduction of the hip. *E* and *F,* Hinged abduction. On abduction of the hip *(F)* the femoral head is displaced further laterally with increase in the medial joint space.

(From Tachdjian MO: Pediatric Orthopedics, ed 2, Vol 1. Philadelphia, WB Saunders Company, 1990, reprinted with permission.)

acetabular osteotomy to improve congruity prior to deformation. The treatment for the older child with an already deformed hip is highly controversial!

In general, the prognosis is good for the younger children, whereas many of those diagnosed after age 9 years require total hip replacement in their forties.

Slipped Capital Femoral Epiphysis

Hip pain in the adolescent should always raise suspicion of this entity. In fact, many of these patients present with pain in the medial thigh radiating to the knee, since referred pain in the obturator nerve distribution is quite typical. These children also share a common body habitus—they tend to be quite obese, with delayed secondary sex characteristics. Many have been limping for several months before they present for evaluation.

Pathologically, the capital femoral epiphysis has "slipped" or translated posteriorly and inferiorly relative to the femoral neck (Fig. 6–38). There are those who prefer to emphasize the fact that the neck is actually moving anteriorly and superiorly relative to the head. The effect of this movement is an irritated hip, manifested by a limp, pain, and an external

rotational deformity of the leg, which should be apparent on clinical examination. There have been multiple suggestions as to etiology. Many feel that these children are hormonally predisposed and, with the stress of obesity, the perichondral ring is no longer able to "girdle" the physis; hence, it begins to move. Typically, the slip is said to occur through the hypertrophic zone of the physis.

Frequently, SCFE is divided into three clinical groups:

1. Chronic slips: symptoms have been present for more than 3 weeks
2. Acute slips: history of acute injury in recent past
3. Acute on chronic slip: acute injury superimposed on child who has been limping for several weeks

The treatment approach is very straightforward: stop the slipping and avoid the complications of doing so. In order to stop the slipping, an "in situ" pinning with a centrally placed screw crossing the physis is employed (Fig. 6–39). It is important to note that *no* attempt should be made to reduce the slipped epiphysis—to do so would subject the head to

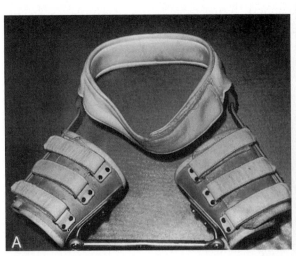
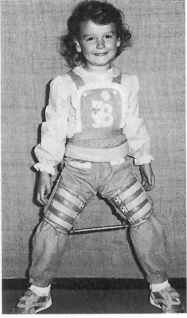

FIGURE 6–37 ■ Scottish-Rite hip orthosis. *A,* Anteroposterior view of the orthosis. *B,* Anteroposterior view of a patient wearing the orthosis.
(From Tachdjian MO: Pediatric Orthopedics, ed 2, Vol 1. Philadelphia, WB Saunders Company, 1990, reprinted by permission.)

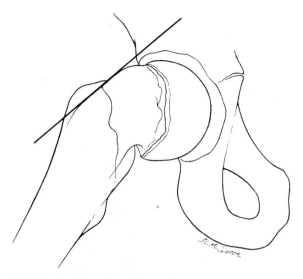

FIGURE 6–38 ■ Slipped capital femoral epiphysis is most reliably seen on the lateral radiograph. Posterior migration of the femoral head relative to the neck is seen. A line drawn up the anterior or lateral margin of the femoral neck does not intersect the epiphysis.

(From Sabiston DC Jr: Essentials of Surgery. Philadelphia, WB Saunders Company, 1987, p 780; reprinted by permission.)

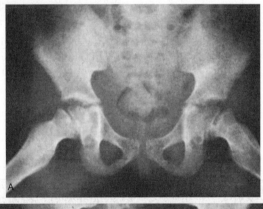

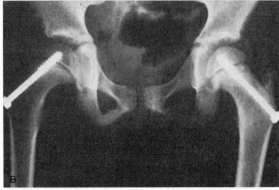

FIGURE 6–39 ■ Slipped capital femoral epiphysis of both hips in a 10-year-old girl with hypothyroidism. *A* and *B,* Anteroposterior and lateral views of both hips.

(From Tachdjian MO: Pediatric Orthopedics, ed 2, Vol 1. Philadelphia, WB Saunders Company, 1990, reprinted by permission.)

a high risk of avascular necrosis. Should severe slipping have occurred resulting in excessive deformity, it is best corrected as a second stage once the physis has fused.

The complications of the disease and its treatment can be devastating. Avascular necrosis is primarily a complication of the treatment, rather than the slip itself. Aggressive reduction maneuvers and femoral neck osteotomies have been implicated. The other concern is chondrolysis. This phenomena may complicate the disease and the treatment. It appears to be a major concern in African-Americans, leading many to suggest an immunologic link. Slowly the articular cartilage is degraded, with resultant joint space narrowing and severe hip stiffness.

As stated before, this condition primarily affects adolescents; when it is diagnosed in a younger child, one should consider specific endocrine abnormalities such as hypothyroidism or chronic renal failure.

Transient Synovitis of the Hip

By far and away, the MOST COMMON cause of limp and hip pain in a child is the "irritable hip syndrome," also called "transient" or "toxic synovitis." Frequently, these children will have a history of an Upper Respiratory Infection (URI) or ear infection in the recent past, leading many to believe that this condition is a postinfectious inflammation of the hip.

Clinically, such children are not sick; they remain active, feed well, and are afebrile. Their lab studies, including x-rays, are usually normal. On a typical exam, the hip is irritable, with additional findings of an antalgic limp, decreased range of motion, and pain with log rolling of the leg.

The treatment is supportive and includes NSAIDs and activity reduction, the latter being key. Normally, the process is self-limited, with the limp disappearing in 5 to 7 days. If it persists longer, one should suspect that the child has remained too active.

The Pediatric Knee

Unlike the hip, the affectations that one sees about the knee in a child are, for the most part, all benign and generally respond to simple treatment measures.

Osgood-Schlatter's Disease

Osteochondritis of the tibial tuberosity (Fig. 6–40) is one of the more common causes of

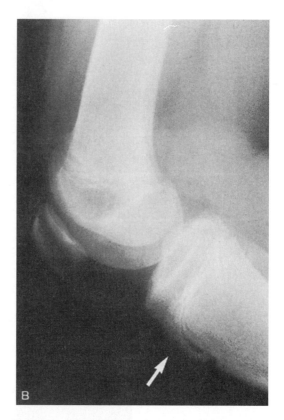

FIGURE 6–40 ■ Osgood-Schlatter disease of the left proximal tibia with free ossicle lying anterior to the proximal tibial tubercle. (From Tachdjian MO: Pediatric Orthopedics, ed 2, Vol 1. Philadelphia, WB Saunders Company, 1990, reprinted by permission.)

knee pain, especially in the preadolescent age group. Although the name implies inflammation, there generally is relatively little present. Essentially this is a "traction apophysitis,"— namely, a powerful muscle group pulls on an open growth plate producing an overload strain and resulting irritation of the local tissues.

These children have local swelling and tenderness over the tibial tuberosity without other findings. The key to successful treatment is activity restriction observed acutely at first, followed by activity modification until the plate closes. It is important for the children to accept responsibility for their knee care: decreasing activity, using ice after activity, and occasionally using a lightweight knee sleeve primarily for psychological support. It is equally important to reassure the parents that, no matter how much pain their child has, he or she is not damaging the knee in any permanent way.

Osteochondritis Dissecans

Another osteochondrosis, osteochondritis dissecans, is felt to be an avascular necrosis of a portion of the subchondral bone (Fig. 6–41). Typically, it most commonly affects the medial side of the lateral femoral condyle, adjacent to the intercondylar notch. However, it can occur on any of the condylar surfaces.

Clinically, the child presents with vague knee pain, which is poorly localized. Occasionally, an effusion will be present. The diagnosis is usually made radiographically, especially if an intercondylar notch view is obtained. Generally short-term activity restriction, ice, and NSAIDs are adequate to relieve acute symptoms. Many can then be returned to sports. If symptoms continue unabated or recur, arthroscopy should be considered; should a loose fragment be identified, it can be removed or pinned into place.

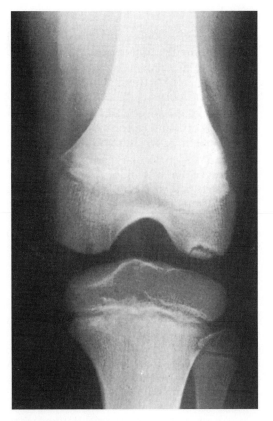

FIGURE 6–41 ■ Osteochondritis dissecans of the knee.

(From Tachdjian MO: Pediatric Orthopedics, ed 2, Vol 1. Philadelphia, WB Saunders Company, 1990, reprinted by permission.)

The Discoid Meniscus

The menisci develop embryologically from a cartilaginous plate referred to as the interzone. The cartilage plates normally thin out to become shaped like the letter "C" on the medial side and the letter "O" on the lateral side of the knee. Should this hollowing out NOT occur on the lateral side, a thick cartilage plate persists as a discoid meniscus (Fig. 6–42). This structure causes the child to have knee pain and occasional effusion beginning about age 3 to 5 years. Most dramatic is a prominent audible and palpable "clunk" seen when the knee is flexed and extended with some rotation applied. If symptoms warrant, arthroscopic removal of the central portion of the disc is required, contouring it to the normal shape. Complete excision is NOT desirable.

Popliteal Cysts

A localized mass in the popliteal space (Fig. 6–43) occurs more than infrequently in small children. Typically, this is a cyst containing gelatinous fluid. As with any mass, these cysts are a source of great concern to the parents, who can benefit a great deal from reassurance as to the correct diagnosis. These can be seen at a young age, frequently just after the child begins to walk.

Typically, the cyst presents between the tendon of the semitendinosus and the medial head of the gastrocnemius; thus it lies medial in the popliteal space. An x-ray should be negative, and an ultrasound will confirm a cystic structure. A more extensive work-up should be considered if the mass is atypical—that is, on lateral side, painful, and enlarging.

Because most of these cysts will disappear in time, surgical excision should be reserved for the ones that cause symptoms. It is important to note that in children these are rarely associated with intra-articular pathology, whereas in the adult that association is the norm.

The Pediatric Foot

There are as many developmental variations in foot configuration as there are children who have feet. It seems that no two pairs of feet are exactly alike. The challenge then for the physician is to determine which of these feet are pathologic and which are essentially normal. Although a number of guidelines have been suggested, none is as helpful as the axiom, "Feel the foot." The pathologically deformed

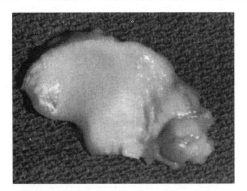

FIGURE 6–42 ■ Discoid lateral meniscus.
(From Tachdjian MO: Pediatric Orthopedics, ed 2, Vol 1. Philadelphia, WB Saunders Company, 1990, reprinted by permission.)

foot cannot be positioned normally by manual manipulation, hence, it is rigid. Conversely, if the abnormally positioned foot can be reduced to a normal configuration with only modest manual pressure, the foot should be considered flexible and the result of excessive intra-uterine molding. It is generally true that most flexible "deformities" are considered "non-disease" and as such require no specific treatment. On the other hand, rigid deformities usually present a definite therapeutic challenge. Foot deformities in children are common and a frequent cause for orthopaedic referrals.

The Flatfoot

As the name implies, the longitudinal arch is low to nonexistent. Officially, the foot is pro-

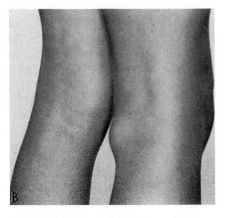

FIGURE 6–43 ■ Popliteal cyst. Clinical appearance.
(From Tachdjian MO: Pediatric Orthopedics, ed 2, Vol 1. Philadelphia, WB Saunders Company, 1990, reprinted by permission.)

nated, and the heel is typically in valgus or everted. Flatfeet can be flexible or rigid, and the difference is critical. Besides feeling the foot, the other technique that is helpful in differentiating the two is simply to examine the child sitting, standing, and standing on the toes. The rigid flatfoot will remain flat in all three positions, whereas the flexible foot is only flat when standing. When seated (not weight-bearing) and when toe-standing, the arch reconstitutes itself and the foot appears to normalize.

Congenital Hypermobile Flatfoot

This is no longer considered an abnormality and is not a cause for exclusion from military service as it once was. Rather, this genetic trait currently is viewed as a normal variant, and the mere finding of it is not an indication for treatment as in years past.

Three pain syndromes do occasionally occur which generally respond to simple therapeutic measures:

1. Arch pain: The child with flatfoot will occasionally develop a strain pattern in the arch. This is easily treated with simple, inexpensive, commercially available supports.
2. Calf pain: Typically, this is caused by tight heel cords and can be treated simply with stretching exercises and arch supports.
3. Accessory navicular syndrome: A modest percentage of children will have a separate ossicle in the posterior tibial tendon adjacent to the tarsal navicular. The prominence of this bone may cause symptoms, which generally respond to padding or occasionally excision of the accessory navicular.

The Rigid Flatfoot

The pronated foot that does not correct on toe-standing should be studied for the presence of a tarsal coalition. These bony, cartilaginous, or fibrous bridges are genetically determined and usually can be diagnosed by appropriate x-rays and a CT scan. Treatment is based on location and severity of symptoms.

Another cause of a rigid flatfoot when seen in a newborn is congenital vertical talus. This germ plasm defect results in abnormal positioning of the talus, with the navicular dorsally dislocated onto the talar neck. As a result, the foot is beyond flat—the arch ac-

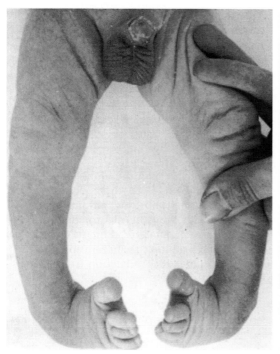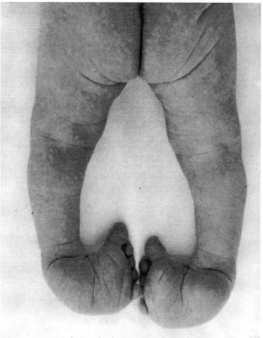

FIGURE 6–44 ■ Bilateral talipes equinovarus in a newborn infant.
(From Tachdjian MO: Pediatric Orthopedics, ed 2. Vol 4. Philadelphia, WB Saunders Company, 1990, p 2449; reprinted by permission.)

tually is convex (rather than concave) and frequently referred to as a "rocker bottom deformity." This uncommon pathologic foot requires surgical correction.

Congenital Clubfoot

Similar to DDH, this deformity is multifactorial in origin. Environmental factors applied to a genetically predisposed individual result in this pathologic deformity. As with DDH, it is important to make it clear to the parents that this is NOT a postural deformity. Rather, there is an anatomic abnormality of the talus. Due to the abnormal medial and plantar deviation of the talar neck, there are a number of secondary deformities. The tarsal navicular is dislocated dorsally onto the talar neck; soft tissue contractures develop, and the resultant configuration is characteristic. The forefoot is adducted, the hind foot is in varus (inverted), and the entire foot is in equinus.

A clubfoot, as is the case with most pathologic feet, is rigid on clinical exam (Fig. 6–44). X-rays can be used to confirm the diagnosis. Since clubfeet are frequently seen in association with other abnormalities, every effort should be made to evaluate the whole child.

Myelodysplasia, arthrogryposis, and diastrophic dwarfism are only a few examples of conditions that may manifest clubfeet. The associated anomalies will determine the type of treatment.

In the case of "standard" congenital clubfoot, the recommended initial treatment is stretching and serial casting. This approach will be adequate to correct about 30 to 40 percent of clubfeet. The remainder will usually require a surgical procedure to complete the correction initiated with close manipulation. Early surgical correction (3 to 6 months of age) has significantly decreased the need for multiple late procedures for residual deformities. If correction is achieved prior to the age of walking, an excellent prognosis can be anticipated.

Metatarsus Adductus

The most common problem seen in the child's foot is metatarsus adductus. Many cases are actually a form of "non-disease" and represent the result of excessive uterine cramming of the newborn. Since most of these cases are normal variants, they will correct without specific treatment. The clinical problem is that some are pathologic, rather than postural, and therefore do need appropriate care.

The child's foot manifests forefoot adduction (Fig. 6–45) and supination. When viewed from the plantar surface, the foot with metatarsus adductus has a typical "kidney bean" appearance. Again, it is essential to "feel the foot." By doing so, these feet can be grouped into three clinical types:

■ Type I (mild): Foot is supple and easily corrects with digital stroking of the lateral side of the foot.
■ Type II (moderate): Gentle manual pressure is required on the medial forefoot for correction.
■ Type III (severe): Moderate force is required for correction; even so, some cases may not be correctable.

The mild and moderate deformities usually correct spontaneously and do not require treatment. A simple way to monitor improvement is to stand the child on a copying machine at each follow-up visit and reproduce a copy of the plantar surface of the feet. The severe feet and some of the "tighter" moderate feet are best treated with serial casting to correct the deformity. Should this approach fail, several surgical procedures are available.

For the vast majority of cases, the prognosis is excellent. Even those children with mild persistent deformity have virtually no problems with their feet. Unfortunately, persistent severe metatarsus adductus (Fig. 6–46) causes such problems as shoe-fitting pain and cosmesis. Late reconstruction requires osteotomies through the midfoot.

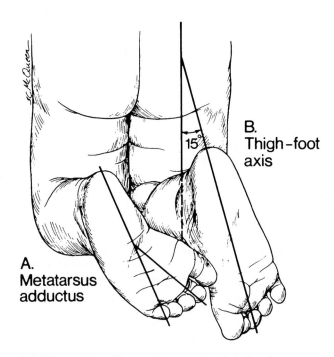

FIGURE 6–45 ■ The heel bisector line is utilized in determining the severity of metatarsus adductus *(A)*. Deviation of the forefoot causes this line to extend lateral to the second toe. The deviation of the forefoot causes the lateral border of the foot to be convex and the medial border to be concave. The thigh-foot axis *(B)* is used to determine tibial version. The normal thigh-foot axis is external 15 degrees, as demonstrated.

(From Sabiston DC Jr: Essentials of Surgery. Philadelphia, WB Saunders Company, 1987, p 784; reprinted by permission.)

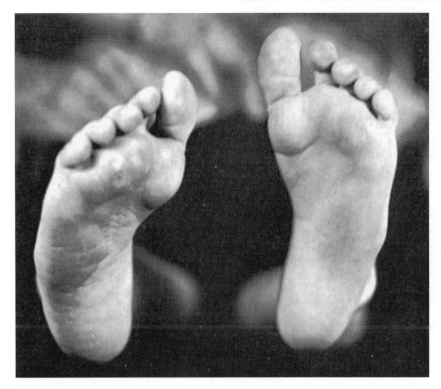

FIGURE 6–46 ■ Untreated metatarsus deformity in young boy.
(From Gartland JJ: Fundamentals of Orthopaedics, ed 4. Philadelphia, WB Saunders
Company, 1987, p 59; reprinted by permission.)

The Pediatric Upper Extremity and Neck

In general, the vast majority of upper extremity problems in children that require orthopaedic evaluation are traumatic in origin. Fractures of the elbow and forearm are relatively common and represent some of the most challenging problems in orthopaedics. Nontraumatic conditions of the upper extremity are far less common, and those worthy of note are primarily congenital in nature.

Sprengel's Deformity

Congenital elevation of the scapular (Fig. 6–47) is generally due to persistence of a fibrous, cartilaginous, or bony bar that persists between the spine and the superior medial border of the scapula—that is, an omovertebral bar. This structure prevents the scapula from migrating interiorly from its embryologic position adjacent to the cervical spine to the normal adult position.

Sprengel's deformity usually presents as asymmetry of the neck or shoulder, and physi-cal examination is generally adequate for diagnosis. Since most children have no significant functional deficits, surgical treatment is usually not required. Cosmesis is an occasional complaint and can be managed by simple excision of the upper portion of the scapula. If a functional deficit does exist, several operative procedures have been developed to reduce the scapula to its normal position.

Congenital Muscular Torticollis

Although not truly an upper extremity problem, children with this condition present with a wry neck and asymmetry. Physical examination is usually adequate to make the diagnosis and differentiate it from some of the other causes of asymmetry in this region: Klippel Fiel anomaly, congenital scoliosis, and Sprengel's deformity (Fig. 6–48).

Essentially, the problem is a contracture within the sternocleidomastoid muscle. The exact etiology of this contracture has been the subject of some controversy. Intrauterine hemorrhage within the muscle, local com-

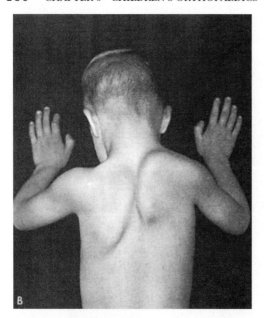

FIGURE 6–47 ■ Sprengel's deformity of the right shoulder. The scapula is elevated and hypoplastic, its horizontal diameter being greater than the vertical.

(From Tachdjian MO: Pediatric Orthopedics, ed 2, Vol 1. Philadelphia, WB Saunders Company, 1990, reprinted by permission.)

partment syndrome, and fibrotic bands have all been proposed. Despite the etiology, the net result is a newborn presenting with a torticollis and facial asymmetry. Typically, the head is tilted TO the side of the lesion and the face and chin are turned AWAY from the side of the lesion.

The deformity usually responds to simple physical therapy, stretching by the parents, and positioning the crib to encourage the infant to look TO the side of the lesion, thereby stretching the tight sternocleidomastoid. Occasionally, nonsurgical treatment is not adequate, and operative release is required. This should be done before the child is 18 months to 2 years of age—most importantly to level the eyes.

Worthy of note, is the coincidence of this condition and developmental hip dysplasia. Since 20 percent of these children have abnormal hips, careful screening in this group is strongly recommended.

Radial Anomalies

The most common long-bone deficiencies in the upper extremity involve the radius (Fig. 6–49). Partial or complete absence of this bone, with or without adjacent hand deficien-

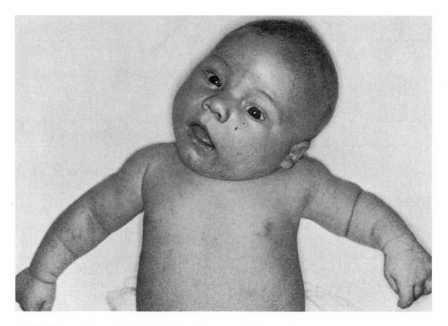

FIGURE 6–48 ■ Congenital muscular torticollis on the left. The head is tilted to the left and the chin rotated to the right.

(From Tachdjian MO: Pediatric Orthopedics, ed 2, Vol 1. Philadelphia, WB Saunders Company, 1990, reprinted by permission.)

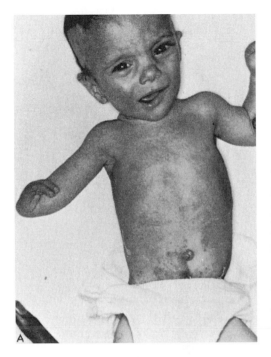

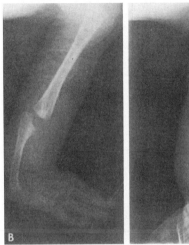

FIGURE 6–49 ■ Congenital absence of the radius in an infant. *A,* Clinical appearance. *B,* Preoperative radiograms.
(From Tachdjian MO: Pediatric Orthopedics, ed 2, Vol 1. Philadelphia, WB Saunders Company, 1990, reprinted by permission.)

cies, can be seen as an isolated finding or in association with several syndromes. Franconi's and Vater syndromes should be considered when the radial dysplasia is bilateral. Further work-up will usually reveal the renal defect or the thrombocytopenia.

The hand tends to deviate to the radial side and is referred to as "radial clubhand." Early treatment is nonoperative and based on stretching and bracing. Later surgical reconstruction of the extremity to improve wrist function is appropriate.

Congenital Trigger Thumb

Perhaps it is best not to use the term "congenital" since the defect is rarely noticed at birth or, for that matter, in the first 6 months. It is usually appreciated when the child begins using the hand for grasping. At this point, the flexed attitude of the interphalangeal joint is noticed by the parents. Initially, stretching will straighten the digit, but as the tendinous nodule of the flexor pollicis longus enlarges, it will no longer slide under the flexor pulley. The thumb is then "stuck" in flexion.

Some will respond to simple stretching, but most require surgical tenolysis after 6 to 9 months of age. The vast majority of those

treated in this way have an excellent result and no recurrence.

PEDIATRIC TRAUMA

The basic principles of injury to the immature skeleton have been discussed in part elsewhere. The unique features of pediatric fractures are primarily due to the biologic differences between child and adult. Specifically, the presence of an open growth plate, the periosteum, the ability of pediatric bone to plastically deform, and the ability to remodel this deformity are the bases for the fracture patterns typically seen.

The physis is clearly an internal "flaw" in the bone and thus, a point of mechanical weakness. Many loading modes are capable of causing failure through the physis. These fractures were classified many years ago by Salter and Harris (Fig. 6–50). Their classification was based on the direction that the fracture line took through the physis and adjacent osseous structures. Purportedly, this classification correlates with prognosis—the higher the number of the fracture type, the poorer the prognosis. Although true within certain limits, this

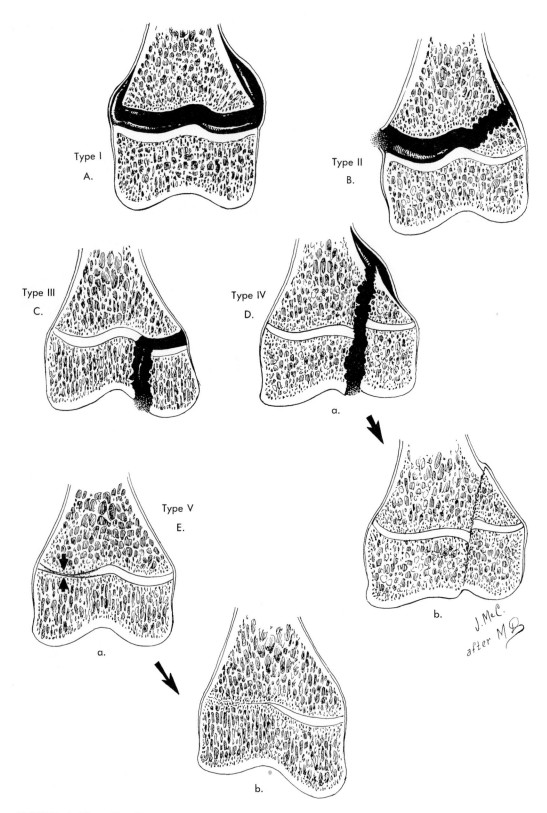

FIGURE 6–50 ■ Classification of epiphyseal plate injuries according to Salter and Harris.

(Redrawn after Salter RB, Harris WR: Injuries involving the epiphyseal plate. J Bone Joint Surg 45-A:587, 1963. In Tachdjian MO: Pediatric Orthopedics, ed 2. Vol 4. Philadelphia, WB Saunders Company, 1990, p 3023; reprinted by permission.)

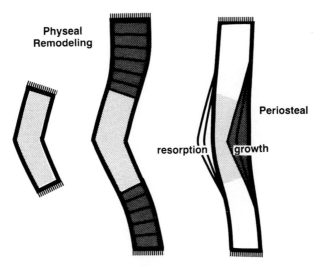

Physeal Remodeling

Periosteal

resorption   growth

FIGURE 6–51 ■ The basis of remodeling.
(From Rang M: In Rang M [ed], Children's Fractures, ed 2.
Philadelphia, JB Lippincott Company, 1983, p 8; reprinted by
permission.)

is not always the case. For example, a Salter II fracture of the distal radius is a common, benign injury, whereas a Salter II fracture of the distal femur is complicated by a partial physeal arrest in more than 50 percent of cases. Fractures of the physis heal rapidly in 3 to 4 weeks, but parents should be warned about potential growth plate arrest. Physeal fractures that cross the plate and/or enter the joint require operative restoration of normal anatomy in an effort to minimize the risk of this complication.

The periosteum (Fig. 6–51), as previously noted, is thicker, more vascular, and more osteogenic than that of an adult. The mechanical benefits provided by the periosteum tend to minimize fracture displacement, act as an aid in reduction, and assist in maintenance of reduction. Biologically, the active osteogenic potential allows fractures to heal in half the time required for a similar bone in the adult.

The biologic plasticity of pediatric bone is responsible for the typical fracture patterns seen in the pediatric diaphysis. The incomplete fractures—greenstick and torus—represent the ability of these bones to bend but not break all the way through. In general, this phenomena is not seen in adult bone, due to the progressive stiffening of cortical bone that occurs with aging. Occasionally, this feature presents a therapeutic dilemma. In the fore-

arm, a plastically deformed ulna will act as a spring to redeform the already fractured radius. The solution is to complete the fracture of the ulna by osteoclasis. This will allow one to align the forearm acceptably and prevent redeformation.

Finally, the extensive remodeling ability of pediatric bone has corrected many seemingly unacceptable reductions without the need for multiple closed reductions. There are limits to the amount of correction that can be anticipated (Fig. 6–52). One should not be overly secure, expecting "Mother Nature" to correct all malposition. In general, angular deformity will remodel to variable degrees. Greater correction can be expected if the deformity is in the plane of motion of the joint; similarly, the closer the fracture to the joint, the more complete will be the correction. Translational deformity (i.e., displacement) at all levels tends to completely remodel. Rotational malalignment does NOT remodel; therefore, it is important to correct all rotary deformity. Complications of pediatric fractures are uncommon with adequate treatment; however, when they do occur, management is frequently problematic. The reason for this is the growth remaining in the skeleton. Any injury compromising the growth mechanics of a long bone will only compound itself over time as the deformity appears to worsen. Periarticular fractures and

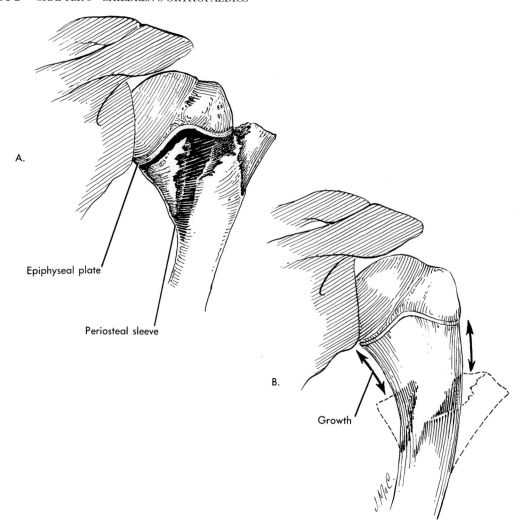

Epiphyseal plate

Periosteal sleeve

Growth

FIGURE 6–52 ■ Diagram showing remodeling process of a malunited fracture involving the proximal humeral physis.

(From Tachdjian MO: Pediatric Orthopedics, ed 2. Vol 4. Philadelphia, WB Saunders Company, 1990, p 3050; reprinted by permission.)

physeal fractures tend to present more problems in this regard than do those in the diaphysis.

The treatment principles, then, are directed toward fracture reduction and maintenance while avoiding complications—goals similar to those in the adult. Operative treatment of certain physeal injuries is common, and there is now current interest in operative treatment of more diaphyseal fractures, especially of the femur, in an effort to decrease length of hospital stay. Regardless of the reduction approach, the need for immobilization is undisputed. Children by definition are noncompliant; premature removal of immobilizing devices usually has disastrous results. One need *not* be concerned about joint stiffness or a cast induced atrophy in children. It is far more important to continue the immobilization until the fracture is healed. Physical therapy following cast removal is rarely needed since the activity level of a normal child, unhampered by a cast, is more than adequate to mobilize the extremity. It is especially important NOT to subject the child with an elbow injury to a well-meaning but overaggressive physical therapist. This will only aggravate the joint stiffness and retard resolution.

In summary, children's fractures mandate management goals similar to the adult: reduction, maintenance, and avoidance of complications. However, due to generally permissive biologic mechanisms, the tolerances in treatment are much greater. Successful results require adequate recognition of the unique qualities of the pediatric skeleton and the special problems that may follow trauma to it.

Battered Child Syndrome

No discussion of pediatric skeletal trauma would be complete without mention of this syndrome. The sociologic implications are extensive for the patient, the family, and the physician. Child abuse rarely occurs as an isolated event, and the result of returning the child to the home may be disastrous. It then becomes important to recognize the signs and symptoms of "nonaccidental" trauma. Failure to recognize or suspect this syndrome has often resulted in continued abuse.

As the name implies, this is a "syndrome," meaning the diagnosis is usually based on finding a constellation of manifestations. The diagnosis rarely can be made on the basis of an isolated fracture; rather, several fractures in multiple stages of healing will more reliably indicate abuse over time. The syndrome typically presents with findings in multiple areas, including:

1. *General neglect.* Beware the child who fails to make eye contact with parents or physician. The child who is dirty and uncared for and who exhibits evidence of psychological and nutritional neglect should raise one's suspicions.
2. *Skin and soft tissue injury.* "Imprinting" of the skin due to blows with specific objects, such as belt buckles, coat hangers, ropes, etc., should be searched out. Evidence of cigarette and radiator burns can commonly be found. Eye-ground hemorrhages and forehead hematomas indicate "shaken baby syndrome."
3. *Craniocerebral injury.* Subdural or epidural hematomas with or without nonparietal skull fractures are highly suggestive of abuse.
4. *Skeletal injury* (Fig. 6–53)
   a. Rib fractures. Multiple fractures especially in a line typically indicate a kicking injury.
   b. Metaphyseal–epiphyseal fractures. "Bucket-handle" and "teardrop" fractures of the metaphyseal region generally suggest shaking the child while holding the limb.
   c. Diaphyseal fractures. Spiral fractures of the distal humerus and fractures of the femoral shaft in a nonambulatory child are the most typical of abuse. Other long-bone injuries occurring as an isolated finding should not generate a referral to child protective services.

This tragic problem is becoming more commonly diagnosed in recent years, primarily due to heightened societal awareness of the problem. Physicians need to be vigilant and knowledgeable of the hallmarks of the syndrome; only then can they meet their legal reporting requirements, thereby saving a child from return to an abusive environment.

Evaluation of a Limp

The limping child is a relatively common problem, and yet one that is difficult to evaluate. Multiple etiologies, the child's difficulty in localizing pain, and a vague history make it essential that the physician has a systematic approach to this problem. Rather than order multiple unpleasant and expensive diagnostic studies, it is usually more valuable to carefully observe and examine the child, especially in a sequential fashion.

Generically, a limp is any uneven or laborious gait or, for that matter, any alteration in normal gait sequence. Normal gait classically occurs with two phases for each extremity: stance and swing. The stance phase is initiated at heel strike for a given limb and terminated with toe-off of that extremity. Stance accounts for 60 percent normally, leaving 40 percent of the cycle for swing—the foot is off the ground. Three classic aberrations of the gait cycle have been described:

1. Antalgic limp: Pain is the etiology of this gait aberration. Due to pain in the limb with ground contact, the stance phase is shortened and the patient unloads the extremity more quickly. Many etiologies will cause an antalgic limp such as a

fracture in the foot or toxic synovitis of the hip.

2. Trendlenberg limp: (gluteus medius lurch). Frequently referred to as an abductor lurch, this pattern is due to the incompetence of the abductor lever arm to stabilize the pelvis (Fig. 6–54). If one remembers that a moment is created by a force acting over a distance, it can be appreciated that altering either factor will cause a Trendlenberg limp:

   a. Force alteration: Muscle weakness, as seen in polio

   b. Distance alteration: Shortened lever arm, as seen in DDH or malunited femoral neck fracture

3. Short leg limp: Leg-length discrepancy of significance will be manifested as an apparent limp with the pelvis dropping on the short side (Fig. 6–55).

A careful history should investigate a past traumatic event, systemic symptoms, and the effect on activity. Physical findings such as fever, focal findings of swelling, limitation of motion, and muscle spasm should be sought. Age itself may be a clue to the etiology since each group seems particularly prone to certain ailments.

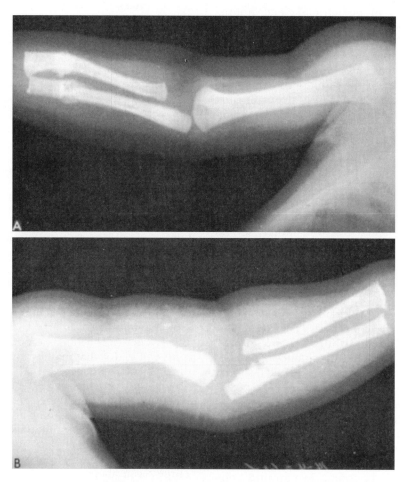

FIGURE 6–53 ■ Multiple fractures in different stages of healing. *A,* Fractures of the distal end of the right radius and ulna with callus at the fracture site and smooth periosteal new bone formation along the shaft. *B,* Fracture of the left humerus and proximal end of the ulna with minimal reaction. There is also a metaphyseal avulsion of the distal end of the radius.

(From Akbarnia BA, Akbarnia NO: The role of [the] orthopedist in child abuse and neglect. Orthop Clin North Am 7[3]:739, 1976; reprinted by permission.)

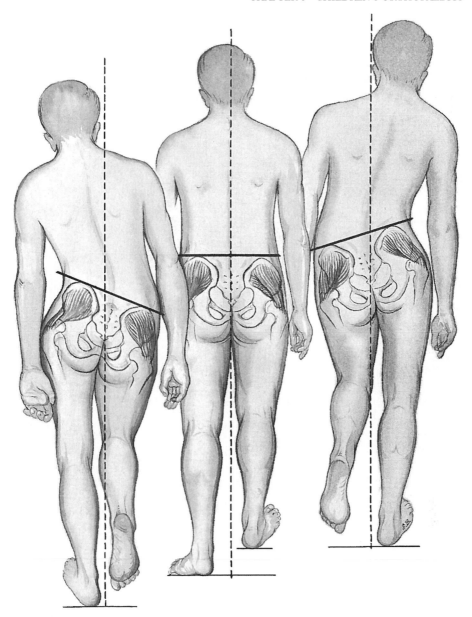

FIGURE 6–54 ■ Gluteus medius lurch.

(From Tachdjian MO: Pediatric Orthopedics, ed 2, Vol 1. Philadelphia, WB Saunders Company, 1990, reprinted by permission.)

1 to 3-year-old: trauma, infection, DDH, new shoes

5 to 9-year-old: transient synovitis, Perthes' disease, JRA, Lyme disease

over 12 years: SCFE

Extending the diagnostic work-up, one should first consider standard x-rays, especially of the hips. Routine hemogram is frequently beneficial. A three-phase bone scan is a reasonable second-line study, especially if localization is necessary. Unfortunately, it is not possible to specifically outline the studies to be routinely obtained. Reaching the correct diagnosis is all too often the result of coinciding historical data, physical findings, laboratory data, and a "gut" sense. Several diagnostic algorithms have been proposed that emphasize the basic factors in evaluating pediatric limp:

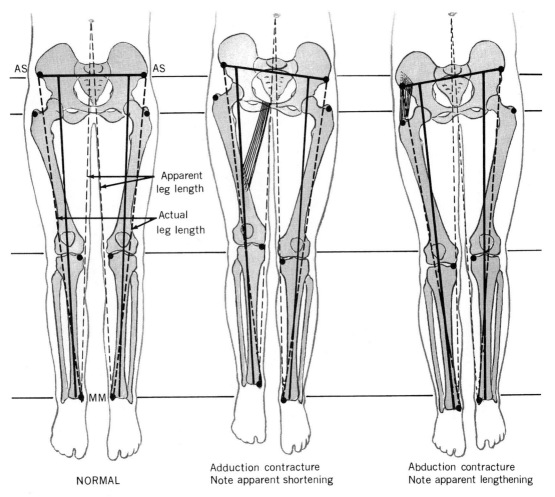

Apparent
leg length

Actual
leg length

NORMAL

Adduction contracture
Note apparent shortening

Abduction contracture
Note apparent lengthening

FIGURE 6–55 ■ Measurement of actual and apparent leg lengths. AS, anterior iliac spine; MM, medial malleolus.

(From Tachdjian MO: Pediatric Orthopedics, ed 2, Vol 1. Philadelphia, WB Saunders Company, 1990, reprinted by permission.}

Is there a history of trauma?
Are there systemic symptoms?
Are there focal findings?

By answering these questions, a work-up can be fashioned that should ultimately reveal the etiology.

CONCLUSIONS

Children are different. They are not small adults. Biologically and mechanically their musculoskeletal system predisposes them to patterns of injury and disease unique to their age group. By understanding these differences, one can anticipate some of the patterns, thereby permitting appropriate treatment and minimizing complications.

The seven categories of disease—vascular, infections, tumor, arthritis, metabolic, injury, and neurodevelopmental—all produce changes in the skeleton that reflect the unique feature of childhood: *growth*. Simple insults can be made worse over time due to aberrational growth and conversely potentially disastrous insults can be palliated by the innate remodeling potential of the pediatric skeleton.

Pediatric Spine
William Lauerman

SCOLIOSIS

Scoliosis refers to abnormal curvature of the spine when viewed in the coronal plane. The human spine is normally straight when viewed from behind, but because of the potential implications of unnecessarily labeling a child as "having" scoliosis, minor deviations from normal (less than ten degrees) may be considered within normal limits. Scoliosis has been discussed in the medical and orthopaedic literature since antiquity and is widely believed, by individuals in the medical profession as well as the lay population, to be a debilitating or disabling condition, resistant to treatment, and with a grave prognosis. Advances in both operative and nonoperative treatment in the last 40 years, as well as a better understanding of the natural history of scoliosis, however, have removed much of the stigma from this condition.

A variety of conditions may cause or be associated with scoliosis (see Table 6–2). The most common type of scoliosis is referred to as idiopathic, meaning simply that the cause of the disorder is unknown. Hereditary factors have been implicated, and research is ongoing as to other possible causes of idiopathic scoliosis. While it is likely that the development of idiopathic scoliosis is multifactorial, genetic, hormonal, biochemical, biomechanical, and neuromuscular abnormalities continue to be investigated. Idiopathic scoliosis has been broken down by age; curvature of the spine that has its onset before the age of 3 years is defined as infantile idiopathic scoliosis, curvature identified between the ages of 3 and 10 as juvenile idiopathic scoliosis, and curvature occurring after the age of 10, or the onset of adolescence, as adolescent idiopathic scoliosis. Most cases of idiopathic scoliosis are identified during the adolescent growth spurt and are therefore considered adolescent curves.

Numerous other conditions either cause or are associated with scoliosis and must be considered when evaluating a patient. Congenital abnormalities of the vertebrae, resulting in congenital scoliosis or congenital kyphosis, represent some of the more common etiologies of spinal deformity. Neuromuscular disorders such as polio, cerebral palsy, muscular dystrophy, spinal muscular atrophy, or myelomeningocele are frequently associated with scoliosis. Other conditions such as neurofibromatosis, Marfan's syndrome, arthrogryposis, osteogenesis imperfecta, and Friedreich's ataxia may also result in scoliosis. There is also a known association between scoliosis and certain congenital conditions such as congenital heart disease, congenital limb deficiency, and congenital or postsurgical thoracic cage defects.

Estimates of the prevalence of scoliosis depend on the threshold for definition. While 1.5 to 3 percent of the population are believed to have curves over 10 degrees, only 0.2 to 0.3 percent of the normal population have curves over 30 degrees, a magnitude where treatment is typically required. The natural history of idiopathic scoliosis has been well established. Most curves are identified in early adolescence. Progression is variable and is more

TABLE 6–2 ■ Etiology of Scoliosis

Idiopathic
Congenital
Neuromuscular
  Polio
  Cerebral palsy
  Posttraumatic (spinal cord injury)
  Spinal muscular atrophy
  Muscular dystrophy
  Friedreich's ataxia
  Charcot-Marie-Tooth disease
  Syringomyelia
  Myelomeningocele
  Arthrogryposis
Neurofibromatosis
Marfan's syndrome
Ehlers-Danlos syndrome
Juvenile rheumatoid arthritis
Spine or spinal cord tumor
Postlaminectomy
Thoracic cage defect/deficiency
Osteochondrodystrophy (dwarfism)
Osteogenesis imperfecta

likely in younger patients, in skeletally imma-ture patients (including premenarchal girls), and in larger curves. Finally, while mild curves are as common in boys as in girls, progressive curves, and curves requiring treatment are far more common in girls.

The implication of scoliosis in adult-hood entails consideration of curve progres-sion, pain, disability, and mortality. It has been established that idiopathic curves of greater than 50 degrees, particularly right thoracic curves, are at significant risk for progression in adulthood. While curve progression is a possibility, the presence of scoliosis does not necessarily place the patient at risk for back pain. Some patients with scoliosis appear to have pain related to the curve, but it has been demonstrated that patients with idiopathic scoliosis are not at any increased risk, when compared to the general population, for the development of disabling low back symptoms. Similarly, pulmonary dysfunction and signif-icant functional disability are relatively rare occurrences.

The mortality rate of individuals with idiopathic scoliosis does not differ significantly from that of the general population when the curve magnitude is less than 90 to 100 degrees. Finally, scoliosis does not have an adverse impact on a woman's ability to bear children, nor is the curve more likely to progress during pregnancy than at other times.

Management

The management of the child with docu-mented or suspected scoliosis begins with a thorough evaluation. Most cases are picked up during school screening, wherein a school nurse or another allied health professional utilizes the Adam's forward bend test to evalu-ate for possible asymmetry of the spine and trunk (Fig. 6–56). This test is performed with the observer seated behind the patient, and the child is asked to bend forward at the waist with the knees straight and the hands hanging towards the floor. Asymmetry of the ribs from right to left is considered a positive test and merits further evaluation by an orthopaedist. Other possible signs of scoliosis include pelvic or shoulder asymmetry. This test, which should

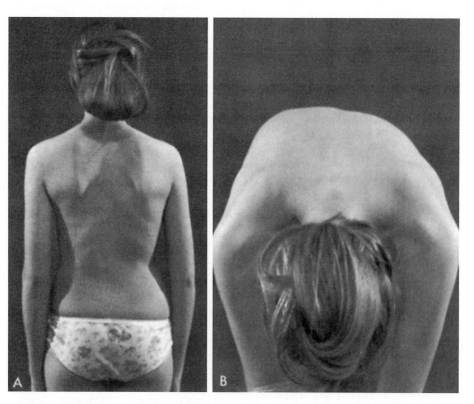

FIGURE 6–56 ■ Careful examination by a school nurse resulted in early diagnosis of this curvature (10 degrees). Note the spine asymmetry in the flexed position (B).

be a routine part of a pediatrician's well child physical examination, is extremely sensitive for picking up most cases of scoliosis and the proven benefits of school screening are now well accepted.

In evaluating the patient with possible scoliosis, important historical points include a family history of spinal deformity, any abnormality or delay in reaching developmental milestones, and associated neurologic symptoms of the lower extremities or urogenital system, including gait abnormalities, paresthesias, recent onset of enuresis, etc. In addition to the above described evaluation of the spine and trunk, the physical examination includes: a thorough inspection of the skin, looking for cafe-au-lait spots; palpation of the spine, looking for an occult spina bifida; examination of the lower extremities, looking for calf or foot atrophy or asymmetry; or any neurologic abnormalities. Careful testing of the deep tendon reflexes, as well as the superficial skin reflexes, and testing for Babinski's sign is essential. Any physical finding suggestive of central nervous system abnormality merits more detailed work-up, possibly including imaging of the brain stem, spinal cord, or cauda equina.

Radiographic evaluation is carried out on any patient suspected of having scoliosis. A standing posteroanterior view (PA) view of the full spine, including the pelvis, will demonstrate the presence or absence of significant deformity. The pelvis is inspected for evidence of skeletal maturity, manifested by closure of the iliac apophysis. In some cases obtaining a wrist film for bone age may be helpful. Because there is a known association between scoliosis and spondylolisthesis (see below), a lateral x-ray of the spine should be obtained, including visualization down to the sacrum.

Treatment options available for the growing child with scoliosis include observation, bracing, and surgery. Previous attempts at curve control utilizing physical therapy, exercises, and electrical stimulation have proved ineffectual and have been abandoned. Observation, with repeat radiographs every 4 to 6 months, is appropriate in the child with scoliosis less than 25 to 30 degrees. Curves that have been documented to progress beyond 25 degrees or curves measuring beyond 30 degrees at first presentation, in a child with significant growth remaining, are commonly treated with a brace.

For many years the standard orthosis for the treatment of scoliosis has been the Milwaukee brace. The Milwaukee brace has been documented to be effective in controlling curves measuring between 25 and 40 degrees, and its use is successful in avoiding surgery in approximately 80 percent of cases. Patient resistance to the use of the Milwaukee brace, including the neck and chin ring, has resulted in the now widespread use of underarm orthoses such as the Boston or Wilmington brace. These braces have proven equally effective in controlling most thoracic and thoracolumbar idiopathic curves and have become the current standard for the management of curves of moderate magnitude in skeletally immature patients.

When a curve exceeds 40 or 45 degrees it becomes increasingly difficult to control with an external orthosis. Because of this, as well as the increasing risk of progression into adulthood with curves greater than 50 degrees, surgery is generally recommended for curves that progress into the range of 40 to 50 degrees. The commonly accepted indications for surgical treatment of scoliosis include adolescents with curves documented to progress beyond 40 to 45 degrees, adolescents with curves at presentation exceeding 45 to 50 degrees, and, on occasion, adults with either documented curve progression, disabling pain, or both. The goals of the surgical treatment of scoliosis include the arrest of progression, achievement of a solidly fused spine, and improvement in the curve with associated improvement in cosmetic appearance. While upwards of 50 percent curve correction can routinely be obtained in the adolescent, the more important goals of surgery are achieving a solid fusion, well balanced over the sacrum, and extending from the top to the bottom of the curve.

The surgical treatment of scoliosis constitutes, first and foremost, a spinal fusion. The standard approach to this fusion is posterior, although certain curves are amenable to anterior fusion. Since the introduction of the Harrington rod in the 1950s instrumentation of the spine at the time of fusion has become well accepted. Improved rates of correction and fusion, as well as a lessened need for postoperative immobilization, have more than offset the risks incurred. Spinal instrumentation has evolved over the last two decades. Newer implants utilize multiple points of fixation along the spine, are more easily contoured to help the surgeon restore physiologic alignment in three planes, and have, in many cases, eliminated the need for postoperative immobilization (Fig. 6–57).

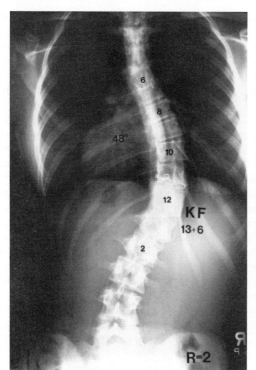
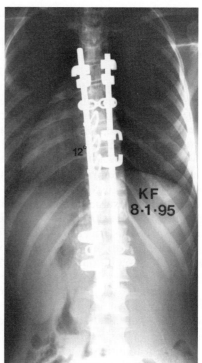

FIGURE 6–57 ■ A 13 year-old girl with progressive idiopathic scoliosis measuring 48°. Following surgery, a posterior spinal fusion with segmental instrumentation and iliac crest bone graft, her curve corrected to 12°. She went on to a solid fusion with no loss of correction.

In the adolescent with idiopathic scoliosis, curve correction using modern techniques averages 50 to 70 percent. Ninety-five to 98 percent of patients go on to solid fusion with less than 10 percent loss of correction. Infection and thromboembolic disease are occasional complications of spinal instrumentation and fusion for scoliosis, and they are seen more commonly in adults than in adolescents. The most feared complication of surgery for scoliosis, paraplegia, is rare in the absence of a known risk factor such as kyphosis, congenital scoliosis, or a preoperative neurologic deficit, but it is a recognized occurrence.

Congenital Scoliosis

Individuals with congenital abnormality of the spine represent an unusual but well-defined subset of patients with spinal deformity. Failures of formation (hemivertebrae), failures of segmentation (bars), and mixed deformities are seen. The prognosis varies depending on the type of anomaly present, but the patient with congenital scoliosis is certainly at higher risk for progression than the patient with an idiopathic curve. There is a known association between congenital scoliosis and congenital anomalies of the urogenital system, and all patients with congenital spine deformity should be referred for imaging of the GU system. Congenital heart disease is also more common in this population, although a normal history and physical examination of the heart is considered sufficient to rule out a significant cardiac abnormality.

In addition to an increased risk of progression, which approaches 100 percent in curves involving a unilateral unsegmented bar, congenital curves are widely held to be resistant to bracing. While progressive congenital scoliosis in a growing child is still routinely treated with an orthosis, the orthopaedic surgeon and the pediatrician need to be aware that there is a high risk of further progression necessitating surgical intervention. Congenital deformities can, on occasion, result in quite severe curves in very young children, but postponing surgery in this setting only results in a more difficult reconstructive problem at a later date.

Neuromuscular Deformity

Neuromuscular or paralytic causes for scoliosis include polio, cerebral palsy, muscular dystrophy, posttraumatic paraplegia, and myelomeningocele. At one time polio was the most common cause of scoliosis in this country, and it continues to be in much of the third world. Neuromuscular curves have a characteristic long, C-shaped appearance. Extension of the curve into the pelvis, with pelvic obliquity on sitting or standing, is common and complicates both surgical and nonsurgical treatment. The risk of scoliosis varies among these conditions, but may be as high as 60 to 70 percent. All neuromuscular curves have a propensity, once progression ensues, for rapid collapse of the spine into a severe curve. Because of the respiratory difficulty associated with many of these conditions, it is imperative to screen patients carefully for scoliosis, to monitor them closely for progression, and to institute early treatment when indicated.

Brace treatment with a well-molded, total contact TLSO is instituted for curves measuring beyond 30 degrees in the growing patient. Progression despite adequate bracing, resulting in progressive loss of function, is believed in most cases to be an indication for surgery in this patient population. In these patients surgical treatment is fraught with a high rate of complications, including instrumentation failure secondary to osteoporosis, as well as increased rates of infection and postoperative respiratory failure.

KYPHOSIS

Kyphosis refers to forward curvature, or rounding, of the spine when viewed from the side. Kyphosis is normal in the thoracic spine, with a range of thoracic kyphosis from 20 to 45 degrees in children and adolescents. Excessive kyphosis, as measured on a standing lateral radiograph exceeding 45 to 50 degrees, has several possible etiologies.

The child or adolescent presenting with hyperkyphosis of the thoracic spine is frequently accompanied by a parent giving a long history of "poor posture." While postural kyphosis is not uncommon, other causes of the deformity should be considered. The most prominent among these is juvenile kyphosis, known as "Scheuermann's disease." Although the etiology of Scheuermann's disease remains unknown, several theories have been proposed, including avascular necrosis of the cartilaginous ring apophysis of the vertebral body, the presence of Schmorl's nodes (herniation of intervertebral disc material through the end plate), endocrine or nutritional abnormalities, and metabolic bone disease. Congenital kyphosis is a rare condition that must be ruled out, due to the possibility of severe progression and subsequent neurologic abnormality. As in congenital scoliosis, congenital kyphosis can result from failure of formation or failure of segmentation. In contrast to congenital scoliosis, however, congenital kyphosis secondary to failure of formation (congenital hemivertebrae) is the more malignant type, with an exceedingly high rate of progression. Congenital kyphosis in association with a hemivertebrae has the highest rate of neurologic involvement of any of the spinal deformities. Tuberculosis should also be considered in the child or adolescent with excessive kyphosis, particularly if there is a history of travel outside the United States or a positive family history.

Scheuermann's kyphosis is the most common form of nonpostural kyphosis. The criteria for diagnosis in the thoracic spine include excessive thoracic kyphosis with associated radiographic abnormalities. The characteristic radiographic findings of Scheuermann's disease include vertebral wedging of greater than five degrees at three consecutive vertebrae, endplate irregularity, and the presence of Schmorl's nodes (Fig. 6–58).

The reported prevalence of this disorder varies among authors but is approximately one percent. The female to male ratio varies from 1.4:1 to 2:1. Although the postural abnormality may be identified earlier, radiographic changes are usually not seen until 11 to 12 years of age.

Most cases of excessive thoracic kyphosis represent primarily cosmetic abnormalities. Mild postural kyphosis will frequently resolve spontaneously, or following a thoracic extension exercise program. The natural history of Scheuermann's disease has only recently been elucidated. Most patients with Scheuermann's kyphosis lead normal lives, with no functional limitations and an incidence of back pain that is not increased over the normal population. There is some evidence, however, that adults with kyphosis in excess of 65 to 70 degrees may have an increased incidence of thoracic back pain and some functional limitations. Neurologic complications secondary to Scheuermann's disease are rare but have been reported. There is no convinc-

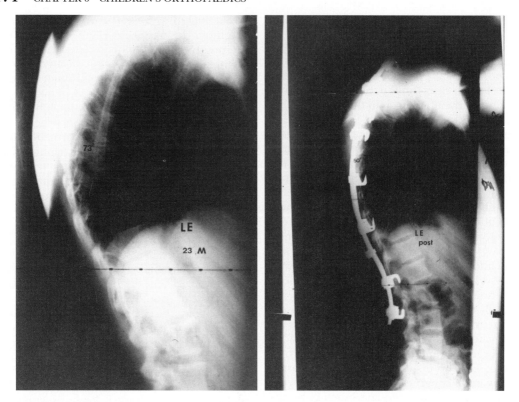

FIGURE 6–58 ■ A 23 year-old young man with persistent thoracic back pain secondary to Scheuermann's kyphosis. Because of failure to improve after a 1 year course of exercises and NSAIDs, he underwent a posterior fusion with segmental instrumentation and bone grafting, which resulted in excellent pain relief.

ing evidence that cardiopulmonary dysfunction is a complication of this condition.

Management of the patient with hyperkyphosis begins with a thorough physical examination. The increase in normal thoracic kyphosis is best appreciated when viewed from the side and frequently coexists with increased lumbar lordosis. Differentiation between Scheuermann's disease and postural kyphosis is facilitated by viewing the patient, in the forward flexed position, from the side. Patients with postural kyphosis have a smooth, round curve, which reverses on voluntary extension. The typical deformity in Scheuermann's kyphosis involves a sharp, angular gibbus that does not correct on extension of the spine. A minimal scoliosis of the spine may also be noticed on forward bending and is a common finding in patients with juvenile kyphosis. A thorough neurologic examination is mandatory to rule out spastic paraparesis, which would suggest other possible diagnoses, including congenital kyphosis, intraspinal

anomaly, or thoracic disc herniation. Standing PA and lateral radiographs of the entire spine are obtained. Kyphosis is measured using the Cobb technique and the lateral x-ray is scrutinized for the characteristic findings of Scheuermann's disease, as described above. A mild scoliosis is frequently observed. In addition, it is important to check for the presence of lumbosacral spondylolisthesis, which has been reported to be increased in prevalence in patients with Scheuermann's kyphosis.

Patients with hyperkyphosis can be treated with observation, bracing, or surgery. Observation, frequently accompanied by a program of thoracic extension exercises, is utilized in patients with postural kyphosis or without evidence of clear-cut progression in cases of Scheuermann's disease. Bracing is indicated for patients with structural kyphosis who have clear-cut evidence of progression of the curve and have at least 18 months of growth remaining. Because underarm orthoses are ineffective in this condition, Milwaukee brace treatment is required in most cases. Unlike scoliosis, Scheuermann's kyphosis responds in many cases with long-lasting curve improvement, following successful brace treatment. It should be noted, however, that patients with large curves, in excess of 70 to 75 degrees, frequently lose correction following cessation of bracing.

Because of the usually benign natural history of Scheuermann's kyphosis, surgery is rarely indicated. Bracing should be attempted in most patients with adequate growth remaining, since long-lasting curve improvement may result. Surgery is usually reserved for individuals who do not respond to brace treatment, who have curve progression in the brace, or who have severe curves, usually in excess of 80 to 90 degrees, which are not likely to respond to bracing and represent a significant functional and cosmetic deformity. Surgery is also undertaken, on occasion, in adults with fixed thoracic back pain that does not respond to a nonoperative program of exercise and nonsteroidal anti-inflammatory medication. These individuals usually have curves in excess of 65 to 70 degrees.

Surgery for the patient with Scheuermann's kyphosis consists of a spinal fusion with instrumentation. The fusion extends from just above to just below the area of kyphosis, typically over 10 to 12 levels. Flexible curves, which can be reversed to 55 degrees or less on hyperextension, are treated with a posterior spinal fusion with compression instrumentation. More severe curves are treated with anterior discectomies and release of the hypertrophied anterior longitudinal ligament, followed by posterior fusion with instrumentation. Surgery typically results in excellent curve correction, ranging from 30 to 50 percent in most series of combined anterior and posterior surgery. Cosmetic improvement is significant, but when surgery is undertaken for pain relief, the results are uncertain. Complications of surgery include infection, implant failure, and neurologic injury. Junctional kyphosis, the development of kyphosis above or below the end of the fusion, may be seen as well. It should be stressed that the surgical treatment of Scheuermann's kyphosis is rarely employed, and the surgeon, the patient, and the patient's parents need to view the natural history of this disorder in the context of the magnitude of surgery required, usually including a combined anterior and posterior approach.

SPONDYLOLISTHESIS

"Spondylolisthesis" refers to the forward slippage of one vertebra on that below it. First described by Herbiniaux, a Belgian obstetrician, this condition has been extensively studied and reported. Spondylolisthesis is most common in the lower lumbar spine, particularly at L5/S1, and is a common cause of back pain in children and adolescents (Fig. 6–59).

Spondylolisthesis has been classified by Newman (See Table 6–3). The most common types are type II, isthmic, and type III, degenerative. Degenerative spondylolisthesis occurs in middle-aged and older adults as a result of degenerative changes in the discs and facet joints allowing subluxation. It most commonly occurs at L4-L5 and may be associated with spinal stenosis. The most common type of spondylolisthesis is type II or isthmic spondylolisthesis. This is caused by a defect in the pars interarticular at L5, resulting in slippage at L5/S1. The pars defect, referred to as spondylolysis, is believed to be a stress fracture and occurs in most affected individuals when they

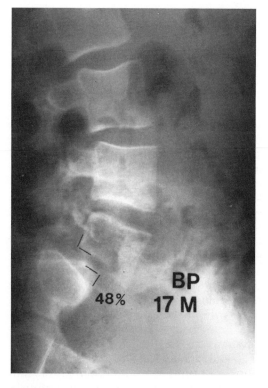

FIGURE 6–59 ■ A 17 year-old boy with a 48% (Grade II) isthmic L5-S1 spondylolisthesis.

TABLE 6–3 ■ *Classification of Spondylolisthesis*

Type I:	Dysplastic—congenital dysplasia of the S1 superior articular facet, or L5 inferior facet.
Type II:	Isthmic—a defect in the pars interticularis a. stressor fatigue fracture b. elongated but intact pars c. acute traumatic pars fracture
Type III:	Degenerative—degenerative changes in the disc and facet joints allowing subluxation
Type IV:	Traumatic—acute fracture, other than in the pars (e.g. facet, pedicle, etc.), allowing anterolisthesis.
Type V:	Pathologic—attenuation of the posterior elements, with subluxation, secondary to abnormal bone quality (e.g. osteogenesis imperfecta, neurofibromatosis, etc.).
Type VI:	Postsurgical—anterolisthesis that occurs or worsens following compressive laminectomy.

are between the ages of 4 and 7. Spondylolysis is present in 5 to 6 percent of the adult population; 75 to 80 percent of these individuals also demonstrate spondylolisthesis. Spondylolisthesis is twice as common in males as in females and is more common in whites than in blacks.

In children and adolescents, spondylolysis or spondylolisthesis may present as back pain, frequently associated with hamstring spasm. Other, less common causes of back pain in the pediatric population include disc space infection, benign tumors such as osteoid osteoma, or lumbar disc herniation. Isthmic spondylolisthesis can also be a cause of back pain in the adult. Patients with isthmic spondylolisthesis are reported to have an increased prevalence of disc degeneration, back pain, and sciatica, with the onset of symptoms occurring anywhere during adulthood. Because back pain is such a ubiquitous complaint, the relationship between a patient's complaint of back or leg pain and the presence of spondylolisthesis is often difficult to determine.

Evaluation of the patient with spondylolisthesis begins with a thorough history and physical. In the adult, a history of back pain during adolescence may be helpful. While acute pars fractures are seen, there is not usually a distinct history of trauma. The patient

typically presents with low back pain, which radiates into the buttock and, on occasion, down the leg in a dermatomal distribution. Physical examination may demonstrate tenderness in the area of the L5/S1 facet joints. Often a characteristic, painful, "catch" in extension is elicited. The most telltale sign in the adolescent is hamstring spasm, which can be quite severe. In patients with a high-grade slip, flattening of the buttocks and a transverse abdominal crease may be seen. Neurologic findings are rare, although in more advanced cases L5 findings are seen.

Plain radiographs should be obtained in the standing position. Most pars defects are visible on the lateral radiograph. If the diagnosis is uncertain, oblique views increase the sensitivity of plain radiography. The posterior arch has been described as a "Scotty dog" on the oblique view, and a pars defect appears as a "collar" on the neck of the Scotty dog (Fig. 6–60). Radionuclide bone scanning or fine cut CT scanning may be used to diagnose occult defects in the pars interarticular, and MR scan-

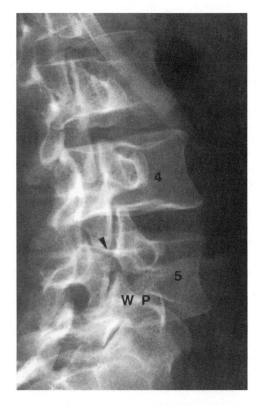

FIGURE 6–60 ■ A pars defect (spondylolysis) at L4, seen on this oblique radiograph as a "collar" on the neck of the "Scotty-dog."

ning is useful to identify nerve root compression in the L5/S1 foramen in patients with significant leg pain.

The treatment of patients with spondylolysis or spondylolisthesis depends on the degree of slippage, as well as the patient's symptoms. The percent slip ranges from zero to 100% and has been broken down as Grades I (0% to 25%), II (25% to 50%), III (50% to 75%), and IV (75% to 100%). It is not uncommon for pediatric patients to be diagnosed with spondylolisthesis following an episode of minor trauma and then to become asymptomatic. In these patients, activity guidelines are based on the degree of slippage. In patients with spondylolysis alone, or with a Grade I slip, full activity is allowed with annual radiographic follow-up. Skeletally immature individuals with Grade II spondylolisthesis, but who are asymptomatic, are advised to avoid contact sports or repetitive hyperextension activities such as are seen in gymnastics. Operative treatment is usually recommended for skeletally immature patients with progressive slippage or with Grades III or IV spondylolisthesis.

Symptomatic patients are initially treated with activity modification and nonsteroidal anti-inflammatory medication. Since many of these patients are athletes, temporarily holding them out of their sport will frequently result in improvement in symptoms. The patient is then begun on a program of Williams' flexion exercises and gradually increased activity. Persistent symptoms sometimes respond to bracing, and treatment with a brace or cast is advocated by some when an acute pars fracture is suspected. The majority of patients, both pediatric and adult, respond quite well to nonoperative treatment, although a return to high-level competitive sports is sometimes impossible.

Operative treatment is recommended for patients with progressive spondylolisthesis, for skeletally immature patients with spondylolisthesis exceeding 50 percent, and for patients with persistent, incapacitating pain. The overwhelming majority of surgical candidates fall into the last category. The hallmark of the surgical treatment of spondylolisthesis is spinal fusion. Inter-transverse fusion between the transverse processes of L5 and the sacral alae, utilizing iliac crest bone graft, has a high rate of success with a low complication rate. In adult patients with significant buttock and leg pain, or in individuals with neurologic deficits secondary to root compression, removal of the loose posterior arch of L5 and decompression of the exiting L5 nerve roots is recommended. Fusion is routinely performed in addition to decompression in these cases. Some authors recommend pedicle screw instrumentation as an adjunct to spinal fusion in patients with higher grades of spondylolisthesis (greater than 25%) or with documented instability. Finally, operative reduction of the spondylolisthesis is advocated by some in cases of severe spondylolisthesis, usually exceeding 75 percent slippage, with a concomitant cosmetic deformity. The results of surgery are usually quite rewarding, particularly in the pediatric population. Complications of surgery include failure of fusion, progressive slippage, persistent or recurrent pain, and neurologic injury. Complication rates are higher in adults, in higher grades of spondylolisthesis, and when reduction is attempted.

SUGGESTED READINGS

MacEwen GD: Pediatric Fractures. Malvern, PA, Williams & Wilkins, 1993.

Staheli L: Fundamentals of Pediatric Orthopaedics. New York, Raven Press, 1992.

Wenger D, Rang M: Art and Practice of Children's Orthopaedics. New York, Raven Press, 1993.

Chapter 7

SPORTS MEDICINE

Benjamin S. Shaffer

INTRODUCTION

The history of sports medicine is as old as human language itself, with the Smith Papyrus, the world's oldest written record, documenting instability of the shoulder as early as 2500 BC. But the development of sports medicine into a subspecialty awaited the late 20th century. Interest and participation in fitness has led to an exponential increase in the number of individuals actively engaged in athletic endeavors at both recreational and competitive levels. Breakthrough medical applications including magnetic resonance imaging (MRI) and arthroscopy have revolutionized our ability to visualize, understand, and reconstruct injured joints.

Unprecedented financial compensation of elite athletes has created demands for developing prevention strategies, improved evaluation methods, and definitive treatment techniques for sports injuries. A number of skilled and trained physicians and other health professionals have developed specific interests in the care of athletes. The goal of sports medicine as a specialty is the prevention of injury, diagnosis and treatment of athletic injury, and returning patients to pre-injury activity, with little or no risk of re-injury. The purpose of this chapter is to present an overview of evaluation and management considerations in sports medicine.

EVALUATION OF COMMON SPORTS MEDICINE PROBLEMS

The principles of evaluation include a thorough history and physical exam, supplemented by appropriate radiographic evaluation when necessary. Prompt "on-the-field" evaluation allows examination of the injured area prior to the onset of joint and soft-tissue swelling, muscle spasm, and reflex guarding. Such sideline evaluation is part of the reason for game and event coverage by team physicians. Delay by even a few hours may preclude early diagnosis, necessitating either more sophisticated diagnostic tests or an otherwise unnecessary delay in definitively establishing a diagnosis and initiating treatment while awaiting resolution of pain and swelling.

History

The history in many sports injuries is straightforward and related to acute trauma. Examples include twisting the ankle when coming down from a rebound, feeling the shoulder "go out" during an overhand throw, or hearing a "pop" after twisting their knee when cutting cross-field. Even when the complaint and offered history seem obvious, however, the clinician should ask about other symptoms, because one may not initially consider the possibility of injury to associated structures (e.g., the axillary nerve may be stretched during an anterior shoulder dislocation). Sometimes, input from players, trainers, coaches, or a review of the actual game film may help determine the mechanism of injury.

Determine if this problem has ever occurred before, and if so, how it happened, what type of treatment was rendered, and what the outcome was up until this re-injury. Previous problems may alert the clinician to the need for a different treatment approach (e.g., treatment of first-time versus recurrent shoulder dislocation).

Some sports medicine problems are unrelated to a specific "event." Rather than a history of injury, the patient reports the gradual onset of pain, stiffness, weakness, giving way, or instability. Problems related to so-called "microtrauma," also known as "overuse" injuries, are common, particularly in un- or inadequately conditioned athletes (e.g., weekend warriors), whose athletic demands outstrip their bodies' structural capability.

For example, shin splints are very common amongst runners, and often are insidious in onset. Determine if there has been a recent change in weekly mileage, shoe wear, or training conditions (track to road, flat surface to uneven terrain). By determining *when* during the course of a throw or swim stroke an athlete experiences symptoms, the examiner may be able to identify the cause of symptoms.

Symptoms that occur with activity and improve with rest are typical of overuse injuries. Nocturnal awakening usually indicates more serious injury or an underlying systemic disorder. Are there specific activities that cause symptoms? In the athlete with intermittent knee symptoms, pain in the front of the knee that is worse with stair-climbing or with prolonged sitting suggests problems of the patellofemoral joint. Symptoms that occur predictably only with pivoting and cutting activities, accompanied by swelling and giving way, suggest an internal derangement such as a meniscus or anterior cruciate ligament (ACL) tear. Are there any associated symptoms, such as upper extremity numbness (common with shoulder instability episodes) or lower extremity giving way (common with patellofemoral pain and ACL instability)?

Has the condition been previously treated, or have the athletes taken any medication or modified their activity in a way that has influenced their symptoms? In athletes whose previous symptoms have recurred or persist

despite seemingly "adequate" nonoperative treatment, it is important to elicit the details of such previous treatment. Did they truly rest? How did they modify their activities during this time? What specific exercises did they do and how frequently? Have they been on an anti-inflammatory medication, and if so, was it effective?

Physical Examination

The specific examination depends on the nature of the symptoms and the region affected. Each anatomic region and orthopaedic condition has pertinent special tests.

Observe the joint or area of interest under dynamic conditions. For example, inspection of the gait of runners with shin splints may reveal that their feet over-pronate (become exaggeratedly flat-footed) during walking. In an athlete whose shoulder is injured, observing elevation of the shoulder for either pain or abnormal scapulohumeral rhythm is helpful.

Static inspection is, of course, important. In addition to skin changes such as ecchymosis, abrasions, and swelling, look for evidence of asymmetry with respect to the opposite extremity, such as the prominent distal clavicle and drooped shoulder girdle of the acromioclavicular (AC) joint-injured patient (Fig. 7-1).

After palpation of the soft and skeletal tissues for tenderness, palpate for tissue integrity, examining for evidence of any defects in underlying fascia, muscle, tendon, or bone.

Evaluate joint motion both actively and passively. First have patients move their joints and observe for evidence of pain or asymmetry. Inability to actively extend the knee or lift it off the examining table may suggest quadriceps or patellar tendon rupture. Failure to completely straighten the knee may occur acutely due to either swelling or a mechanical block (most commonly, a torn meniscus interposed within the joint). Restricted subtalar motion (limited motion when trying to invert and evert the hindfoot) is common in adolescents with foot or heel pain, in whom abnormal persistent tarsal coalition may exist.

Ligament assessment is dependent on applying a force to a joint and determining the amount that joint "opens up" in comparison to the opposite normal joint. Because of variability in the populations' laxity, distinguishing normal excessive *laxity* from abnor-

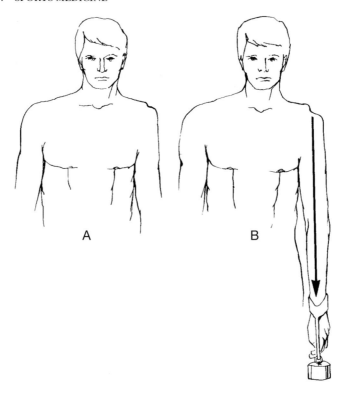

FIGURE 7–1. ■ *A,* Note the slight deformity at the acromioclavicular (AC) joint of this patient's left shoulder, sustained from landing directly on the point of the shoulder. *B,* Note that with the application of weights to the patient's wrists, the slight deformity is exaggerated, and the AC joint displacement is easily seen. This is known as a stress view of a "separated shoulder."
(From Rockwood CA, Green DP (eds). Fractures, ed 2, Vol 3. Philadelphia, JP Lippincott, 1984, reprinted by permission.)

mal *instability* is at times challenging. For ligaments that are subcutaneous, palpation for tenderness and actual ligament integrity is possible (for example, in the medial collateral ligament of the elbow and the lateral collateral ligament of the knee).

Most ligaments however, are not subcutaneous and therefore not palpable. For example, the ACL of the knee is intra-articular, and its integrity can only be assessed by examining the joint for abnormal laxity (the Lachman exam). In general, when joint motion or translation reproduces the patient's symptoms, causes displacement to a degree or amount greater than that of the opposite side, or both, ligament injury is likely.

During strength assessment, weakness may be due to pain, guarding, or reflex inhibition of muscular contraction. Although relatively uncommon, injuries to nerve and vascu-

lar structures can and do occur. Palpation of pulses is always performed, particularly following traumatic injury.

Physical examination is completed by applying special examination techniques specific to the area and suspected diagnosis. Examples of special tests include impingement signs in cases of shoulder pain, the apprehension signs for recurrent patellar, or shoulder instability (Fig. 7–2), or the Tinels' sign for entrapment neuropathies.

X-rays

X-rays are mandatory in the athlete with a history of trauma. As a general rule, overuse conditions, such as lateral epicondylitis (tennis elbow), iliotibial band friction syndrome (runners' knee), and posterior tibial tendinitis (shin splints) rarely demonstrate X-ray findings.

Stress Views

Specially obtained stress X-rays are occasionally useful in assessing joint integrity. Common examples include stress views taken for Grade III sprains of the AC joint, the medial collateral ligament (MCL) of the elbow, and the anterior talofibular ligament (ATFL) of the ankle.

Bone Scan

Bone scans generate images based on dynamic physiology rather than static structure. Increased tracer uptake can occur due to a number of conditions and is not pathognomonic of any one specific entity. Interpretation should be carried out in the context of the patient's history, physical, and X-ray findings. For example, in the runner with progressively increasing leg pain, in whom bone scan shows focal uptake in the mid-tibia, a stress fracture is overwhelmingly likely (Fig. 7–3).

Magnetic Resonance Imaging

Revolutionizing our ability to visualize soft tissues and establish diagnoses noninvasively, MRI is a remarkable investigative and diagnostic tool. In addition to demonstrating precise anatomic detail, MRI gives us a physiologic window with which to see various inflammatory, metabolic, and traumatic conditions. Variation in software allows the radiologist and clinician to distinguish scar from conventional soft tissue, identify effusions (fluid in joints), and confirm ligament injury and tendon avulsion (Fig. 7–4). Newer techniques even permit assessment of the articular cartilage covering the joint's subchondral surfaces. Unfortunately, MRI is very expensive, and in the current climate of cost-effective resource allocation, must be used judiciously.

Electrodiagnostic Tests

In patients with atypical pain or neurologic complaints, evaluation of their neurologic function is carried out via electromyography and nerve conduction velocity tests. Through

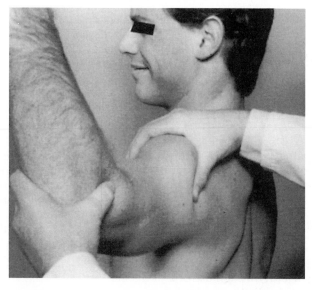

FIGURE 7–2. ■ Examining for anterior instability, the apprehension test is performed by placing the shoulder in a provocative position of abduction and external rotation. Gentle anterior pressure is placed on the humeral head in this position, seeking to elicit patient apprehension as an indication of shoulder instability.

(From Clinical Evaluation of Shoulder Problems, Rockwood CA, Matsen (eds): The Shoulder, Vol 1, p. 170.)

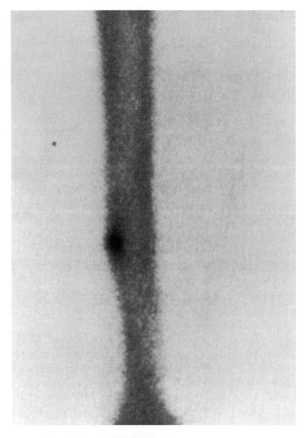

FIGURE 7–3. ■ Bone scan of the tibia in a runner with leg pain reveals focal uptake at the junction of the mid and distal third tibia, consistent with a stress fracture.
From DeLee JC, Drez Jr D (eds): Orthopaedic Sports Medicine: Principles and Practice, vol 2. Philadelphia, WB Saunders Company, 1994, p 1011; reprinted by permission.)

analysis of the exact pattern of electrical activity and nerve speed, inference regarding etiology and site of nerve involvement is possible.

Arthroscopy

Arthroscopy literally derives from *oscopy* (visualization) of *arthros* (joints) and refers to the technique of imaging a joint through use of a camera. Most commonly applied to the knee, shoulder, ankle, and elbow, arthroscopy is the gold-standard diagnostic tool for evaluation of joint problems and injuries. In addition to avoiding the complications of open joint surgery (arthrotomy), arthroscopy actually provides visualization that is superior to conventional open techniques (Fig. 7–5). This is because of the magnification afforded by the

optics and because the joint is evaluated in situ. Normal anatomic relationships are appreciated rather than severed or sacrificed. Despite its substantial uses and benefits, however, arthroscopy is an invasive technique and is a surgical resource. It should only be indicated for diagnostic purposes when other evaluative methods have not successfully afforded the diagnosis.

PATTERNS OF SPORTS MEDICINE INJURIES

Sports medicine injuries can be divided into two patterns—*macrotrauma* and *microtrauma*. In contact and collision sports such as football, rugby, hockey, and downhill skiing, macrotrauma from a specific discrete traumatic event is common. Conversely, in noncontact, endurance sports such as running, cycling, swimming, and throwing, microtrauma, or *overuse* is the most common cause of injury. Microtraumatic injury occurs due to repetitive stresses leading to structural breakdown. Overuse injuries occur when physical stresses temporarily exceed the body's reparative potential.

Macrotrauma

Ligaments

Discrete traumatic events from direct collision, contact, or from sudden and abrupt stopping or deceleration, can affect a number of different structures. When applied to the skeleton, trauma can cause a bone bruise or fracture. When the stress is applied to a ligament (the organized discrete fibrous structures connecting one bone to another), a *sprain* occurs, whose severity (grades I-III) depends on the amount of stress applied.

In a grade I sprain, some ligament fibers are torn on a microscopic level, accompanied by hemorrhage and edema, but overall there is normal structural integrity. A grade I sprain of the ATFL (anterior talofibular ligament) of the ankle (lateral ankle sprain) is one of the most common sprains encountered.

In a grade II sprain, some of the fibers are macroscopically disrupted, with a stretching out of the remaining ligament. Applying a valgus stress to the grade II MCL sprain of the

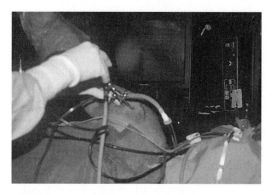

FIGURE 7–5. ■ In this photograph, an arthroscope is being used to examine the left shoulder. The patient is lying on his right side, with the camera inserted into the traditional posterior shoulder portal. Note the television screen in the foreground upon which the image of the shoulder joint is projected for viewing.

knee, for example, will slightly "open up" the joint. Some of the ligament, however, remains intact.

In a grade III sprain, the ligament structure fails, usually in its midportion. On examination of a grade III MCL, for example, results in the medial aspect of the joint "opening up" which when compared to the normally tight end point of the opposite knee MCL, is especially obvious. Grade III sprains are relatively common, and are seen in the ACL of the knee, the ATFL of the ankle, the anterior capsule of the shoulder, and the MCL of the elbow.

Complete ligament tears may render the joints which they normally protect unstable. Despite this, even severe sprains sometimes have excellent healing potential, such as in the MCL of the knee or the ATFL of the ankle. Other ligaments heal much less successfully, with a high likelihood of progressing to joint instability patterns. Common examples would be the anterior shoulder capsule and the ACL of the knee. Instability can occur with either *subluxation* or *dislocation*. In a subluxation, there is partial separation of the normal articular surfaces. Usually the joint returns to its normal position spontaneously. In a dislocation, the articular surfaces are completely displaced from one another and reduction is often necessary.

Muscle Tendons

Muscles and/or their tendinous insertions can be injured by either direct (blunt or sharp force causing bruise, contusion or laceration).

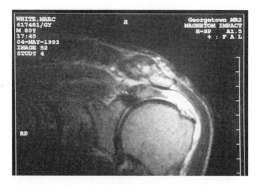

FIGURE 7–4. ■ An MRI scan taken of the left shoulder of this 46-year-old man with persistent shoulder pain demonstrated a full thickness rotator cuff tear. Note the presence of fluid (white signal) in the space normally occupied by the retracted cuff.

The more common type of muscle injury is indirect, known as a *strain,* and results when the stress generated from contraction exceeds the strength of the muscle. Seen most commonly in the hamstrings and achilles, strains are classifiable into three grades. In a grade I, there is some microscopic injury but no loss in overall continuity. There may be pain and local tenderness but no actual palpable defect in the muscle belly and little in the way of weakness. A grade II injury is more severe, with compromise of some fibers, but overall continuity remains. In a grade III strain, there is complete disruption of the muscle, which usually occurs at the musculo-tendinous junction (rather than within the muscle belly or at the tendinous attachment to bone). The athlete is unable to actively move the joint normally powered by the affected muscle. Complete tears of the gastrocnemius-achilles complex, the pectoralis major muscle, and the quadriceps muscle are examples seen clinically.

A relatively infrequent complication of direct trauma is that of *myositis ossificans.* A blow to the muscle (usually the quads) stimulates differentiation of normally reparative mesenchymal cells into osteoblasts, which generate bone. Normal bone formation in abnormal soft tissue area results and leads to a disquieting hard lump in the athlete's leg. Occasionally this same phenomenon can occur in the anterior soft tissues (brachialis) of the elbow following trauma.

Periarticular Structures

Trauma can impact any of the periarticular structures. Structures common to all joints include the articular cartilage, the synovial lining, and the surrounding neurovascular structures. Other structural injuries can only occur in the specific joint in which they exist, for example the meniscus of the knee and the labrum of the shoulder.

Cartilage

Cartilage injury occurs as a consequence of either excessive compression or shear stresses. Chondral injury can be in the form of softening, fibrillation, cracks and fissures, or actual detachment of fragments—with or without the underlying bone. Cartilage lesions are classified on the basis of appearance. In grade I chondral damage, there is softening of the normally firm and smooth articular surface. Grade II lesions demonstrate some surface roughening, appearing fibrillated and shaggy.

Grade III changes are deeper and often involve areas of cracks and/or fissures. In grade IV, subchondral bone is exposed, with full-thickness articular cartilage loss.

When an underlying fragment of bone is detached with a piece of cartilage, this is known as an osteochondral injury. Such injuries can occur in any joint, may become painful and loose, and are most commonly seen in the ankle and knee. In the knee, the load-bearing, shock-absorbing, crescent-shaped, fibrocartilaginous medial and lateral menisci are usually torn as a consequence of a twist or hyperflexion. In the shoulder, trauma may tear the labrum, a fibrous lip of tissue surrounding the bony glenoid.

Microtrauma (Overuse)

Responsible for perhaps the majority of sports-related injuries, overuse occurs whenever the degree of stress generated by the activity exceeds the body's ability to tolerate the stress. The breakdown that occurs most commonly affects the muscle-tendon units and the bones.

Overuse can occur in both the highly trained athlete and the poorly conditioned nonathlete. It most commonly occurs in the poorly conditioned recreational athlete who neglects warm-ups and stretching and then proceeds to do in 1 hour what he or she has not done for months. Repetitive stresses subject various structures to cyclic loading and eventually fatigue failure.

In bone, repetitive stresses can result in structural failure of the bone. An example is that of a *stress fracture* of the femur, tibia, fibula, or foot, seen commonly in distance runners. In the tendon, repetitive tensile stresses are thought to initiate a similar breakdown of tissue, which initiates the inflammatory cascade, causing local tissue edema and pain, referred to as "tendinitis." Such conditions are particularly common around the elbow (medial and lateral epicondylitis).

TREATMENT OF SPORTS INJURIES

Treatment of macrotraumatic and microtraumatic (overuse) injuries follows an algorithmic approach. The goals of treatment are to reduce pain, inflammation, swelling; prevent atrophy and stiffness; and return to normal function and activity. Treatment can be divided into three distinct but overlapping phases: immediate, early, and definitive.

Traumatic Sports Injuries

Immediate

Immediate treatment begins at the time of injury, and involves the mnemonic RICE (rest, ice, compression, and elevation). Rest means the cessation of activity that causes or exacerbates the symptoms and protects the extremity or joint from further injury. After an acute twisting injury to the knee, for example, the person may be unable to bear weight and should be placed on crutches. Ice is used immediately and applied directly to the affected area. Compression and elevation further decrease local tissue edema, swelling, and pain.

Early

Early treatment involves establishing a working diagnosis and minimizing the complications of trauma (joint stiffness and muscle atrophy). Muscular atrophy occurs rapidly in the absence of normal physiologic stress.

Definitive

Most traumatic sports injuries are successfully treated nonoperatively, with rehabilitation to restore motion and strength. Specific indications for operative management vary with the injury, its natural history, patient goals and activity level, and response to nonoperative treatment. Surgery may involve traditional open techniques or, more commonly, arthroscopic evaluation and repair or reconstruction.

Treatment of Microtraumatic (Overuse) Injuries

Immediate

Rest, in the treatment of overuse injury, does not necessarily require crutches, cast, or sling, but means activity modification. Any activities which cause the patient's symptoms should be avoided. This means no running for the track star with unrelenting shin splints, and no tennis for the player with recurrent tennis elbow. The tissues must be allowed to heal and resolve their inflammatory process. This is only achievable through a temporary interruption of the repetitive stress pattern.

Early

During the period of activity modification a number of techniques can be helpful to further relieve pain, inflammation, and to restore function. This can begin immediately with the use of nonsteroidal anti-inflammatory drugs (NSAIDs). Various *modalities* (local agents such as ice, heat, electrical stimulation, and massage) are often useful in decreasing pain, inflammation and swelling.

Definitive

Although rest in and of itself is sometimes the mainstay of treatment, symptoms frequently recur on resumption of activity. Definitive treatment, through rehabilitation in a physical therapy program, is usually required to prevent this inevitability.

The goal of rehabilitation is to restore normal function, including flexibility, motion, strength, conditioning and endurance. Supervised by a physical therapist or a trainer, specific phases of treatment include local modalities to the affected area, followed by passive (by the therapist/trainer) and active (by the patient) stretching and strengthening techniques. As symptoms resolve, surrounding, supporting muscles are strengthened and the mechanics of the sport are examined. Alignment problems are often identified in this phase, allowing fabrication of a shoe lift orthotic for previously unrecognized leg-length discrepancy or a medial arch support for over-pronation during gait. Sometimes videotape analysis of the activity or technique (by coaching staff) is helpful to identify, correct, and prevent poor mechanics.

Occasionally, despite rest, modalities, NSAIDs, and rehabilitation, symptoms persist. In these instances, injection of a corticosteroid preparation may be effective. Care is taken to avoid intra-tendinous injection because of potential weakening of the collagen and subsequent rupture. For this reason, cortisone is rarely, if ever, injected near the achilles or patellar tendons.

Occasionally, overuse injuries do not respond to nonoperative measures, and surgical intervention may be necessary. Some conditions seem to be more refractory to rehabilitation than others. Conditions that will occasionally lead to operative treatment include lateral epicondylitis and rotator cuff impingement (shoulder tendinitis). Rarely, stress fractures will fail to heal with rest or immobilization, and require fixation surgically.

CONCLUSION

As the numbers of active individuals continue to grow, so too does the demand for knowledgeable and skilled care of the recreational and elite level athlete. Focus on injury prevention, evaluation and treatment has become subspecialized into the specific field of sports medicine, whose goal is comprehensive care of the athlete, and prompt treatment for return to activity without risk of re-injury. The two most common mechanisms of injury involve acute trauma and overuse. In acute injury, treatment strategies include RICE, early exercises to avoid atrophy and stiffness, and definitive treatment through rehabilitation or occasionally, surgery. Overuse injuries occur due to repetitive stresses which outstrip the body's structural integrity, and are usually successfully treated with activity modification, identification and treatment of underlying malalignment, and return to activity.

SUGGESTED READINGS

DeLee JC, Drez Jr D (eds): Orthopaedic Sports Medicine: Principles and Practice. Philadelphia, WB Saunders Company, 1994.

Garrick JG, Webb DR: Sports Injuries: Diagnosis and Management. Philadelphia, WB Saunders Company, 1990.

Griffin LY (ed): Orthopaedic Knowledge Update: Sports Medicine. American Academy of Orthopaedic Surgeons. Philadelphia, WB Saunders Company, 1994.

Chapter 8

The Spine

Sam W. Wiesel and William C. Lauerman

A large proportion of the adult population is affected by disorders involving some area of the spine. Every physician should have a working knowledge of the potential pathology and be able to recognize a serious problem when it arises. Disastrous sequelae such as paralysis can occur if these conditions are overlooked. This chapter will first address the cervical spine and then present the lumbar spine. In each area the history, physical, and appropriate diagnostic studies will be reviewed. Next a standardized protocol or algorithm for the diagnosis and management of these patients will be described. Finally, several of the most common conservative treatment modalities will be presented, with special attention given to their efficacy.

CERVICAL SPINE

Neck pain is a very common problem that is familiar to most individuals. Pain can occur secondary to *spondylosis,* which is a term used to describe the sequence of degenerative changes in the cervical spine with increasing age or after trauma. The outcome of an injury is usually recovery; but poor results can occur, with paraplegia and/or death the most disastrous. Every clinician should be familiar with the signs and symptoms of the various diagnostic entities that occur in the cervical spine and be able to identify the serious problems that require immediate attention.

History

The main point to obtain from a patient's history is the location of the pain. The majority of patients complain of localized symptoms in the neck, with or without referral to pain between the scapulae or shoulders. The pain is described as vague, diffuse, axial, nondermatomal, and poorly localized. The pathogenesis of this type of complaint is attributed to structures innervated by the sinuvertebral nerve or the nerves innervating the paravertebral soft tissues, and it is generally a localized injury.

Another group of patients will complain of neck pain with the addition of arm involvement. This arm pain is secondary to nerve root irritation and is termed "radicular pain." The degree of nerve root involvement can vary from a monoradiculopathy to multiple levels of involvement. It is described as a deep aching, burning, or shooting arm pain, often with associated paresthesias. The pathogenesis of radicular pain can derive from soft tissue (herniated disc), bone (spondylosis), or a combination of the two.

Finally, a third group of patients will complain of symptoms secondary to cervical myelopathy, which is compression of the spinal cord and usually secondary to degenerative changes. The clinical complaints vary considerably. The onset of symptoms begins after 50 years of age, and males are more often affected. Onset is usually insidious, although there is occasionally a history of trauma. The natural history is that of initial neurologic deterioration followed by a plateau period lasting several months. The resulting clinical picture is often one of an incomplete spinal lesion with a patchy distribution of deficits. Disability varies with the number of vertebrae involved and with the degree of involvement at each level.

Common presenting symptoms of cervical myelopathy include numbness and paresthesias in the hands, clumsiness of the fingers, weakness (greatest in the lower extremities), and gait disturbances. Abnormalities of micturition are seen in about one third of cases and indicate more severe cord involvement. Symptoms of radiculopathy can coexist with myelopathy and confuse the clinical picture. Sensory disturbances may show a patchy distribution. Spinothalamic tract (pain and temperature) deficits may be seen in the upper extremities, the thorax, or the lumbar region and may be in a stocking or glove distribution. Posterior column deficits (vibration and proprioception) are more commonly seen in the feet than in the hands. Usually there is no gross sensory impairment but a diminished sense of appreciation of light touch and pinprick. A characteristic broad-based, shuffling gait may be seen, signaling the onset of functionally significant deterioration.

Physical Examination

The physical examination should begin with observation of the cervical spine and upper torso unencumbered by clothing. The physical findings are of two different types. One set can be categorized as nonspecific and found in most patients with neck pain, but will not help to localize the type or level of the pathological process. A decreased range of motion is the most frequent nonspecific finding. It can be secondary to pain or, structurally, to distorted bony and soft tissue elements in the cervical spine. Hyperextension and excessive lateral rotation, however, will usually cause pain— even in a normal individual.

Tenderness is another nonspecific finding that can be quite helpful. There are two types of tenderness that must be considered. One is diffuse, elicited by compression of the paravertebral muscles, and is found over a wide area of the posterolateral muscle masses. The second type of tenderness is more specific and may help localize the level of the

pathology. It can be localized by palpation over each intervertebral foramen and spinous process.

The next goal of the physical exam is to isolate the level or levels in the cervical spine responsible for the symptomatology. The exam is also important to rule out other sources of pain, which include compressive neuropathies, thoracic outlet syndrome, and chest or shoulder pathology.

The major focus of the exam is directed at finding a neurologic deficit (Table 8–1). A motor deficit (most commonly weak triceps, biceps, or deltoid) or diminished deep tendon reflex is the most likely objective finding in a patient with a radiculopathy. Although less reproducible, manual tests and maneuvers that increase or decrease radicular symptoms may be helpful. In the neck compression test, the patient's head is flexed laterally, slightly rotated toward the symptomatic side, and then compressed to elicit reproduction or aggravation of the radicular symptoms. The axial manual traction test is performed in the presence of radicular symptoms in the supine position. With 20 to 20 lbs. of axial traction, a positive test is the decrease or disappearance of radicular symptoms. All of these tests are highly specific (low false-positive rate) for the diagnosis of root compression, but the sensitivity (false-negative rate) is less than 50 percent.

Myelopathic physical findings should also be specifically checked. These patients can have a gait disturbance, so they should be observed walking. The extent of motor disability can vary from mild to severe. Pyramidal tract weakness and atrophy are more commonly seen in the lower extremities and are the most common abnormal signs. The usual clinical findings in the lower extremities are spasticity and weakness.

Weakness and wasting of the upper extremities and hands may also be due to combined spondylotic myelopathy and radiculopathy. In this situation the patient usually complains of hand clumsiness. A diminished or absent upper-extremity deep tendon reflex can indicate compressive radiculopathy superimposed on spondylotic myelopathy.

Sensory deficits in spinothalamic (pain and temperature) and posterior column (vibration and proprioception) function should be documented. Usually there is no gross impairment of sensation; rather, a patchy decrease in light touch and pinprick is seen. Hyperreflexia, clonus, and positive Babinski's

TABLE 8–1 ■ *Cervical Radiculopathy Symptoms and Findings*

Disc Level	Nerve Root	Symptoms and Findings
C2-3	C3	*Pain:* Back of neck, mastoid process, pinna of ear *Sensory Change:* Back of neck, mastoid process, pinna of ear *Motor Deficit:* None readily detectable except by EMG *Reflex Change:* None
C3-4	C4	*Pain:* Back of neck, levator scapula, anterior chest *Sensory Change:* Back of neck, levator scapulae, anterior chest *Motor Deficit:* None readily detectable except by EMG *Reflex Change:* None
C4-5	C5	*Pain:* Neck, tip of shoulder, anterior arm *Sensory Change:* Deltoid area *Motor Deficit:* Deltoid, biceps *Reflex Change:* Biceps
C5-6	C6	*Pain:* Neck, shoulder, medial border of scapula, lateral arm, dorsal forearm *Sensory Change:* Thumb and index finger *Motor Deficit:* Biceps *Reflex Change:* Biceps
C6-7	C7	*Pain:* Neck, shoulder, medial border of scapula, lateral arm, dorsal forearm *Sensory Change:* Index and middle fingers *Motor Deficit:* Triceps *Reflex Change:* Triceps
C7-T1	C8	*Pain:* Neck, medial border of scapula, medial aspect of arm and forearm *Sensory Change:* Ring and little fingers *Motor Deficit:* Intrinsic muscles of hand *Reflex Change:* None

From Boden S, Wiesel SW, Laws E, et al: The Aging Spine. Philadelphia, WB Saunders Company, 1991, p 46; reprinted by permission.

signs are seen in the lower extremities. Hoffman's sign and hyperreflexia may be observed in the upper extremities.

Diagnostic Studies

In evaluating any pathologic process one will usually have a choice of several diagnostic tests. The cervical spine is no exception. This section will deal with the most common ones that are routinely used. In general, all of these tests play a confirmatory role. In other words, the core of information derived from a thorough history and physical examination should be the basis for a diagnosis; the additional tests are obtained to confirm this clinical impression. Trouble develops when these tests are used for screening purposes since most of them are overly sensitive and relatively unselective. Thus, the studies discussed should never be interpreted in isolation from the overall clinical picture.

Plain Radiographs

Radiographic evaluation of the cervical spine is helpful in assessing patients with neck pain, and the routine study should include anteroposterior, lateral, oblique, and odontoid views. Flexion-extension x-rays are necessary in defining stability. The generally accepted radiographic signs of cervical disc disease are loss of height of the intervertebral disc space, osteophyte formation, secondary encroachment of the intervertebral foramina, and osteoarthritic changes in the apophyseal joints.

It should be stressed that the identification of "some pathology" on plain cervical x-rays does not, per se, indicate the cause of the patient's symptoms. In several series large numbers of asymptomatic patients have shown radiographic evidence of advanced degenerative disc disease. At approximately age 40 some disc degeneration (narrowing) can be expected, particularly at the C5-6 and C6-7 levels. This is considered to represent a normal aging process. The difficult problem with regard to radiographic interpretation is not in the identification of these changes but rather in determining how much significance should be attributed to them.

Radiographic abnormalities of alignment in the cervical spine may also be of clinical significance but they need to be correlated with the whole clinical picture; listhesis or slipping forward or backward (retrolisthesis) of one vertebra upon the vertebra below it is such a finding.

If "instability" is suspected, functional x-rays may be taken. These view the spine from the side, with the head flexed (bent forward) or extended (arched back); the spine normally flexes equally at each spinal level. If one vertebral level is "unstable," that particular vertebra moves more or less and disrupts the symmetry of motion. Again, this finding must be correlated with the whole clinical picture, as its mere presence may be asymptomatic.

Myelography

A myelogram is performed by injecting a water-soluble dye into the spinal sac so that the outline of the sac itself, as well as each nerve root sleeve, can be evaluated (Fig. 8–1). If there is pressure upon the nerve root or dural sac from either a bony spur or disc herniation it will be seen as a constriction on the x-ray picture.

Complications from myelography are rare, and it can be performed on an outpatient basis. The major disadvantages are its invasive nature, radiation exposure, and the lack of diagnostic specificity. Water-soluble myelography does provide excellent contrast for subsequent examination by computerized tomography (CT).

The myelogram should be used as a confirmatory test to substantiate a clinical impression. It should not be used as a screening test since there are many false-positive as well as false-negative results. This means that some normal people will have abnormal myelographic findings, whereas other abnormal people will be found to have normal myelograms.

Computerized Tomography

Computerized tomography permits one to create cross-sectional imaging of the cervical spine at any desired level. It is currently used after the instillation of water-soluble dye, which is termed a "CT-myelogram." The advantages of CT-myelography include excellent differentiation of bone and soft tissue (disc or ligament) lesions, direct demonstration of spinal cord and spinal cord dimensions, assessment of foraminal encroachment, and visualization of regions distal to a myelographic blockade.

Unfortunately, when combined with myelography, it becomes an invasive procedure and involves radiation exposure. It does, however, provide very good information and is especially useful for patients who, for a variety of reasons, cannot undergo a magnetic resonance imaging (MRI) investigation.

Magnetic Resonance Imaging

The MRI technique provides an image on film that is obtained by measuring the differences in proton density between the various tissues evaluated. With the use of the computer, multiplanar images are obtainable. It is a safer test than either the CT scan or myelogram since it uses neither ionizing radiation nor invasive contrast agents.

The technical modifications of MRI are rapidly changing. The distinction between soft tissues and bone and the relationship of both to the neural foramen are clearer. Magnetic resonance imaging accurately detects rare conditions such as infection or tumor of the spine and can identify intrinsic abnormalities of the cord. An excellent test, MRI can be combined with plain films to permit an accurate noninvasive evaluation of cervical radiculopathy and myelopathy. It is currently the diagnostic test of choice in the cervical spine.

Electromyography

Electromyography (EMG) is an electric test that confirms the interaction of nerve to muscle. The test is performed by placing needles into muscles to determine if there is an intact nerve supply to that muscle. The EMG is particularly useful in localizing a specific abnormal nerve root. It should be appreciated that it takes at least 21 days for an EMG to show up as abnormal. After 21 days of pressure on a nerve root, signs of denervation with fibrillation can be observed. Before 21 days, the EMG will be negative in spite of nerve root damage. It should also be noted that there is no quantitative interpretation of this test. Thus, it cannot be said that the EMG is 25 or 75 percent normal.

The EMG is an electronic extension of the physical examination. Although it is 80 to

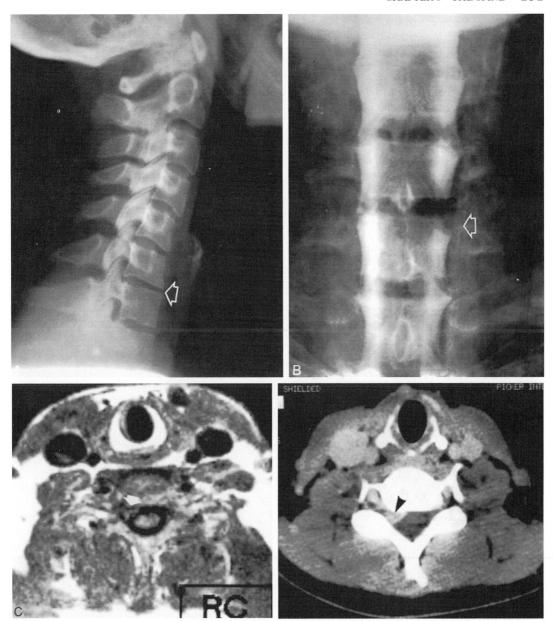

FIGURE 8–1 ■ This 33-year-old male presented with right triceps weakness, C7 radicular pain, and absent triceps reflex. *A,* Lateral radiograph of C6-7 shows loss of disc height *(arrow).* B, Anteroposterior myelogram confirms right C7 root sleeve cut-off. *C,* Axial magnetic resonance imaging *(left)* and computerized tomography *(right)* show occlusion of the right C6-7 foramen *(arrows).*

(From Boden S, Wiesel SW, Laws E, et al: The Aging Spine. Philadelphia, WB Saunders Company, 1991, p 58; reprinted by permission.)

90 percent accurate in establishing cervical radiculopathy as the cause of pain, false-negative results do occur. If cervical radiculopathy affects only the sensory root, the EMG will be unable to demonstrate an abnormality.

A false-negative examination can occur if the patient with acute symptoms is examined early (4 to 28 days from onset of symptoms). A negative study should be repeated in 2 to 3 weeks if symptoms persist. The accuracy of the

EMG increases if both the paraspinal and extremity muscles innervated by the suspected root demonstrate abnormalities.

The EMG is not part of the routine evaluation of the cervical spine. It is indicated to confirm a clinical impression or to rule out other sources of pathology such as peripheral neuropathies or compressive neuropathies in the upper extremities.

Clinical Conditions

There are many conditions that may present as neck pain, with or without arm pain, in any particular individual. However, there are several that are quite common and will be presented in detail.

Neck Sprain–Neckache

Neck sprain, while a misnomer, describes a clinical condition involving a non-radiating discomfort or pain about the neck area associated with a concomitant loss of neck motion (stiffness). While the clinical syndrome may present as a headache, most often the pain is located in the middle to lower part of the back of the neck. A history of injury is rarely obtained but the pain may start after a night's rest or on simply turning the head. The source of the pain is most commonly believed to be the ligaments about the cervical spine and/or the surrounding muscles. The axial pain may also be produced by small annular tears without disc herniation, or from the facet joints.

The pain associated with a neck sprain is most often a dull aching pain, which is exacerbated by neck motion. The pain is usually abated by rest or immobilization. The pain may be referred to other mesenchymal structures derived from a similar sclerotome during embryogenesis. Common referred pain patterns include the scapular area, the posterior shoulder, the occipital area, or the anterior chest wall (cervical angina pectoris). Those referred pain patterns do not connotate a true radicular pain pattern and are not usually mechanical in origin.

Physical examination of patients with neckache usually reveals nothing more than a locally tender area(s) usually just lateral to the spine. The intensity of the pain is variable and the loss of cervical motion correlates directly with the pain intensity. The presence of true spasm, defined as a continuous muscle contraction, is rare except in severe cases where the head may be tilted to one side (torticollis).

Since the radiograph in cervical sprain is usually normal, a plain x-ray is usually not warranted on the first visit. If the pain continues for more than 2 weeks or the patient develops other physical findings, then an x-ray should be taken to rule out other more serious causes of the neck pain such as neoplasia or instability. The prognosis for these individuals is excellent since the natural history is one of complete resolution of the symptoms over several weeks. The mainstay of therapy includes rest and immobilization, usually in a soft cervical orthosis. Although medications such as anti-inflammatory agents or muscle relaxants may aid in the acute management of pain, they do not seem to alter the natural history of the disorder.

Acute Herniated Disc

A herniated disc is defined as the protrusion of the nucleus pulposus through the fibers of the annulus fibrosus (Fig. 8–2). Most acute disc herniations occur posterolaterally and in patients around the fourth decade of life when the nucleus is still gelatinous. The most common areas of disc herniation are C5-6 and C6-7, whereas C7-T1 and C3-4 are infrequent. Disc herniation of C2-3 is very, very rare. Unlike the lumbar herniated disc, the cervical herniated disc may cause myelopathy in addition to radicular pain due to the presence of the spinal cord in the cervical region.

The disc herniation usually affects the root numbered lowest for the given disc level; for example, a C3-4 disc affects the C4 root, C4-5 the fifth cervical root, C5-6 the sixth cervical root, C6-7 the seventh nerve root, and C7-T1 the eighth cervical root. Unlike the lumbar region, the disc herniation does not involve other roots but more commonly presents some evidence of upper motor neuron findings secondary to spinal cord local pressure.

Not every herniated disc is symptomatic. The presence of symptoms depends on the spinal reserve capacity, the presence of inflammation, the size of the herniation, as well as the presence of concomitant disease such as osteophyte formation.

Clinically, the patient's major complaint is arm pain, not neck pain. The pain is often perceived as starting in the neck area but then radiates from this point down the shoulder, arm, forearm, and usually into the hand, commonly in a dermatomal distribution. The onset of the radicular pain is often gradual, although there can be a sudden onset associated with a tearing or snapping sensation. As time passes,

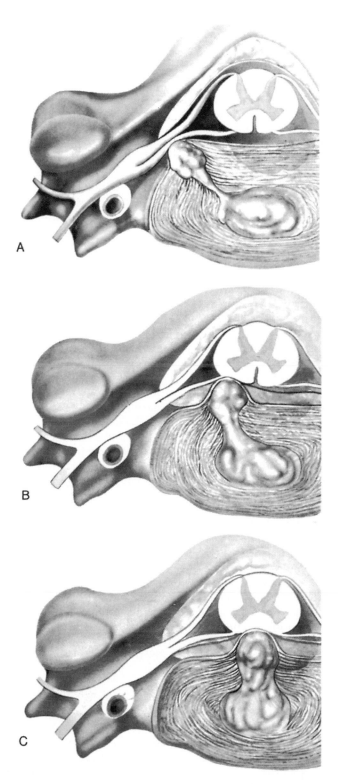

FIGURE 8–2 ■ Types of soft disc protrusion. *A,* Intra-foraminal, most common. *B,* Posterolateral, produces mostly motor signs. *C,* Midline, may manifest as myelopathy.

(Modified from DePalma AF, Rothman RH: The Intervertebral Disc. Philadelphia, WB Saunders Company, 1970, pp 102, 104; reprinted by permission.)

the magnitude of the arm pain will clearly exceed that of the neck or shoulder pain. The arm pain may vary in intensity from severe enough to preclude any use of the arm without severe pain to a dull cramping ache in the arm muscles with use of the arm. The pain is usually severe enough to awaken the patient at night.

Physical examination of the neck usually shows some limitation of motion and on occasion the patient may tilt the head in a "cocked robin" position (torticollis) toward the side of the herniated cervical disc. Extension of the spine will often exacerbate the pain since it further narrows the intervertebral foramina. Axial compression, Valsalva maneuver, and coughing may also exacerbate or re-create the pain pattern.

The presence of a positive neurologic finding is the most helpful aspect of the diagnostic workup, although the neurologic exam may remain normal despite a chronic radicular pattern. Even when a deficit exists it may not be temporally related to the present symptoms but to a prior attack at a different level. To be significant, the neurologic exam must show objective signs of reflex diminution, motor weakness, or atrophy. The presence of subjective sensory changes are often difficult to interpret and require a coherent and cooperative patient to be of clinical value. The presence of sensory changes alone are usually not enough to make the diagnosis firm.

Nerve root sensitivity can be elicited by any method which increases the tension of the nerve root. Radicular arm pain is often increased by the Valsalva maneuver or by directly compressing the head. While these signs are helpful when present, their absence alone does not rule out radicular pain.

The provisional diagnosis of a herniated disc is made by the history and physical examination. The plain x-ray is usually nondiagnostic, although occasionally disc-space narrowing at the suspected interspace or foraminal narrowing on the oblique films will be seen. The value of the films is largely to exclude other causes of neck and arm pain. Tests such as an EMG or MRI are confirmatory examinations and should not be used as screening tests since misinformation may ensue.

The treatment for most patients with a herniated disc is nonoperative since the majority of patients respond to conservative treatment over a period of months. The efficacy of the nonoperative approach depends heavily on the doctor-patient relationship. If a patient is well informed, insightful, and

willing to follow instructions, the chances for a successful nonoperative outcome are greatly improved.

The cornerstone to the management of a cervical herniated disc is rest and immobilization. The use of a cervical orthosis greatly increases the likelihood that the patient will rest. Patients should markedly decrease their physical activity for at least 2 weeks and wear the cervical orthosis at all times (especially at night). After the acute pain begins to abate, patients should gradually increase their activity and wean off the orthosis. Most persons will be able to return to work, or at least to light duty, in a month.

Drug therapy is an important adjunct to rest and immobilization. Anti-inflammatory medications, analgesics, and muscle relaxants have historically been used in the acute management of these patients. Since it is commonly believed that the radicular pain is in part inflammatory, the use of aspirin or other nonsteroidal, anti-inflammatory medications seems to be appropriate. All these medications have gastrointestinal side effects but are generally well tolerated for brief periods.

Analgesic medication is only rarely needed if the patient is compliant. However, if the pain is severe enough, a brief course of oral codeine may be prescribed. In-hospital intramuscular narcotic injections may be required on rare occasions. Muscle relaxants and the benzodiazepines are truly tranquilizers and central nervous system depressants. As such they have at best a limited role in the management of the acute herniated disc patient. While it is true that these medications help patients relax and get their needed rest, the potential for an addictive effect adding to any psychosocial problems patients may have is not, in the majority of patients, worth the long-term risk for the short-term gain.

Cervical Spondylosis

What was once commonly referred to as "cervical degenerative disc disease" more recently has been called "cervical spondylosis." Cervical spondylosis is a chronic process defined as the development of osteophytes and other stigmata of degenerative arthritis as a consequence of age-related disc disease. This process may produce a wide range of symptoms. However, it should be stressed that an individual may have significant spondylosis and be asymptomatic.

Cervical spondylosis is believed to be the

direct result of age-related changes in the intervertebral disc. These changes include desiccation of the nucleus pulposus, loss of annular elasticity, and narrowing of the disc space with or without disc protrusion or rupture. In turn, secondary changes include overriding of facets, increased motion of the spinal segments, osteophyte formation, inflammation of synovial joints, and even microfractures. These macro- and microscopic changes can result in various clinical syndromes (spondylosis, ankylosis, central or foraminal spinal stenosis, radiculopathy, myelopathy, or spinal segmental instability).

The typical patient with symptomatic cervical spondylosis is over the age of 40 and complaining of neckache. Not infrequently, however, these patients will have very few neck pain symptoms and will present with referred pain patterns: occipital headaches; pain in the shoulder, suboccipital, and intrascapular areas and the anterior chest wall; or other vague symptoms suggestive of anatomic disturbances (e.g., blurring of vision, tinnitus). In patients with predominantly referred pain, a past history for neck pain is usually obtained.

Physical examination of the patient with cervical spondylosis is often associated with a dearth of objective findings. The patient will usually have some limitation of neck motion associated with midline tenderness. Not infrequently, palpation of the referred pain areas will also produce local tenderness and should not be confused with local disease. The neurologic examination is normal.

Anteroposterior (AP), lateral, and oblique radiographs of the cervical spine in cervical spondylosis show varying degrees of changes. These include disc space narrowing, osteophytosis, foraminal narrowing, degenerative changes of the facets, and instability. As previously discussed, these findings do not necessarily correlate with symptoms. In large part, the radiograph serves to rule out other more serious causes of neck and referred pain such as tumors. Further diagnostic testing is usually not warranted.

Cervical spondylosis alone is treated by nonoperative measures. The mainstay of treatment for the acute pain superimposed on the chronic problem is rest and immobilization. In addition, oral anti-inflammatory medications like aspirin will be of benefit. Often these medications will need to be administered on a chronic basis or at least intermittently. Trigger-point injections with local anesthetics (lidocaine) and corticosteroids (triamcinolone) may be therapeutic as well as diagnostic. Once the pain abates, the immobilization (usually a soft cervical collar) should be discontinued and the patient maintained on a series of cervical isometric exercises. Further counseling with regard to sleeping position, automobile driving, and work is in order. Manipulation and traction are rarely needed and may, in fact, be deleterious to the patient.

Cervical Spondylosis With Myelopathy

When the secondary bony changes of cervical spondylosis encroach on the spinal cord, a pathologic process called "myelopathy" develops. If this involves both the spinal cord and nerve roots, it is called "myeloradiculopathy." Radiculopathy, regardless of its etiology, causes shoulder or arm pain.

Myelopathy is the most serious sequelae of cervical spondylosis and the most difficult to treat effectively. Less than 5 percent of patients with cervical spondylosis develop myelopathy, and they are usually between 40 to 60 years of age. The changes of myelopathy are most often gradual and associated with posterior osteophyte formation (called "spondylitic bone" or "hard disc") and spinal canal narrowing (spinal stenosis). Acute myelopathy is most often the result of a central soft disc herniation producing a high-grade block on myelography.

The characteristic stooped, wide-based, and somewhat jerky gait of the aged summarizes the chronic effects of cervical spondylosis with myelopathy. The spinal cord changes may develop from single or multiple-level disease and as such may not present in a singular or standard manner. A typical clinical presentation of chronic myelopathy begins with the gradual notice of a peculiar sensation in the hands, associated with clumsiness and weakness. The patient will also note lower-extremity symptoms that may antedate the upper extremity findings, including difficulty walking, peculiar sensations, leg weakness, hyperreflexia, spasticity, and clonus. The upper-extremity findings may start out unilaterally and include hyperreflexia, brisk Hoffmann's sign, and muscle atrophy (especially of the hand muscles). Neck pain per se is not a prominent feature of myelopathy. Sensory changes can evolve at these levels and are often a less reliable index of spinal cord disease. The protean nature of the signs and symptoms of cervical myelopathy, along with its potential for severe functional impairment, merit a high index of suspicion in patient evaluation.

Radiographs of the cervical spine in these patients will often reveal advanced degenerative disease including spinal canal narrowing by prominent posterior osteophytosis, variable foraminal narrowing, disc space narrowing, facet joint arthrosis, and instability. Congenital stenosis of the cervical canal is frequently seen, predisposing the patient to the development of myelopathy. The myelogram is diagnostic, exhibiting a washboard appearance to the dye column with multiple anterior and posterior defects. The posterior defects are secondary to facet arthrosis and buckling of the ligamentum flavum. The MRI is also quite striking and diagnostic.

In general, myelopathy is a surgical disease, but is not an absolute indication for surgical decompression. Conservative therapy consisting of immobilization and rest with a soft cervical orthosis offers the myelopathic patient, who is not a good operative risk, a viable option. The goals of surgery in the myelopathic patient are to decompress the spinal canal to prevent further spinal cord compression and vascular compromise. If the myelopathy is progressive despite a trial of conservative treatment, surgery is clearly indicated. These indications may vary slightly from surgeon to surgeon because of the lack of absolute or definitive clinical data.

Rheumatoid Arthritis

Rheumatoid arthritis affects 2 to 3 percent of the population. About 60 percent of patients with rheumatoid arthritis will exhibit signs and symptoms of cervical spine involvement, whereas up to 86 percent will have radiographic evidence of cervical disease. Cervical spine involvement, secondary to the erosive, inflammatory changes of rheumatoid arthritis (synovitis), is divided into three categories: (1) atlantoaxial instability, (2) basilar invagination, and (3) subaxial instability. Atlantoaxial instability is the most common and most serious of the instability patterns affecting 20 to 34 percent of hospitalized patients. The evaluation of a patient with rheumatoid arthritis is difficult due to the multiple system involvement. The physical examination should start with a careful neurologic evaluation to rule out upper motor neuron disease before moving to neck range of motion or other vigorous maneuvers that may harm the patient.

The patient with cervical spine involvement from rheumatoid arthritis most often has neck pain located in the middle posterior neck and occipital area. The range of motion is decreased, and crepitance or a feeling of instability may be noted. The neurologic changes can be variable and difficult to elicit in the context of diffuse rheumatoid changes. The evaluation of the patient with cervical rheumatoid arthritis begins with plain radiographs of the neck, which may reveal osteopenia, facet erosion, disc-space narrowing, and subluxation of the lower cervical spine (stepladder appearance). To determine that atlantoaxial disease is present, dynamic-flexion extension views of the lateral upper cervical spine are required.

Basilar invagination is defined as upper migration of the odontoid projecting into the foramen magnum. The addition of a CT scan with or without contrast material in the upper cervical spine can provide valuable information as to the relationship of the bony elements to the spinal cord. Subaxial subluxations are identified by dynamic flexion-extension films.

The majority of these patients, despite rather dramatic disease patterns can be successfully managed nonoperatively. While the natural history of rheumatoid arthritis predicts a high incidence of involvement of the cervical spine, it is estimated that only a few patients die from medullary compression associated with significant atlantoaxial disease and that, although atlantoaxial disease worsens with time, only 2 to 14 percent of patients exhibit neurologic progression.

The mainstay in nonoperative therapy is the cervical orthosis (Philadelphia collar). Although this does not fully immobilize the atlantoaxial interval, it does produce symptomatic relief. Some authors have advocated intermittent home traction, but it must be used only with great caution under a physician's direction. Medications have a definite role in the nonoperative management of rheumatoid disease. Initial management includes aspirin in high dosages monitored by serum drug levels. Secondary agents such as methotrexate, chloroquine, or oral steroids are best administered under the direction of a rheumatologist.

Cervical Hyperextension Injuries

Hyperextension injuries of the neck occur most often when the driver of a stationary car is struck from behind by another vehicle. The driver is usually relaxed and unaware of the impending collision. The sudden acceleration of the struck vehicle pushes the back of the car seat against the driver's torso. This pushes the driver's torso forward and his or her head is thrown backward, causing hyperextension of the neck. This occurs very quickly after impact. If no head rest is present, the driver's head is hyperextended past the normal limit of stretch of the soft tissues of the neck. This injury has been descriptively termed "whiplash" because of the hyperextension of the head.

The sternocleidomastoid muscle, the scalenes, and the longus colli muscles may be mildly or severely stretched or, at worst, torn. Muscle tears of the longus colli muscles might involve injury to the sympathetic trunk unilaterally or bilaterally, resulting in Horner's syndrome, nausea, or dizziness. Further hyperextension may injure the esophagus, resulting in temporary dysphagia and injury to the larynx, causing hoarseness. Tears in the anterior longitudinal ligament may cause hematoma formation with resultant cervical radiculitis (arm pain) and injury to the intervertebral disc. In the recoil-forward flexion that occurs when the car stops accelerating, the head is thrown forward. This forward flexion of the head is usually limited by the chin striking the chest and does not usually cause significant injury. However, if the head is thrown forward and strikes the steering wheel or the windshield, a head injury can occur.

The driver is often unaware that he has been injured. He suffers little discomfort at the scene of the accident and often does not even wish to go to the hospital. Later that evening or the next day, 12 to 14 hours after the accident, the patient begins to feel stiffness in the neck. Pain at the base of the neck increases and is made worse by head and neck movements. Soon any movement of the head or neck causes excruciating pain. The anterior cervical muscles are often tender to the touch. The patient may have pain on mouth opening or chewing, hoarseness or difficulty swallowing, and will seek medical care.

The physical examination must be detailed and complete. Abrasions on the forehead would suggest that forward flexion led to the head striking the steering wheel or windshield. A dilated pupil might suggest a case of Horner's syndrome secondary to the injury of the sympathetic chain, or it might be a sign of significant intracranial injury if the patient's level of consciousness is altered. Point tenderness in front of the ear would

suggest injury to the temporomandibular joint, and tenderness to touch in the suboccipital area would suggest the head struck the back of the seat.

A complete neurological examination is crucial. Any evidence of objective neurological deficit merits immediate diagnostic tests to determine the cause. Although by definition, hyperextension cervical injury causes damage only to the soft-tissue structures of the neck, plain radiographs of the cervical spine should be obtained in all cases. Unsuspected fracture—dislocations of the cervical spine, facet fractures, odontoid fractures, or spinous process fractures—might be otherwise missed in the neurologically intact patient. Cervical spondylosis will be demonstrated on plain radiographs as well. Of course, if objective neurologic deficits are present, then further diagnostic aids are necessary, (e.g., head CT, spine CT, myelogram, MRI).

A reasonable medical routine, since the majority of patients have no neurologic deficit, is based on the premise of resting the involved injured soft tissues. A soft cervical collar helps significantly in relieving muscle spasm and preventing quick head turns. The collar should not be worn for more than 2 to 4 weeks, lest the recovering muscles start weakening from nonuse. Heat is helpful and should be applied by a heating pad, hot showers, or hot tub soaks. If neck pain is severe, a short period of bed rest may be necessary. Mild analgesics, nonsteroidal, anti-inflammatory drugs (NSAIDs), and muscle relaxants are all helpful and are generally indicated. Narcotic analgesics should be avoided if at all possible. Activity should be restricted as determined by the severity of the symptoms. Generally, driving should be avoided for the acute symptomatic period. After approximately 2 weeks of this regimen, significant improvement should be noted. If not, 2 more weeks of continued conservative care with the addition of some light home-cervical traction should be employed. If symptoms persist at 4 weeks post injury, some further testing is necessary before emotional overlay is considered the cause. If headaches persist, a cranial CT scan should be done. If normal at 4 weeks, the patient can be assured that no intracranial abnormality is present. If arm or shoulder pain persist, a spine CT scan or MRI should be considered. If these tests are normal, the patient can be assured that no compression of neural structures is present.

Cervical Spine Algorithm

The task of the physician, when confronted with the cervical spine patient, is to integrate his or her complaints into an accurate diagnosis and to prescribe appropriate therapy. Achieving this goal depends on the accuracy of the physician's decision-making ability. Although specific information is not available for every aspect of neck pain, there is a large body of data to guide us in handling these patients. Using this knowledge, which has already been presented, an algorithm for neck pain has been designed.

Webster defines an algorithm as "a set of rules for solving a particular problem in a finite number of steps." It is, in effect, an organized pattern of decision making and thought processes found useful, in this instance, in approaching the universe of cervical spine patients. The algorithm can be followed in sequence (Fig. 8–3) and is also presented in table form (Table 8–2).

The primary objective for the physician is to return patients to their normal function as quickly as possible. In the course of achieving this goal, the physician must be concerned with other circumstances, which include making efficient and precise use of diagnostic studies, minimizing the use of ineffectual surgery, and making therapy available at a reasonable cost to society. The algorithm follows well-delineated rules, established from the consensus of a broad segment of qualified spine surgeons. It allows the patient to receive the most helpful diagnostic and therapeutic measures at optimal times.

The algorithm begins with the universe of patients who are initially evaluated for neck pain, with or without arm pain. Patients with major trauma, including fractures, are not included. After an initial medical history and physical examination—and assuming that the patient's symptoms are originating from the cervical spine—the first major decision is to rule in or out the presence of a cervical myelopathy.

The character and severity of the myelopathy depends on the size, location, and duration of the lesion. Ventrolateral lesions encroach on the nerve roots and lateral aspects of the spinal cord, producing all the manifestations accompanying nerve root compression. The chief radicular signs are weakness, loss of tone, and volume of the muscles of the upper extremity, while the pressure on the spinal cord may produce pyramidal tract signs and spasticity in the lower extremities.

Midline lesions intrude on the central aspect of the anterior portion of the spinal cord. They produce no signs of nerve root compression. Both lower extremities are primarily involved and the most common problem relates initially to gait disturbance. As the disease progresses, bowel and bladder control may be affected.

Once a diagnosis of cervical myelopathy is made, surgical intervention should be considered without delay. The best results are attained in patients with one or two motor units involved and with myelopathy of a relatively short duration. The longer pressure is applied to the neural elements, the poorer the results. A cervical MRI or CT-myelogram should be obtained in these patients to precisely define the neural compression, and an adequate surgical decompression should be performed as soon as possible to achieve the best results.

After cervical myelopathy has been ruled out, the remaining patients, who constitute an overwhelming majority, should be started on a course of conservative management. At this stage of the patient's course a specific diagnosis, whether it be a herniated disc or neck strain, is not important because the entire group is treated in the same fashion.

Conservative Treatment

The primary mode of therapy in both acute and chronic cervical spine disease is immobilization. In the acute neck injuries, immobilization allows for healing of torn and attenuated soft tissues, whereas in chronic conditions immobilization is aimed at reduction of inflammation in the supporting soft tissues and around the nerve roots of the cervical spine.

Immobilization is best achieved by the use of a soft felt collar. It needs to be properly fitted and comfortable for the patient. Initially, the collar is worn 24 hours a day. The patient must understand that during sleep the neck is totally unprotected from awkward positions and movement, and that therefore the collar is most important.

The other mainstay of the initial treatment is drug therapy. It is directed at reducing inflammation—especially in the soft tissues. There are a variety of anti-inflammatory medications available; however, there is no one drug that has proven to be significantly better than

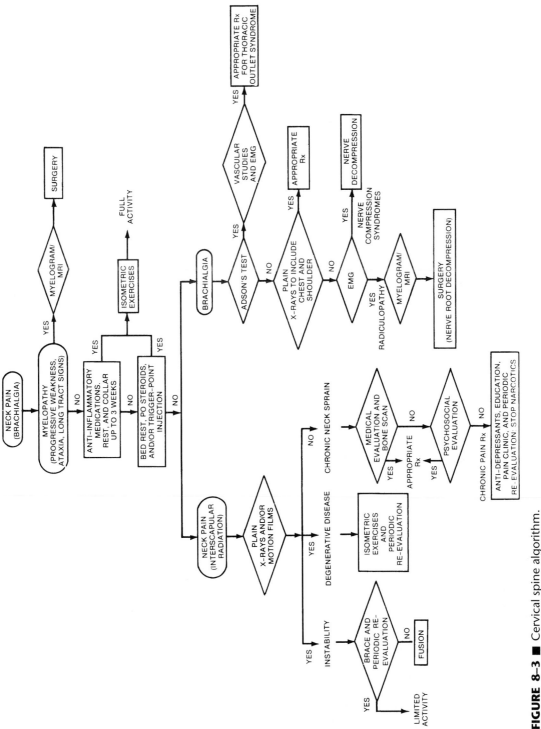

FIGURE 8–3 ■ Cervical spine algorithm.
(From Wiesel SW, et al: Neck Pain. Charlottesville, VA, The Michie Co., 1988; reprinted by permission.)

TABLE 8–2 ■ *Differential Diagnosis of Neck Pain*

Evaluation	Neck Strain	Herniated Nucleus Pulposis	Instability	Degenerative Disc Disease	Myelopathy	Tumor	Spondylo-arthropathy	Metabolic	Infection
Predominant pain (arm vs. neck)	Neck	Arm	Neck	Neck	Neck	Neck	Neck	Neck	Neck
Constitutional symptoms						+	+	±	+
Compression test		+							
Neurologic exam		+			+				
Plain radiographs			±	+	±	±	+	+	±
Lateral motion radiographs			+						
CAT scan		+		+	±	+			+
Myelogram		+			+				
Bone scan						+	+	±	++
ESR							+		+
Ca/P/alk phos						+		+	+

Ca/P/alk phos indicates calcium, phosphate, and alkaline phosphatase; CAT, computerized axial tomography; ESR, erythrocyte sedimentation rate.

all the others. Salicylates have proven to be as effective and safe as the rest and are the least expensive. The dosage must be adequate to achieve a therapeutic blood level. The efficacy of this treatment regimen is predicated on the patient's ability to understand the disease process and the role of each therapeutic modality. The vast majority of patients will respond to this approach in the first 10 days, but a certain percentage will not heal rapidly.

At this juncture a local injection into the area of maximum tenderness should be considered. Localized tender areas in the paravertebral musculature and trapezii will be found in many individuals and are referred to as "trigger points." Marked relief of symptoms is often achieved dramatically by infiltration of these trigger points with a combination of lidocaine (Xylocaine) and 1 mL of a steroid preparation. The object of the injection is to decrease the inflammation in a specific anatomic area. The more localized the trigger point, the more effective this form of therapy.

The patient should be treated conservatively for up to 6 weeks. The majority of cervical spine patients will get better and should be encouraged to gradually increase their activities. The goal is a return to their normal lifestyles. An exercise program should be directed at strengthening the paravertebral musculature, not at increasing the range of motion.

The pathway along this top portion of the algorithm is reversible. Should regression occur—with exacerbation of symptoms—the physician can resort to more stringent conservative measures. These may include additional bed rest and stronger anti-inflammatory medication. The majority of patients with neck pain will respond to therapy and return to a normal life pattern within 2 months of the beginning of their problem. If the initial conservative treatment regimen fails, symptomatic patients are divided into 2 groups. The first is comprised of people who have neck pain as a predominant complaint, with or without interscapular radiation. The second group is made up of those who complain primarily of arm pain (brachialgia).

Neck Pain Predominant

After 6 weeks of conservative therapy with no symptomatic relief, plain roentgenograms with lateral flexion-extension films are carefully examined for abnormalities. One group of patients will have objective evidence of instability. In the lower cervical spine (C-3 through C-7), instability is identified by horizontal translation of one vertebra on another of more than 3.5 mm, or of an angulatory difference of adjacent vertebrae of more than 11 degrees. The majority of patients with instability will respond well to further nonoperative measures, including a thorough explanation of the problem and some type of bracing. In some cases, these measures will fail and a surgical fusion of the involved spinal segments will be necessary.

Another group of patients complaining mainly of neck pain will be found to have degenerative disease on their plain x-ray films. The roentgenographic signs include loss of height of the intervertebral disc space, osteophyte formation, secondary encroachment of the intervertebral foraminae, and osteoarthritic changes in the apophyseal joint. The difficulty is not in identifying these abnormalities on the roentgenogram but in determining their significance.

Degeneration in the cervical spine can be a normal part of the aging process. In a study of matched pairs of asymptomatic and symptomatic patients, it was concluded that large numbers of asymptomatic patients show roentgenographic evidence of advanced degenerative disease. The most significant roentgenographic finding relevant to symptomatology was found to be narrowing of the intervertebral disc space, particularly between C5-6 and C6-7. There was no difference between the two groups as far as changes at the apophyseal joints, intervertebral foraminae, or posterior articular processes.

These patients should be treated symptomatically with anti-inflammatory medication, support, and trigger-point injections as required. In the quiescent stages they should be placed on isometric exercises. Finally, they should be reexamined periodically because some will develop significant pressure on the neurologic elements (myelopathy).

The majority of patients with neck pain will have normal roentgenograms. The diagnosis for this group is neck strain. At this point, with no objective findings, other pathology must be considered. These patients should undergo a bone scan and medical evaluation. The bone scan is an excellent tool, often identifying early spinal tumors or infections not seen on routine roentgenographic examinations. A thorough medical search may also reveal problems missed in the early stages of neck pain evaluation. If these diagnostic studies are positive, the patient is treated appropriately.

If the above workup is negative, the patient should have a thorough psychosocial evaluation. This is predicated on the belief that a patient's disability is related not only to his pathologic anatomy but also to his perception of pain and his stability in relationship to his sociologic environment. Drug habituation, alcoholism, depression, and other psychiatric problems are frequently seen in association with neck pain. If the evaluation reveals this type of pathology, proper measures should be instituted to overcome the disability.

Should the outcome of the psychosocial evaluation prove to be normal, the patient can be considered to have chronic neck pain. One must be aware that other outside factors such as compensation and/or litigation can influence a patient's perception of his subjective pain. Patients with chronic neck pain need encouragement, patience, and education from their physicians. They need to be detoxified from narcotic drugs and placed on an exercise regimen. Many will respond to antidepressant drugs such as amitriptyline (Elavil). All of these patients need periodic reevaluation to avoid missing any new or underlying pathology.

Arm Pain Predominant (Brachialgia)

Patients who have pain radiating into their arm may be experiencing their symptoms secondary to mechanical pressure and inflammation of the involved nerve roots. This mechanical pressure may arise from a ruptured disc or from bone secondary to degenerative changes. Other pathologic causes of arm pain should be carefully considered. Extrinsic pressure on the vascular structures or on the peripheral nerves are the most likely imitators of brachialgia. Pathology in the chest and shoulder should also be ruled out.

A careful physical examination should be conducted. If there is any question about these findings, appropriate roentgenograms and an EMG should be obtained. If any of these are positive for peripheral pressure on the nerves or other pathology, the appropriate therapy should be administered.

Should all of these studies prove negative and the EMG is consistent, the patient is considered to have brachialgia. One must carefully reevaluate the patient who has a neurologic deficit and/or a positive EMG; those who have either should undergo an MRI. If the MRI is positive and is consistent with the physical findings, surgical decompression should be considered at this juncture.

It has been repeatedly documented that for surgery to be effective, unequivocal evidence of nerve root compression must be found at surgery. One must have a strong confirmation of mechanical root compression from the neurologic exam and a confirming study before proceeding with any surgery. The indications for surgery are the subjective complaint of arm pain and a neurologic deficit or positive EMG. If the patient does not have these, there is inadequate clinical evidence of root compression to proceed with surgery, regardless of the radiographic findings. For individuals who have met these criteria for cervical decompression, the results will usually be satisfactory: 95 percent of them can expect good or excellent outcomes.

Conservative Treatment Modalities

Most patients with neck pain will achieve relief from a conscientious program of conservative care. As the algorithm indicates, all patients with either chronic or acute neck pain (except those with myelopathy) deserve an initial period of conservative therapy. There are a multitude of treatment modalities available but many of them are based on empiricism and tradition. The purpose of this section is to discuss the rationale behind the use of some of the more common nonoperative therapeutic measures.

Immobilization

The cornerstone of conservative therapy is immobilization of the cervical spine. The goal of immobilization is to rest the neck so that healing of torn and/or attenuated soft tissues in acute cervical injuries can take place. In the chronic situation, the purpose of immobilization is to reduce any inflammation.

Immobilization can best be achieved by the use of a soft cervical collar that holds the head in a neutral or slightly flexed position. It is very important that the collar is fitted properly. If the neck is held in hyperextension the patient is usually quite uncomfortable and does not derive any benefit from its use. In acute neck injuries, the collar should be worn on a full-time basis, night and day, until the acute pain subsides. This may sometimes take as long as 4 to 6 weeks, and the patient should be aware of this time course from the outset of treatment so that the physician will not feel pressured to discontinue immobilization before the proper time.

In some instances, patients fail to attain adequate pain relief with ambulatory use of the soft collar. These people should be put to bed to relieve the cervical spine from the burden of supporting the weight of the head. While at bed rest, these patients should be instructed to continue using their collar on a full-time basis. The amount of immobilization prescribed varies for each patient; such patients should not be mobilized until they are reasonably comfortable, at which time isometric exercises can be considered.

Drug Therapy

There are three different groups of medications that have proved helpful in the treatment of neck pain: anti-inflammatory drugs, analgesics, and muscle relaxants. They are used as an important adjunct to adequate immobilization.

Anti-inflammatory drugs are used because it is felt that inflammation in the soft tissues is a major contributor to pain production in the cervical spine. This is especially true for those patients with symptoms secondary to a herniated disc. The arm pain that these people experience is due not only to the mechanical pressure from the ruptured disc, but also to the inflammation in and around the involved nerve roots. Usually, if one can get rid of the inflammation, the patient's pain will markedly decrease.

There is a spectrum of anti-inflammatory agents available but none has been proven superior. The author's usual treatment plan is to begin the patient on adequate doses of aspirin, which is effective and inexpensive. If the response is not satisfactory, other anti-inflammatory agents such as naproxen or indomethacin are tried. Most patients will get significant relief from one of the agents presently available. It should be stressed that anti-inflammatory medications are utilized in conjunction with immobilization; they do not replace adequate rest.

Analgesic medication is also very important during the acute phase of neck pain. The goal is to keep the patient comfortable. Most patients will respond to the equivalent of 30 to 60 mg of codeine every 4 to 6 hours. If stronger medication is required the patient should be monitored very closely and in some instances admitted to the hospital for observation. In some cases, narcotics will be abused by the patient and addiction will become a problem to some degree. The treating physician must maintain control of the patient's drug use at all times.

Injuries to the cervical spine frequently result in painful muscle spasm. A vicious cycle is established, whereby pain leads to muscle spasm, which leads to ischemia and a further increase in pain. Once the cycle is established, it tends to be self-perpetuating. An effective muscle relaxant frequently breaks this painful cycle and allows more comfort and an increased range of motion in the cervical spine. Methocarbamol or carisoprodol in adequate doses are the drugs recommended. They are safe and quite effective.

Traction

Cervical traction has been used for many years. Today, opinions regarding its effectiveness range from that of it being a valuable clinical therapy to the conclusion that it is either ineffective and/or potentially harmful.

There is no uniform idea as to how traction actually works and there are a number of methods of actually applying the traction. The three major ways of administering traction are mechanical, manual, and home traction. Many feel that manual traction is preferred due to the interaction between the therapist and patient and the potential specificity of individually varying the traction.

In certain situations cervical traction is contraindicated. Malignancy, cord compression, infectious disease, osteoporosis, and rheumatoid arthritis are the major disorders for which cervical traction should *not* be employed. It is also felt that when there is a herniated disc present, either in the midline or laterally, traction should not be considered.

The author feels that cervical traction is useful when a collar has proved ineffective in those patients with a cervical strain or a hyperextension injury. The major benefit is felt to be continued rest, and a home traction device is preferred. When used in this situation, only minimal amounts of weight (4 to 6 lbs.) should be utilized and the direction of pull should be in slight flexion. As already mentioned, there are other ways of applying traction, but to date there is no valid scientific evidence available that traction in and of itself is effective.

Trigger-Point Injection

Many patients will complain of a very localized tender spot in the paravertebral area. In some of these cases relief of the discomfort can be achieved with the infiltration of the trigger point with a combination of Xylocaine and a steroid preparation or Xylocaine by itself. There have been no true randomized clinical trials to study the efficacy of trigger-point injections, but from empirical evidence they seem to work on some patients. It is interesting to note that although the pharmacologic effects of these drugs may wear off in 2 to 3 hours, the relief may last indefinitely.

Before actually injecting a patient, a history of allergy to the drugs to be used should be obtained. The more localized the trigger point, the more effective the injection tends to be. An area of diffuse tenderness does not respond very well to this approach.

Manipulation

Manipulation of the cervical spine should be approached very carefully. In the United States this is mainly performed by chiropractors although other health care professionals are involved. The goal of manipulation is to correct any malalignment of the spinal structures, which is assumed to be the etiology of the patient's pain. There is no real scientific evidence that manipulation of the cervical spine is effective in the treatment of acute or chronic neck problems.

Unfortunately, there have been a number of tragic complications associated with the use of cervical manipulation. In one clinical study the morbidity was as high as 7 percent. Injuries from manipulation include joint injury, nerve damage, vascular injury, and fracture-dislocation. Although some patients receive a good symptomatic response after cervical manipulation, it is the authors' feeling that the hazards are too great to warrant its use and that manipulation at this time has no place in the treatment of cervical spine disorders.

Exercises

After a patient's acute symptoms have cleared and there is no significant pain or spasm, an exercise regimen is reasonable. The exercises should be directed at strengthening the paravertebral musculature and not at increasing the range of motion. Motion will return with the disappearance of pain.

The exercises are isometric in nature. They are performed once each day with increasing repetitions. It should be appreciated that at present there are no scientific studies demonstrating that isometric exercises or any other type of cervical exercises will reduce the frequency of recurrent neck pain episodes.

Empirically, they do appear to have a positive psychologic effect and give the patient an active part in his treatment program.

LUMBAR SPINE

Low back pain occurs much more commonly than neck pain. The lifetime incidence of low back pain is estimated to be 65 percent. Every physician will either be personally affected (family/friends) or professionally challenged by this problem.

History

A general medical review, especially in the older patient, is imperative. Metabolic, infectious, and malignant disorders may initially present to the physician as low back pain.

The location of the pain is one of the most important historical points. The majority of patients just have back pain with or without referral into the buttocks or posterior thigh. Referred pain is defined as pain in structures which have the same mesodermal origin. These patients have a localized injury, and the referral of pain into the buttocks or thigh does not signify any compression on the neural elements. This type of pain is described as dull, deep, and/or boring.

Another group of patients complains of pain that originates in their back but travels below the knee into the foot. It is described as sharp and lancinating. It may be accompanied by numbness and tingling. This pain is termed "radicular pain" or a "radiculopathy." A radiculopathy is defined as a mechanical compression of an inflamed nerve root where the pain travels along the anatomic course of the nerve. The compression can be secondary to either soft tissue (disc) or bone. The most common nerve roots affected are L5 and S1—levels that account for pain traveling below the knee.

Finally, one should inquire about changes in bowel or bladder habits. Occasionally, a large midline disc herniation may compress several roots of the cauda equina (Fig. 8-4). This is termed "cauda equina compression (CEC)" syndrome. Urinary retention or incontinence of bowel and bladder are, along with severe pain, the major symptoms. This is a surgical emergency. Spontaneous neurologic recovery has not been observed. Only surgery undertaken promptly can offer any hope of neurologic recovery.

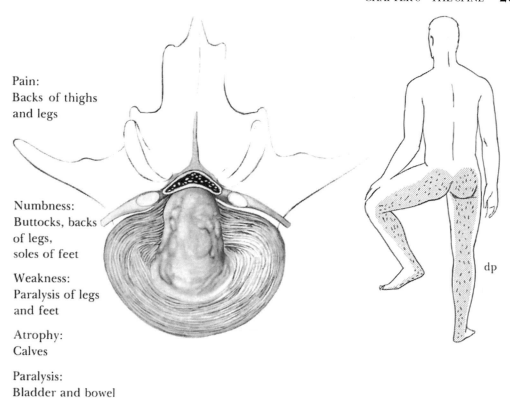

Pain:
Backs of thighs
and legs

Numbness:
Buttocks, backs
of legs,
soles of feet

Weakness:
Paralysis of legs
and feet

Atrophy:
Calves

Paralysis:
Bladder and bowel

FIGURE 8–4 ■ Massive herniation at the level of the third, fourth, or fifth disc may cause severe compression of the cauda equina. Pain is confined chiefly to the buttocks and the back of the thighs and legs. Numbness is widespread from the buttocks to the soles of the feet. Motor weakness or loss is present in the legs and feet with loss of muscle mass in the calves. The bladder and bowels are paralyzed. DP indicates distribution of pain and paresthesia. (From DePalma, AF, Rothma, RH: The Intervertebral Disc. Philadelphia, WB Saunders Company, 1970, p 194; reprinted by permission.)

Physical Examination

The physical examination is directed at finding the location of the pain. All patients with low back pain can have some nonspecific findings which vary in degree depending on the severity of the condition. These include a list to one side, tenderness to palpation and percussion, and a decreased range of motion of the lumbar spine. The above findings can be present in both radiculopathy and referred pain patients. Their presence denotes that there is a problem but does not identify the etiology or level of the problem.

The neurologic examination may yield objective evidence of nerve root compression if present (Table 8–3). A thorough neurologic evaluation of the lower extremities should be conducted on each patient, particularly to check the reflexes and motor findings. Sen- sory changes may or may not be present but because of overlap in the dermatomes of spinal nerves, it is difficult to identify specific root involvement.

In patients with radiculopathies there are several maneuvers that tighten the sciatic nerve, and in so doing, further compress an inflamed lumbar root against a herniated disc or bony spur. These maneuvers are generally termed "tension signs" or a "straight leg-raising test (SLRT)." The conventional SLRT is performed with the patient supine. The examiner slowly elevates the leg by the heel with the knee kept straight (Fig. 8–5). This test is positive when the leg pain below the knee is reproduced or intensified; the production of back and/or buttock pain does not constitute a positive finding. The reliability of the SLRT is age-dependent. In a young patient, a negative test most probably excludes the possibility of a

TABLE 8–3 ■ *Clinical Features of Herniated Lumbar Discs*

L3-4 Disc: L4 Nerve Root

Pain	Lower back, hip, posterolateral thigh, across patella, anteromedial aspect of leg
Numbness	Anteromedial thigh and knee
Weakness	Knee extension
Atrophy	Quadriceps
Reflexes	Knee jerk diminished

L4-5 Disc: L5 Nerve Root

Pain	Sacroiliac region, hip, posterolateral thigh, anterolateral leg
Numbness	Lateral leg, first webspace
Weakness	Dorsiflexion of great toe and foot
Atrophy	Minimal anterior calf
Reflexes	None, or absent posterior tibial tendon reflex

L5-S1 Disc: S1 Nerve Root

Pain	Sacroiliac region, hip, posterolateral thigh/leg
Numbness	Back of calf; lateral heel, foot, and toe
Weakness	Plantar flexion of foot and great toe
Atrophy	Gastrocnemius and soleus
Reflexes	Ankle jerk diminished or absent

From Boden S, Wiesel SW, Laws E, et al: The Aging Spine. Philadelphia, WB Saunders Company, 1991, p 177; reprinted by permission.

PRACTICALLY NO FURTHER DEFORMATION OF ROOTS OCCURS DURING FURTHER STRAIGHT-LEG-RAISING.

SCIATIC ROOTS TENSE OVER THE I.V. DISC DURING THIS RANGE. RATE OF DEFORMATION DIMINISHES AS THE ANGLE INCREASES.

over 70°

35-70°

TENSION APPLIED TO THE SCIATIC ROOTS AT THIS ANGLE.

0-35°

SLACK IN SCIATIC ARBORIZATION TAKEN UP DURING THIS RANGE.

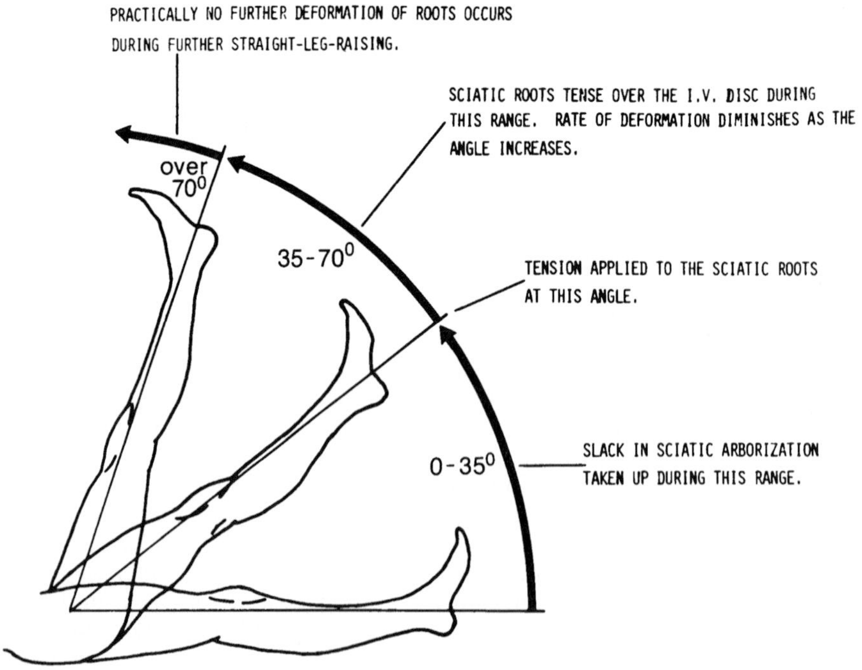

FIGURE 8–5 ■ The dynamics of the straight leg-raising test.

(Modified from Fahrni WH: Observations on straight leg-raising, with special reference to nerve root adhesions. Can J Surg 9:1966; reprinted by permission.)

herniated disc. After the age of 30, however, a negative SLRT no longer reliably excludes the diagnosis.

Finally, the physical examination should evaluate some specific problems that can present as low back pain. This includes a peripheral vascular examination, hip joint evaluation, and abdominal examination.

Diagnostic Studies

As in the cervical spine, diagnostic tests should be used to confirm the core of information gathered from a thorough history and physical examination. Several lumbosacral imaging modalities are currently available including plain films, myelography, CT, and MRI.

To evaluate the true clinical value of any diagnostic study, one must know its sensitivity (false-negatives) and specificity (false-positives). The specificity, or false-positive rate, is usually measured in a population of symptomatic patients who have undergone surgery; however, often there is a much higher rate of false-positives when an asymptomatic group is studied. The accuracy of any single test increases when it is combined with a second or third diagnostic study. The physician's challenge is to select diagnostic tests on the basis of their performance characteristics so that the correct diagnosis is obtained with the least cost and morbidity. The studies most frequently utilized in the diagnostic assessment of low back pain will be described and critically analyzed with this in mind.

Plain Radiographs

The diagnosis of disc herniation can usually be made on the basis of a history and physical examination. Plain radiographs of the lumbosacral spine will rarely add any information, but must be obtained in the appropriate setting to rule out other pathologic conditions such as infection or tumor. Plain radiographs are valuable for seeking the diagnosis of spinal stenosis, spondylolisthesis, gross segmental instability, or fracture.

The radiograph must be of excellent quality and taken with attention to detail. In general, three views are all that are required to assess the lumbosacral spine: an AP view, a lateral view, and a coned-down lateral view of the lower two interspaces. On occasion, two oblique views are also taken to identify subtle spondylolysis or pars interarticularis defects.

However, oblique views provide limited information and should not be routinely included.

Although plain films are useful for surveying the bony elements of the spine and paraspinal soft tissues, the contents of the spinal canal, including cord, dura, ligaments, and encroaching disc, are not visualized. In addition, bony lesions may not be apparent until 50 percent of the cancellous bone has been destroyed.

Finally, degenerative changes such as disc-space narrowing, traction osteophytes, vacuum-disc phenomenon, and end-plate sclerosis, are quite prevalent in older individuals. Unfortunately, these radiographic findings have been shown to correlate poorly with clinical symptoms.

Myelography

Myelography has long been the "gold standard" for evaluating neural compression. Dye is injected into the dural sac and mixes with the spinal fluid. The outline of the contents of the spinal canal can be visualized on x-ray; any extradural mass such as a herniated disc will show up as a filling defect in the dye column (Fig. 8–6), while an intrathecal mass will appear as an outward protrusion. Myelography is unable to differentiate disc protrusion from bony or other encroachment on the spinal canal. The diagnostic accuracy of myelography is also questionable in cases of far lateral disease and at the L5-S1 level where the epidural space may be quite large.

The myelogram is an invasive procedure and should not be taken lightly. Complications include severe headache, nausea, vomiting, and, although rare, even seizures. Prior to the utilization of the water-soluble dye metrizamide, the oil-based agent Pantopaque had a much higher incidence of complications and was known to cause a crippling arachnoiditis. Newer contrast agents are now available that are reported to have fewer side effects.

Despite the role of myelography historically as the standard, more recent data indicate that 24 percent of asymptomatic people have an abnormal myelogram. For this reason, when the myelogram is used as a "screening test" in the absence of objective clinical findings, exploratory surgery and disaster frequently result. A particular advantage of the myelogram over conventional CT is that it can evaluate the lower thoracic spine without additional radiation. Acute radiculopathies can be

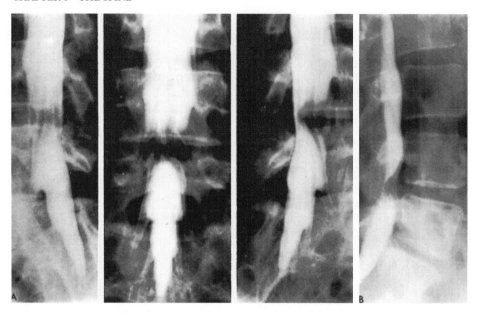

FIGURE 8–6 ■ This metrizamide myelogram illustrates a large central disc herniation at the L4-5 level. *A,* Anterior-posterior and oblique views reveal this prominent defect more marked on the right. *B,* This lateral view illustrates a "double density" prominent ventral indentation of the dye column.

(From Rothman RH, Simeone FA: The Spine, ed 2. Philadelphia, WB Saunders Company, 1982, p 551; reprinted by permission.)

caused by intradural extramedullary tumors in the lower thoracic area. However, new multiplanar CT and MRI can also image this area.

Computed Tomography

Computed tomography is a very versatile and widely available noninvasive modality for evaluating abnormalities of the lumbosacral spine. Multiple cross-sectional (axial) images of the spine are made at various levels and, with reformatting, coronal, sagittal, and three-dimensional images may be created. The CT scan demonstrates not only the bony spinal configuration but also the soft tissue in graded shading, so that ligaments, nerve roots, free fat, and intervertebral disc protrusions can be evaluated as they relate to their bony environment (Figs. 8–7 and 8–8).

Several prospective comparisons of CT with myelography have demonstrated that CT is at least as sensitive (97% vs. 93%) and specific (80% vs. 76%) in the diagnosis of herniated lumbar discs. The sensitivity of CT appears to be enhanced by the addition of intradural metrizamide contrast, which has been shown to demonstrate additional pathology in up to 30 percent of cases. The primary weakness of CT scanning remains its inability

to reliably demonstrate intrathecal pathology (e.g., tumors).

The CT scan is an extremely valuable diagnostic tool when it is used appropriately to confirm the patient's clinical findings. However, recent studies reveal the pitfalls of making clinical decisions on the basis of isolated CT scan findings. Despite many reports in the literature indicating that CT scanning has a mean accuracy of 90 percent in symptomatic patients, 34 percent of asymptomatic patients had abnormal CT scans when reviewed by three independent expert interpreters. The implication is that a patient with a negative history and physical examination for a spinal lesion has a 1-in-3 chance of having an abnormal CT scan. If the decision for surgery is based only on scan results, there is a 30 percent chance that the patient will undergo an unnecessary and unsuccessful operation. However, if the patient's clinical picture correlates with the CT scan abnormalities, CT can be a useful confirmatory diagnostic tool.

Magnetic Resonance Imaging

Magnetic resonance imaging is the newest diagnostic imaging modality for the spine. The image of different tissues is obtained by the detection of extremely small differences in proton density in a magnetic field bombarded with short pulses of radio waves causing atoms to vibrate at an angle out of the field. Variations in proton density, radio frequency, and relaxation time in the nonexcited state will modify the MRI scan to highlight different tissues. Unlike CT and myelography, this approach does not require ionizing radiation or contrast agents. Multiplanar images are directly available (Fig. 8–9).

The MRI has proved to be an excellent imaging modality for the lumbar spine. It is especially good for evaluating disc pathology. Since it provides a "static" picture, it is not as useful for spinal stenosis. Magnetic resonance imaging, especially with gadolinium-DTPA contrast enhancement, is superb for demonstrating intraspinal tumors and for distinguishing recurrent disc herniation from scar tissue.

As with the other diagnostic imaging modalities discussed, MRI also has been shown to have a significant clinical false-positive rate in asymptomatic individuals. In one prospective and blinded study, 22 percent of the

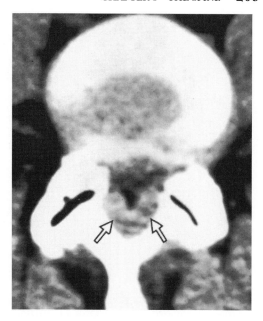

FIGURE 8–8 ■ Spinal stenosis. The size of the thecal sac is diminished owing to thickening of the ligamenta flava *(arrows)*. Gas within the facet joints (vacuum facet) is evident.

(From Kricun ME: Imaging Modalities in Spinal Disorders. Philadelphia, WB Saunders Company, 1988; reprinted by permission.)

asymptomatic subjects under age 60 and 57 percent of those over age 60 had significantly abnormal scans. In addition, the prevalence of disc degeneration on the T2-weighted MRI scans was found to approach 98 percent in subjects over the age of 60.

Electrodiagnostic Testing

The EMG is performed by placing needles into muscles to determine if there is an intact nerve supply to that muscle. An abnormal EMG can demonstrate impaired nerve transmission to a specific muscle and isolate the nerve root involved. Initially, the EMG will be negative in spite of nerve entrapment and will only show muscle irritability. After 3 weeks of significant pressure on a nerve root, signs of denervation with fibrillation can be observed.

The EMG, like all of the other confirmatory tests already discussed, is not a screening tool. In fact, when dealing with the average low back problem, the EMG rarely provides any information that cannot be derived from a careful physical examination. It may even confuse the picture, since an EMG may be abnormal from diabetic neuropathy, previous pe-

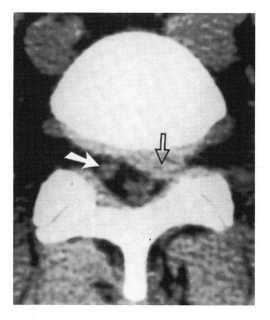

FIGURE 8–7 ■ Posterolateral disc herniation. A posterolateral disc herniation at L5-S1 on the left *(open arrow)* is encroaching on epidural fat and compressing the S1 nerve root. Notice the uninvolved S1 nerve root on the right *(white arrow)*, which is surrounded by epidural fat.

(From Kricun ME: Imaging Modalities in Spinal Disorders. Philadelphia, WB Saunders Company, 1988; reprinted by permission.)

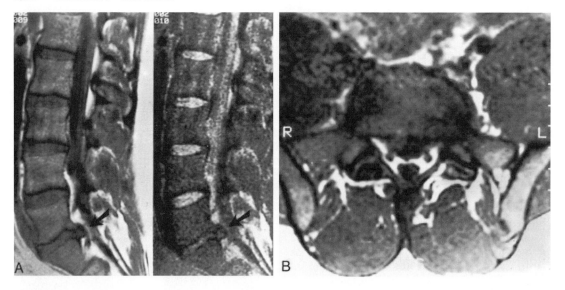

FIGURE 8–9 ■ *A*, Magnetic resonance imaging (MRI) scan of a herniated disc, sagittal view. T_1-weighted image *(left)* demonstrates a herniated disk *(arrow)* at the L5-S1 level. The T_2-weighted image *(right)* shows loss of the normal white signal within the nucleus pulposus *(arrow)*, a sign of degenerative disc disease.

(From Boden SD, Davis DO, Dina TS, et al: Abnormal lumbar spine MRI scans in asymptomatic subjects: A prospective investigation. J Bone Joint Surg 72-A:403–408, 1990; reprinted by permission.)

B, MRI scan of a herniated disc, axial view. T_1-weighted image at the L5-S1 disc space demonstrates a large, central herniated disc with lateral displacement of both S1 nerve roots and posterior displacement of the cauda equina.

(From Boden S, Wiesel SW, Laws E, et al: The Aging Spine. Philadelphia, WB Saunders Company, 1991, p 147; reprinted by permission.)

ripheral nerve entrapment, or trauma. In cases in which the correlation of clinical signs and imaging is equivocal—especially with chronic unexpected sciatica—nerve conduction studies and EMG may be helpful. Electromyography can also detect the involvement of a secondary nerve root in cases of complex back injury preoperatively, sometimes prompting a more extensive operation.

Clinical Conditions

There are a number of conditions that can present as low back pain in any particular individual. However, the following four are the most common of those typically evaluated by orthopaedic surgeons and will be discussed in detail: back strain, herniated disc, spinal stenosis, and spondylolisthesis.

Back Strain–Lumbago

The vast majority of people who have low back discomfort suffer from a non-radiating type of low back pain called "back sprain" or "lumbago." The etiology is not always clear, but it probably is a ligamentous or muscular strain secondary to either a specific traumatic episode or the continuous mechanical stress of a postural inadequacy. These may also include patients with a small tear in the annulus fibrosus, which would account for the frequent prior history of low back pain in patients with a ruptured disc.

These patients' main complaint is back pain, and it can be limited to one spot or cover a diffuse area of the lumbosacral spine. At times there may be a referral of pain to the buttocks or posterior thigh since the lower back, buttocks, and posterior thigh all originate from the same embryonic tissue, or mesoderm. Such referral of pain does not necessarily connote any mechanical compression of the neural elements and should not be called "sciatica."

The usual physical findings are limited to local tenderness over the involved area and muscle spasm; however, the attacks will vary in intensity and can conveniently be divided into three categories: mild, moderate, and severe. Those placed in the mild group have subjective pain without objective findings and should be able to return to customary activity in less than a week. The moderate group is characterized by a limited range of spinal motion and paravertebral muscle spasm as well as pain, and these patients should be able to resume full activity in <2 weeks. The severe group includes those patients who are tilted forward or to the side. They have trouble ambulating and can take up to 3 weeks to become functional again.

Since a normal x-ray is a standard occurrence with a patient complaining of back strain, a radiographic study is usually not necessary on the first visit if the physician feels comfortable with the diagnosis; however, if the response to treatment does not proceed as expected, films should be taken to rule out other more serious problems such as spondylolisthesis or tumor. The authors' usual recommendation is that if a patient fails to respond to conservative treatment for an acute attack of low back pain after a period of 2 weeks, then a routine lumbosacral spine x-ray series is clinically indicated.

The authors' preferred treatment for low back strain is the functional restorative approach. The mainstay of treatment is controlled physical activity, with the judicious use of trunk flexibility and strengthening exercises as the acute phase subsides. Often, particularly in the obese patient with weak abdominal muscles, a light-weight lumbosacral corset is useful in helping to mobilize those encumbered by low back strain.

Herniated Disc

A herniated disc can be defined as the herniation of the nucleus pulposus through the torn fibers of the annulus fibrosus. Most disc ruptures occur during the third and fourth decade of life while the nucleus pulposus is still gelatinous. The perforations usually arise through a defect just lateral to the posterior midline where the posterior longitudinal ligament is weakest. The two most common levels for disc herniation are L4-5 and L5-S1. These two discs account for 95 percent of all lumbar disc herniations; pathology at the L2-3 and L3-4 levels can occur but is relatively uncommon.

Disc herniations at L5-S1 will usually compromise the first sacral nerve root. A lesion at the L4-5 level will most often compress the fifth lumbar root, while a herniation at the L3-4 more commonly involves the fourth lumbar root. It should be pointed out, however, that variations in root configuration as well as in the position of the herniation itself can modify these relationships. An L4-5 disc rupture can at times affect the first sacral as well as the fifth lumbar root and, in extreme lateral herniations, the nerve exiting at the same level as the disc will be involved.

Not everyone with a disc herniation has significant discomfort. A large herniation in a capacious canal may not be clinically significant since there is no compression of the neural elements, while a minor protrusion in a small canal may be crippling since there is not enough room to accommodate both the disc and the nerve root.

Clinically, the patient's major complaint is pain. Although there may be a prior history of intermittent episodes of localized low back pain, this is not always the case. The pain not only is present in the back but also radiates down the leg in the distribution of the affected nerve root. It will usually be described as sharp or lancinating, progressing from the top downward in the involved leg. Its onset may be insidious or sudden and associated with a tearing or snapping sensation in the spine. Occasionally when the sciatica develops, the back pain may resolve since once the annulus has ruptured, it may no longer be under tension. Finally, the sciatica may vary in intensity; it may be so severe that patients will be unable to ambulate and will feel that their back is "locked." Conversely, the pain may be limited to a dull ache that increases in intensity with ambulation.

On physical examination, there is usually a decreased range of motion in flexion, and patients will tend to drift away from the involved side as they bend. On ambulation, the patient walks with an antalgic gait, holding the involved leg flexed so as to put as little weight as possible on the extremity.

Although neurologic examination may yield objective evidence of nerve root compression, these findings are often undependable since the involved nerve is often still functional. In addition, such deficit may have little temporal relevance since it may relate to a prior attack at a different level. To be significant, reflex changes, weakness, atrophy, or sensory loss must conform to the rest of the clinical picture.

When the first sacral root is compressed, the patient may have gastrocnemius-soleus weakness and be unable to repeatedly raise up on the toes of that foot. Atrophy of the calf may be apparent and the ankle (Achilles) reflex is often diminished or absent. Sensory loss, if any, is usually confined to the posterior aspect of the calf and lateral side of the foot.

Involvement of the fifth lumbar nerve root can lead to weakness in extension of the great toe and, less often, to weakness of the everters and dorsiflexors of the foot. An associated sensory deficit can appear over the anterior leg and the dorsomedial aspect of the foot down to the great toe. There are usually no primary reflex changes, but on occasion a diminution in the posterior tibial reflex can be elicited. The absence of this reflex, however, must be asymmetrical for it to have any clinical significance.

With compression of the fourth lumbar nerve root, the quadriceps muscle is affected. The patient may note weakness in knee extension, and it is often associated with instability. Atrophy of the thigh musculature can be marked. A sensory loss may be apparent over the anteromedial aspect of the thigh and the patellar tendon reflex is usually diminished.

Nerve root sensitivity can be elicited by any method that creates tension; however, the SLRT is the one most commonly employed. As discussed before, a positive test reproduces the patient's pain down the leg. The reproduction of back pain is not considered positive.

The initial diagnosis of a herniated disc is ordinarily made on the basis of the history and physical examination. Plain x-rays of the lumbosacral spine will rarely add to the diagnosis but should be obtained to help rule out other causes of pain such as infection or tumor. Other tests such as the EMG, the computerized axial tomography (CAT) scan, and MRI are confirmatory by nature and can be misinformative when they are used as screening devices.

The treatment for most patients with a herniated disc is nonoperative since 80 percent of them will respond to conservative therapy when followed over a period of 5 years. The efficacy of nonoperative treatment, however, depends upon a healthy relationship between a capable physician and a well-informed patient. If a patient has insight into the rationale for the prescribed treatment and follows instructions, the chances for success are greatly increased.

One of the most important elements in the nonoperative treatment is controlled physical activity. Patients should markedly decrease their activity. This will sometimes require bed rest and in most cases can be accom-

plished at home. An acute herniation usually takes at least 2 weeks of significant rest before the pain substantially eases.

Drug therapy is another important part of the treatment and three categories of pharmacological agents are commonly used: anti-inflammatory drugs, analgesics, and muscle relaxants or tranquilizers. Inasmuch as the symptoms of low back pain and sciatica result from an inflammatory reaction as well as mechanical compression, the authors feel that anti-inflammatory medication in the form of two aspirin every 4 hours should be taken in conjunction with rest. It should be stressed, however, that no medication can take the place of controlled physical activity. Buffered aspirin can be used by patients with gastrointestinal intolerance. The patient's pain generally will be relieved once the inflammation is brought under control. There may be some numbness or tingling in the involved extremity but this is usually tolerable. In addition, a large array of NSAIDs are available for the refractory patient.

Analgesic medication is rarely needed if the patient really rests, since the pain is usually adequately controlled by decreased activity. If the pain is severe enough to require hospitalization, however, then morphine sulfate is the drug of choice; codeine is recommended for use when the patient is home.

There is some question as to whether there actually is a muscle relaxant; all drugs that are so designated probably act to some degree as tranquilizers. If one is required, though, methocarbamol and carisoprodol are the ones most frequently used, and they can be employed intravenously as well as orally. The use of diazepam (Valium) for this purpose should be discouraged since it is actually a depressant and often will add to the patient's psychological problems.

Eighty percent of those who follow the above regimen will be markedly improved but it requires patience since frequently at least 6 weeks will have passed before any additional therapy is indicated. Although the noninvasive treatment of a herniated disc can be quite gratifying, it generally takes a significant period of rest, and the patient must be aware of the time constraints from the beginning in order to understand the rationale behind the measures employed.

The long-term prognosis for patients with disc herniation is quite good. It has been shown that between 85 percent and 90 percent of surgically treated and nonsurgically treated patients were asymptomatic at 4 years. Less than 2 percent of both groups were symptomatic at 10 years.

Spinal Stenosis

Spinal stenosis can be defined as a narrowing of the spinal canal, and the mechanical pressure on the neural structures within will depend upon the degree of narrowing. Every person's spine, however, becomes narrower with age due to osteoarthritis. Not everyone with a narrowed spinal canal, however, will have symptoms.

For those who do suffer, the discomfort can vary from mild annoyance to an inability to walk. The symptom complex is well documented. Patients of either sex, usually not before their fifth decade, will first complain of vague pains, dysesthesias, and paresthesias with ambulation but will typically have excellent relief of their symptoms when they are sitting or lying supine. The increased lordotic stance assumed with walking, and particularly walking down grades, is most likely the inciting cause. The hyperextension further narrows the spinal canal and increases the symptoms.

With maturation of the syndrome, symptoms may even occur at rest. Muscle weakness, atrophy, and asymmetrical reflex changes may then appear; however, as long as the symptoms are only aggravated dynamically, neurological changes will occur only after the patient is stressed. The following stress test can be used in an outpatient clinic: after a neurological examination has been performed on the patient, he or she is asked to walk up and down the corridor until symptoms occur or the patient has walked 300 feet. A repeat examination is then done and in many cases the second examination will be positive for a focal neurologic deficit when the first was negative.

Plain x-rays are often helpful in visualizing spinal stenosis, particularly degenerative spinal stenosis. One can see intervertebral disc degeneration, decreased interpedicular distance, a decreased sagittal canal diameter, and facet degeneration. If a patient fails conservative treatment and becomes a surgical candidate, the location and degree of neurological compression can be assessed with MRI or a CT scan/myelogram.

The majority of patients with spinal stenosis, especially the degenerative and combined variety, can be treated nonsurgically. Aspirin has been the drug of choice, but the physician must watch for gastric irritation in what is typically an older patient population.

Finally, a lumbosacral corset is often helpful in reminding the patient to avoid excessive strain. Symptoms are usually intermittent and the individual often needs encouragement in getting through the episode without getting depressed. Nonoperative management is preferable as long as the pain is tolerable.

Spondylolisthesis

Spondylolisthesis is a spinal condition where all or a part of a vertebra has slipped forward on another. The word is derived from the Greek *spondylos,* meaning "vertebra," and *olisthesis,* meaning "to slip." There are several different types of spondylolisthesis, but the most common is that in which the lesion is in the isthmus or pars interarticularis. If a defect can be identified, but no slipping has occurred, the condition is termed "spondylolysis;" if one vertebra has slipped forward on another (horizontal translation), it is referred to as "spondylolisthesis."

The etiology of the defect in spondylolysis is not clear. Although there may be a hereditary component, the lesion is seldom seen in patients under the age of 5 and is found in 5 percent of people over the age of 17. The most attractive explanation is that although these children inherit a potential deficiency in the pars, they are not born with any identifiable defect. Between the ages of 5 and 17, however, they become more active and a stress fracture, caused by repetitive hyperextension stresses, can develop into a spondylolysis. It is likely that most of these fractures occur during the period of rapid growth known as the adolescent growth spurt, and they are particularly prevalent in gymnasts and football players.

Spondylolisthesis has several characteristic features, but the forward displacement is easily recognized radiographically on the lateral projection (Figs. 8–10 and 8–11). The degree of slip varies from patient to patient and can range from minimal displacement to complete dislocation of the vertebral body. Increased slipping rarely occurs after the age of 20 unless there has been a severe superimposed injury or surgical intervention. The period of most rapid progression coincides with the rapid growth spurt between the ages of 9 and 15.

The most common clinical manifestation of spondylolisthesis is low back pain. Although the cause of this type of back pain in the adult has been studied extensively, its origin is still not clear. There is no clear under-

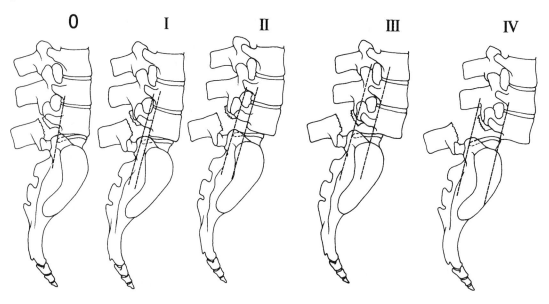

FIGURE 8–10 ■ Grading system for spondylolisthesis.
(From Borenstein DG, Wiesel SW: Low Back Pain: Medical Diagnosis and Comprehensive Management. Philadelphia, WB Saunders Company, 1989, p 166; reprinted by permission.)

standing of how so many patients develop this lesion between the ages of 5 and 17 but still have no back complaints until perhaps age 35, when a sudden twisting or lifting motion will precipitate an acute episode of back and leg pain. Other patients with significant degrees of slipping, however, will go through life with no discomfort.

Although 50 percent of patients overall normally cannot associate an injury with the onset of the symptoms, of those working in industry almost all will report an associated incident. It is possible to sustain an acute fracture of the pars, but it is a very rare occurrence. If the acuity of a pars defect is in question, it can be documented by a bone scan within 3 months of the injury; if the defect is long-standing, the scan will be negative.

There is also frequently a buildup of a fibrocartilaginous mass at the defect, and this can cause pain by irritating the nerve root as it exits. It is thus not unusual in spondylolisthesis to have the patient first complain of back pain, but over time have leg pain develop as the most annoying part of the problem.

Once the symptoms begin, the patient usually has constant low grade back discomfort that is aggravated by activity and relieved by rest. There are some periods during which the pain is more intense than others, but unless the picture is complicated by severe leg pain, total incapacitation is rare. The patients are seldom aware of any sensory or motor deficit. At this point, it should be reemphasized that in some people, even severe displacement is asymptomatic and gives rise to no disability. It is not uncommon to pick up a previously unrecognized spondylolisthesis on a routine gastrointestinal radiological study of a 50-year-old patient.

The physical findings of this syndrome are fairly characteristic. In the absence of any radicular pain, the patient exhibits no postural scoliosis; but there is usually an exaggeration of the lumbar lordosis and a palpable "stepoff" with a dimple at the site of the abnormality. Occasionally mild muscle spasm is demonstrable and, in most instances, some local tenderness can be elicited. Although the range of motion is usually complete, some pain can be expected on hyperextension.

Radiographs, particularly the lateral views, confirm the diagnosis. Even the slightest amount of forward slipping of the body of the involved vertebra is readily discernible, and the oblique views will disclose the actual defect in the pars.

The nonoperative treatment of the adult with spondylolisthesis is much the same as that used for backache from other causes. When the symptoms are acute, rest is indicated. If leg pain is a significant problem, then anti-inflammatory medication can be quite beneficial. Exercises, usually a flexion exercise program, should be started once patients are in remission, and they are usually advised to own a corset for use during occasional strenuous activity. If conservative treatment is not successful, an operative approach can be considered and would include a spinal fusion.

Lumbar Spine Algorithm

As with patients with neck pain, the task of the physician when confronted with low back pain patients is to integrate their complaints into an accurate diagnosis and to prescribe appropriate therapy. This problem (universe of low back pain patients) has been formatted

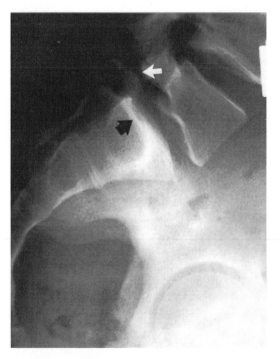

FIGURE 8-11 ■ Lateral spot view of the lumbosacral junction. A grade I spondylolisthesis is present with 25 percent slippage of the superior vertebral body (*black arrow*). This view demonstrates a Type II spondylolisthesis with a pars defect (*white arrow*).

(From Borenstein DG, Wiesel SW: Low Back Pain: Medical Diagnosis and Comprehensive Management. Philadelphia, WB Saunders Company, 1989, p 167; reprinted by permission.)

into an algorithm (Fig. 8–12), the aim of which is to select the correct diagnostic category and proper treatment avenues for each patient with low back pain. A specific patient may fall outside the limits of the algorithm and require a different approach, and the physician must constantly be on the alert for exceptions. The algorithm can be followed in sequence and is also presented in table form (Table 8–4).

The information necessary to use the algorithm is initially obtained through the history and physical examination. The key points in the history are differentiation of back pain that is mechanical in nature from nonmechanical pain that is present at rest, detecting changes in bowel or bladder function, and defining the precise location and quality of the pain. The physical examination must be oriented toward ruling out other medical causes of low back pain, assessing neurologic function, and evaluating for the presence of tension signs.

Following the low back pain algorithm, the first major decision is to make a ruling on the presence or absence of CEC syndrome. Mechanical compression of the cauda equina, with truly progressive motor weakness, is the only surgical emergency in lumbar spine disease. This compression from a massive rupture of the L4-5 disc in the midline is usually due to pressure on the caudal sac, through which pass the nerves to the lower extremities, bowel, and bladder.

The signs and symptoms of CEC are a complex mixture of low back pain, bilateral motor weakness of the lower extremities, bilateral sciatica, saddle anesthesia, and even frank paraplegia with bowel and bladder incontinence or urinary retention. Cauda equina compression can be caused by either bone or soft tissue damage, the latter generally a ruptured or herniated disc in the midline. These patients should undergo an immediate definitive diagnostic test and, if it is positive, emergency surgical decompression. Historically, the myelogram was the study used in this setting; however, the development of MRI has facilitated the noninvasive diagnosis of CEC. The principal reason for prompt surgical intervention is to arrest the progression of neurologic loss; the chance of actual return of lost neurologic function following surgery is small. Although the incidence of CEC syndrome in the entire back pain population is very low, it is the only event that requires immediate opera-

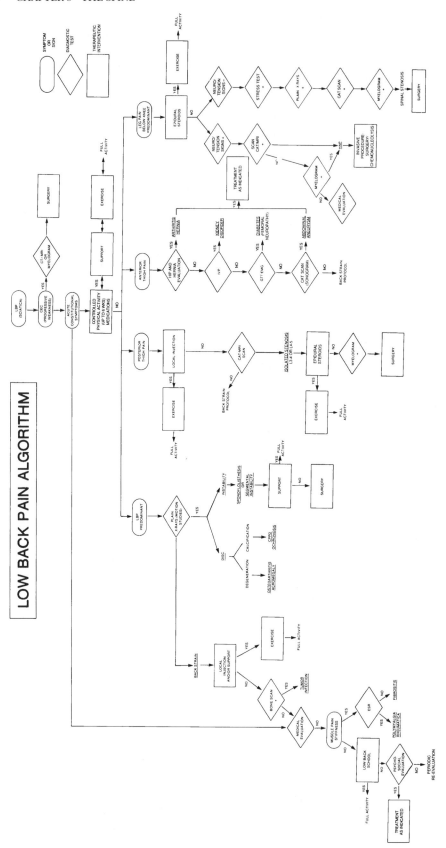

FIGURE 8–12 ■ Algorithm for the differential diagnosis of low back pain.

(From Boden S, Wiesel SW, Laws E, et al: The Aging Spine. Philadelphia, WB Saunders Company, 1991, p 156; reprinted by permission.)

TABLE 8–4 ■ *Differential Diagnosis of Low Back Pain*

Evaluation	Back Strain	Herniated Nucleus Pulposus	Spinal Stenosis	Spondylo-listhesis/Instability	Spondylo-arthropathy	Infection	Tumor	Metabolic	Hemato-logic	Visceral
Predominant pain (back vs. leg)	Back	Leg (below knee)	Back/leg	Back	Back	Back	Back	Back	Back	Back (buttock, thigh)
Constitutional symptoms					+	+	+	+	+	
Tension sign		+		±						
Neurologic exam		±	± after stress							
Plain x-rays		+	+	+	+	±	±	+	+	
Lateral motion x-rays				+						
CT/MRI		+	+			+	+			+
Myelogram		+	+							
Bone scan					+	+	+	+	+	+
ESR					+	+	+		+	+
Serum chemistries							+	+	+	+

ESR indicates erythrocyte sedimentation rate.

From Borenstein DG, Wiesel SW: Low Back Pain: Medical Diagnosis and Comprehensive Management. Philadelphia, WB Saunders Company, 1989, p 534; reprinted by permission.

tive intervention; if its diagnosis is missed, the consequences can be devastating.

The remaining patients make up the overwhelming majority. They should be started on a course of conservative (nonoperative) therapy regardless of the diagnosis. At this stage the specific diagnosis, whether a herniated disc or simple back strain, is not important to the therapy because the entire population is treated the same way. A few of these patients will eventually need an invasive procedure (surgery), but at this point there is no way to predict which individuals will respond to conservative therapy and which will not.

Conservative Treatment

The vast majority in this initial group have nonradiating low back pain, termed lumbago or back strain. The etiology of lumbago is not clear. There are several possibilities, including ligamentous or muscular strain, continuous mechanical stress from poor posture, facet joint irritation, or a small tear in the annulus fibrosis. Patients usually complain of pain in the low back, often localized to a single area. On physical examination they demonstrate a decreased range of lumbar spine motion, tenderness to palpation over the involved area, and paraspinal muscle spasm. Their roentgenographic examinations are usually normal, but if therapy is not successful, films should be obtained to rule out other possible etiological factors. Two exceptions to this rule are patients younger than 20 years of age and patients over age 60; x-rays are important early in the diagnostic process because these patients are more likely to have a diagnosis other than back strain (tumor or infection). Other situations warranting x-rays sooner rather than later include a history of serious trauma, known cancer, unexplained weight loss, or fever.

The early stage of the treatment of low back pain (with or without leg pain) is a waiting game. The passage of time, the use of anti-inflammatory medication, and controlled physical activity are the modalities proven safest and most effective. The vast majority of these patients will respond to this approach within the first 10 days, although a small percentage will not. In today's society with its emphasis on quick solutions and "high technology," many patients are pushed too rapidly toward more complex (i.e., invasive) management. This "quick fix" approach has no place in the treatment of low back pain. The physi-

cian should treat the patient conservatively and wait up to 6 weeks for a response. As already stated, most of these patients will improve within 10 days—a few will take longer.

Once the patients have achieved approximately 80 percent relief, they should be mobilized with the help of a lightweight, flexible corset. After they are more comfortable and have increased their activity level, they should begin a program of isometric lumbar exercises and return to their normal lifestyles. The pathway along this section of the algorithm is a two-way street: should regression occur with exacerbation of symptoms, the physician can resort to more stringent conservative measures. The patient may require further bed rest. Most acute low back pain patients will proceed along this pathway, returning to their normal life patterns within 2 months of onset of symptoms.

If the initial conservative treatment regimen fails and 6 weeks have passed, symptomatic patients are sorted into four groups. The first group is comprised of people with low back pain predominating. The second group complains mainly of leg pain, defined as pain radiating below the knee and commonly referred to as "sciatica." The third group has posterior thigh pain. The fourth group has anterior thigh pain. Each group follows a separate diagnostic pathway.

Refractory Patients with Low Back Pain

Those patients who continue to complain predominantly of low back pain for 6 weeks should have plain x-rays carefully examined for abnormalities. Spondylolysis with or without spondylolisthesis is the most common structural abnormality to cause significant low back pain. Approximately 5 percent of the population has this defect, thought to be caused by a combination of genetics and environmental stress. In spite of this defect, most people are able to perform their activities of daily living with little or no discomfort. When symptoms are present, these patients will usually respond to nonoperative measures, including a thorough explanation of the problem, a back support, and exercises. In a small percentage of such cases, conservative treatment fails and a fusion of the involved spinal segments becomes necessary. This is one of the few times primary fusion of the lumbar spine is indicated, and it must be stressed that it is a relatively infrequent occurrence.

The vast majority of patients with pain

predominantly in the low back will have normal plain x-rays. The diagnosis at this point is back strain. Before there is any additional workup, a local injection of steroids and Xylocaine may be tried at the point of maximum tenderness. This can be quite successful, and if there is a good response the patient is begun on exercises with gradual resumption of normal activity. In some instances, if there are no objective findings, such a "trigger-point" injection can be considered as early as the third week after onset of symptoms.

Should the patient not respond to local injection, other pathology must be seriously considered. A bone scan, along with a general medical evaluation, should be obtained. The bone scan is an excellent tool, often identifying early bone tumors or infections not visible on routine radiographic examinations. It is particularly important to obtain this study in the patient with nonmechanical back pain. If the pain is constant, unremitting, and unrelieved by postural adjustments, more often than not the correct diagnosis will be one of an occult neoplasm or metabolic disorder not readily apparent from other testing.

Approximately 3 percent of cases of apparent low back pain that present at orthopaedic clinics are attributable to extraspinal causes. A thorough medical search also frequently reveals problems missed earlier such as a posterior penetrating ulcer, pancreatitis, renal disease, or an abdominal aneurysm. If these diagnostic studies are positive, the patient should be transferred into a nonorthopaedic treatment mode and would no longer be in the therapeutic algorithm.

Those patients who have no abnormality on their bone scans and do not show other medical disease as a cause for their back pain are then referred for another type of therapy—the low back school. It is believed that many of these patients are suffering from discogenic pain or facet joint pain syndrome. The low back school concept has as its basis the belief that patients with low back pain, given proper education and understanding of their disease, can often return to a productive and functional life. Ergonomics, the proper and efficient use of the spine in work and recreation, is stressed. Back school need not be an expensive proposition. It can be a one-time classroom session with a review of back problems and a demonstration of exercises with patient participation. This type of educational process has proved to be very effective. It is most important, however, that before patients are referred to this type of program, they be thoroughly screened. One does not want to be in the position of treating a metastatic tumor in a classroom.

If low back school is not successful, the patient should undergo a thorough psychosocial evaluation in an attempt to explain the failure of the previous treatments. This is predicated on the knowledge that a patient's ability is related not only to his or her pathologic anatomy but also to the patient's perception of pain and stability in relation to the social environment. It is quite common to see a stable patient with a frank herniated disc continue working—regarding the disability as only a minor problem—while a hysterical patient takes to bed at the slightest twinge of low back discomfort.

Drug habituation, depression, alcoholism, and other psychiatric problems are seen frequently in association with back pain. If the evaluation suggests any of these problems, proper measures should be instituted to overcome the disability. There are a surprising number of ambulatory patients addicted to commonly prescribed medications using complaints of back pain as an excuse to obtain these drugs. Oxycodone (Percodan) and diazepam, alone or in combination, are the two most popular offenders. Oxycodone is truly addictive; diazepam is both habituating and depressing. Since the complaint of low back pain may be a common manifestation of depression, it is counterproductive to treat such patients with diazepam.

Approximately 2 percent of patients who initially present with low back pain will fail treatment and elude any diagnosis. There will be no evidence of any structural problem in the back or criteria for an underlying medical disease or psychiatric disorder. This is a very difficult group to manage. The authors' strategy has been to discontinue narcotics, reassure patients, and periodically reevaluate them. Over time, one third of these patients will be found to have an underlying medical disease; thus, one cannot abandon this group and discontinue treatment. For the remainder, as much physical activity as possible should be encouraged.

Refractory Patients with Sciatica

The next group of patients consists of those with sciatica, which is pain radiating below the knee. These patients usually experience their symptoms secondary to mechanical pressure and inflammation of the nerve roots that originate in the back and extend down the leg. The etiology of the mechanical pressure can be soft tissue—herniated disc, bone, or a combination of the two.

At this point in the algorithm, the patient has had up to 6 weeks of controlled physical activity and medication but still has persistent leg pain. The next therapeutic step is an epidural steroid injection, which is performed on an outpatient basis. An epidural injection is worth trying; the chance of success is 40 percent and morbidity is low, particularly compared with the next treatment step—surgery. The maximum benefit from a single injection is achieved at 2 weeks. The injection may have to be repeated once or twice, and 4 to 6 weeks should pass before its success or failure is judged.

If epidural steroids are effective in alleviating patients' leg pain or sciatica, they are begun on a program of back exercises and encouraged to return promptly to as normal a lifestyle as possible. Should the epidural steroids prove ineffective, and 3 months have passed since the initial injury without relief of pain, some type of invasive treatment should be considered. The patient group is then divided into those with probable herniated discs and those with symptoms secondary to spinal stenosis.

The physician must now carefully reevaluate the patient for a neurologic deficit and for a positive tension sign or SLRT. For those who have either a neurologic deficit or positive tension signs along with continued leg pain, a CT or MRI scan should be obtained. If either the CT or MRI scan is clearly positive and correlates with the clinical findings, there is no need for myelography since it is invasive. If there is any question about the findings, one should proceed with the other noninvasive study not yet done (CT or MRI) or perform a metrizamide myelogram.

As in the cervical spine, there is repeated documentation that for surgery to be effective in the treatment of a herniated disc, the surgeon must find unequivocal operative evidence of a nerve root compression. Accordingly, nerve root compression must be firmly substantiated preoperatively, not only by neurologic examination but also by radiographic data. There is no place for "exploratory" back surgery. Many asymptomatic patients have been found to have abnormal myelograms, EMGs, CT scans, and MRI scans.

If the patient has neither a neurologic deficit nor a positive SLRT, then regardless of radiographic findings there is not enough evidence of root compression to proceed with successful surgery. These patients without objective findings are the ones who have poor results and who have given back surgery a bad name.

If there are no objective findings, the physician should avoid surgery and proceed to the psychosocial evaluation. Exceptions should be few and far between. When sympathy for the patient's complaints outweighs the objective evaluation, surgery is fraught with difficulties. For those who meet these specific criteria for lumbar laminectomy, results will be satisfactory: 95 percent of them can expect a good-to-excellent result.

The second group of patients whose symptoms are based on mechanical pressure on the neural elements are those with spinal stenosis. The diagnosis of spinal stenosis usually can be inferred from the plain x-rays which will demonstrate facet degeneration, disc degeneration, and decreased interpedicular and sagittal canal diameters. A CT scan and/or MRI can confirm the diagnosis (Figs. 8–13 and 8–14). If symptoms are severe, and there is radiographic evidence of spinal stenosis, surgery is appropriate. Age alone is not a deterrent to surgery; many elderly people who are in good health except for a narrow spinal canal will benefit greatly from adequate decompression of the lumbar spine.

Refractory Patients with Anterior Thigh Pain

A small percentage of patients will have pain that radiates from the back into the anterior thigh. This usually is relieved by rest and anti-inflammatory medication. If the discomfort persists after 6 weeks of treatment, a workup should be initiated to search for underlying pathology. Although an upper lumbar radiculopathy can cause anterior thigh pain, several other entities must be considered.

A hip problem or hernia can be ruled out with a thorough physical examination. If the hip examination is positive, radiographs should be obtained. An IV pyelogram is useful to evaluate the urinary tract, because kidney stones often may present as anterior thigh pain. Peripheral neuropathy, most commonly secondary to diabetes, also can present initially with anterior thigh pain; a glucose tolerance test as well as an EMG will reveal the underlying

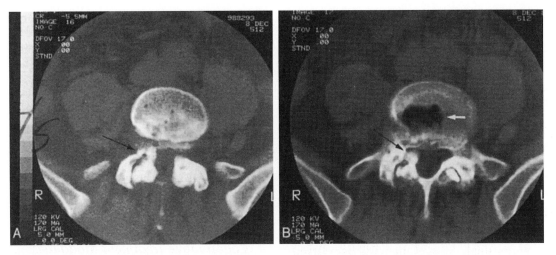

FIGURE 8–13 ■ Computerized tomography scan of a 68-year-old man with back pain that is exacerbated with standing. Cross-sectional views demonstrate vacuum phenomenon in intervertebral disc *(white arrow)* and facet hypertrophy (most prominent on the right), resulting in canal stenosis at multiple levels *(black arrows).* The patient's symptoms responded to epidural steroid injections.

(From Borenstein DG, Boden S, Wiesel SW: Low Back Pain: Medical Diagnosis and Comprehensive Management, ed 2. Philadelphia, WB Saunders Company, 1995, p 203; reprinted by permission.)

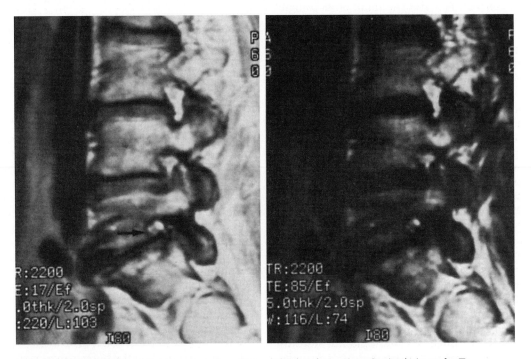

FIGURE 8–14 ■ Magnetic resonance imaging of the lumbar spine. Sagittal view of a T_2-weighted image demonstrating foramenal narrowing at L5-S1 interspace *(black arrow)* with associated intervertebral disc degeneration.

(From Borenstein DG, Boden S, Wiesel SW: Low Back Pain: Medical Diagnosis and Comprehensive Management, ed 2. Philadelphia, WB Saunders Company, 1995, p 204; reprinted by permission.)

problem. Finally, a retroperitoneal tumor can cause symptoms by mechanically pressing on the nerves that innervate the anterior thighs. A CT or MRI scan of the retroperitoneal area will eliminate or confirm this possibility.

If any of the entities reviewed above is diagnosed, the patient is treated accordingly. If no physical cause can be found for the anterior thigh pain, the patient is treated for recalcitrant back strain by the method already outlined.

Refractory Patients with Posterior Thigh Pain

This final group of patients will complain of back pain with radiation into the buttocks and posterior thigh. Most of them will be relieved of their symptoms with 6 weeks of conservative therapy. However, if their pain persists after the initial treatment period, they can be considered to have back strain and given a trigger-point injection of steroids and Xylocaine in the area of maximum tenderness. If the injection is unsuccessful, it is necessary to distinguish between referred and radicular pain.

As noted earlier, referred pain is pain in mesodermal tissues of the same embryologic origin. The muscles, tendons, and ligaments of the buttocks and posterior thigh have the same embryologic origin as those of the low back. When the low back is injured, pain may be referred to the posterior thigh, where it is perceived by the patient. Referred pain from irritated soft tissues cannot be cured with a surgical procedure.

Radicular pain is caused by compression of an inflamed nerve root along the anatomic course of the nerve. A herniated disc or spinal stenosis in the high lumbar area can cause radiation of pain into the posterior thigh. An MRI or CT scan and an EMG may be used in this situation to differentiate radicular etiology from referred pain or a peripheral nerve lesion. If the studies are within normal limits, the patient is considered to have back strain and treated accordingly to the algorithm. If a radicular abnormality is found, the patient is diagnosed as having mechanical compression on the neural elements either from a herniated disc or spinal stenosis. Epidural steroids should be tried first; if these do not provide adequate relief, surgery should be contemplated.

This group of patients with unexplained posterior thigh pain is very difficult to treat. The biggest mistake made is the performance of surgery on people thought to have radicular pain who actually have referred pain. Again, referred pain in this setting is not responsive to surgery.

In most instances the treatment of low back pain is no longer a mystery. The algorithm described here presents a series of easy-to-follow and clearly defined decision-making processes. Use of this algorithm provides patients with the most helpful diagnostic and therapeutic measures at the optimal time. It neither denies them helpful surgery nor subjects them to procedures that are useless technical exercises.

Conservative Treatment Modalities

As the algorithm indicates, all low back pain patients, regardless of diagnosis (except those with CEC syndrome), require an initial period of conservative therapy. At present there are many modalities available, but few have been scientifically validated because of the difficulty in performing a prospective double-blind study in this field. Each treatment plan in popular use today is surrounded by conflicting claims for its indications and efficacy. The purpose of this section is to discuss the rationale behind the use of some of the more common therapeutic measures.

Bed Rest (Controlled Physical Activity)

Decreased activity has evolved over the years as one of the most important elements in the treatment of low back pain. The degree of rest depends on the severity of the symptoms and can vary from complete bed rest to just a decrease in active exercise.

The amount of rest prescribed varies for each patient; these people should not be mobilized until reasonably comfortable. The type of pathology will determine the duration of rest required. Most patients with acute back strain will need only 2 to 7 days of bed rest before they can ambulate. However, a patient with an acute herniated disc may require up to 1 week of complete bed rest with another 10 days for gradual mobilization. Complete bed rest for long periods (more than 2 weeks) has a deleterious effect on the body in general and should be closely monitored. As their discomfort eases, the patient should be strongly encouraged to take short walks, but to do as little sitting as possible. Each patient should be followed carefully and not allowed complete mobility until the objective signs, such as a list and/or paravertebral muscle spasm, disappear. The patient's physical activity is tailored to increase movement without incurring a return of symptoms.

The purpose of controlled physical activity is to allow any inflammatory reaction that is present to subside. Bed rest will not result in the disc's return to its original position. However, as the disc herniates, it causes a secondary inflammatory process responsible for the patient's pain; if this reaction can be brought under control, the patient's symptoms will disappear. This relief may or may not be permanent.

Drug Therapy

The judicious use of drug therapy is an important adjunct in the treatment of low back pain. As in the cervical spine, there are three main categories of drugs in common use: anti-inflammatories, analgesics, and muscle relaxants.

Anti-inflammatory agents are employed because of the belief that inflammation within the affected tissues is a major cause of pain in the low back. This is especially true for those patients with symptoms secondary to a herniated disc.

There are a variety of NSAIDs available. Based on several scientific studies, none of these appear to be superior to the others. The authors' preference is to begin the patient on adequate doses of aspirin, which is effective and inexpensive. If the response is not satisfactory, other anti-inflammatories can be tried. Most patients will get significant relief from one of these agents. Again, all anti-inflammatory medications are utilized in conjunction with controlled physical activity to relieve pain; they do not replace adequate rest. Occasionally, after an initial recovery, a patient will experience intermittent recurrent attacks or complain of a chronic low backache; in some instances these patients will be helped by a maintenance dose of an anti-inflammatory drug.

Analgesic medication is very important during the acute phase of low back pain. The goal is to keep the patient comfortable while in bed. Most of the anti-inflammatory agents also have analgesic properties. In more severe cases, patients will respond to 30 to 60 mg of codeine every 4 to 6 hours. If stronger medication is necessary, it is the authors' feeling that the patient should be admitted to the hospital and given parenteral narcotics as required. As the pain decreases, non-narcotic analgesics may be substituted for the more potent drugs.

The biggest mistake seen is treatment with very strong narcotics such as meperidine (Demerol) or oxycodone (Percodan, Tylox) on an outpatient basis. Many of these patients become addicted to the medication. In other cases, patients try to shortcut the controlled physical activity and use analgesic medication instead. This, of course, will not work, and when the patient tries to stop the drug, the back pain returns.

Muscle relaxants generally are not recommended for the treatment of low back pain. In most cases the muscle spasm is secondary to a primary problem such as a herniated disc. If the pain from the ruptured disc can be controlled, the muscle spasm will usually subside.

Occasionally, muscle spasm will be so severe that some type of treatment is required. Carisoprodol (Soma), methocarbamol (Robaxin), or cyclobenzaprine (Flexeril) are the drugs recommended. Diazepam (Valium) should be discouraged since it is actually a physiological depressant, and depression is often an integral feature of back pain syndromes. Administering diazepam to depressed patients only increases their problems. If anxiety is prominent and a sedative is needed, phenobarbital will alleviate the symptoms.

In summary, drug therapy for low back pain should be viewed as an adjunct to adequately controlled physical activity. Anti-inflammatory medication should be the primary agent employed. Analgesic medication should be used selectively in a controlled environment and not for extended periods. Muscle relaxants are generally not recommended, and if employed should be carefully monitored.

Trigger-Point Injection

Trigger-point therapy is indicated for nonradiating low back pain when a point of maximal tenderness can be identified. This procedure involves the injection of steroids and Xylocaine at an area of maximal tenderness in the low back. The precise mechanism of action is not clear, but may be related to modulation of peripheral nerve stimulation as it affects the afferent input perceived as pain.

Although anecdotal reports claim effectiveness for this technique, it has not been well studied in the setting of acute low back pain syndrome. A prospective randomized double-blind evaluation of trigger-point injection was conducted in 51 acute low back pain patients. Although not statistically significant, the data suggested that the medication injected is not the critical factor, since the patients treated with a needle stick and nothing injected (acupuncture) had a greater improvement in symptoms (61%) than the patients injected with Xylocaine alone (40%) or with steroids (45%). The intended control group received vapocoolant spray followed by pressure from the plastic needle guard, and had the highest frequency of improvement (66%) and the greatest average subjective decrease in pain. Unfortunately, no patients were randomized to a "watch and wait" control group to evaluate for the placebo effect.

Trigger-point therapy is easy to perform, has a negligible risk, and may help certain patients. Further controlled research is required to delineate the true value of this modality in the treatment of acute low back pain.

Epidural Steroid Injection

Epidural steroid injections are indicated for severe lumbar radiculopathy, not in most cases, for nonradiating low back pain. They have generally been viewed as an intermediate form of treatment between conservative and surgical management. It is a more aggressive attempt at pain relief after conservative therapy has failed, yet avoids the disadvantages of surgery. The rationale for this therapy is that lumbar radiculopathy (in the early phase) involves a significant inflammatory component, evoked by chemical or mechanical irritation or an autoimmune response—all of which should be amenable to treatment with corticosteroid drugs in the early stages.

Unfortunately, few studies have systematically and accurately studied the efficacy of this treatment modality. Poorly controlled, nonrandomized studies have yielded controversial results with a range of success rates from 25 to 75 percent. Another problem is that some studies have attempted to determine the efficacy of epidural steroids compared to epidural saline injection, while others have compared their results to a true placebo.

Despite the lack of optimally designed investigations, upon review of the literature, certain trends seem to be evident. Epidural steroids appear to be more beneficial in acute rather than chronic radiculopathy, especially when no neurologic deficit is present. Improvement may not be noted until 3 to 6 days after injection and may be only temporary. No neurotoxicity has been reported in humans or animal models; complications stem from the technique of epidural injection and are rare. Suppression of plasma corticosteroid concentration may occur up to 3 weeks following the injection.

The authors maintain that epidural steroids may be helpful in relieving an irritative component of radicular pain in 40 percent of patients. Until controlled investigations indicate otherwise, this is a treatment worth trying in patients who have failed 6 weeks of conservative management in an effort to avoid a major invasive procedure.

Traction

The application of traction to the lumbar spine is a popular treatment for patients with herniated discs. The theory is that stretching the lumbar spine distracts the vertebrae so that the protruded disc is allowed to return to a more normal anatomic position. In fact, the disc material probably does not change position at all. Scientific evidence indicates that a traction force equal to 60 percent of body weight is needed just to reduce the intradiscal pressure at the third lumbar vertebra by 25 percent. Such a force could not practically be applied to a patient. Furthermore, there has never been any proof that disc material returns to its normal position following herniation.

Traction can be applied as gravity lumbar traction, autotraction, and through motorized techniques. None of these methods has been proven to be more effective than the others. While a few studies have shown traction to have a short-lived benefit on sciatica patients, most double-blind studies have not demonstrated any positive effect. In one study two groups of patients with proven herniated discs (by myelogram) were treated by applying traction apparatuses to each group in the hospital. However, for one group there were weights in the traction bag; for the other, no weights. There was no statistically significant difference between the two groups in terms of relief of symptoms. Traction had no effect on spinal mobility, tension signs, deep tendon reflexes, paresis, or sensory deficit, and although it usually was well tolerated, it made some patients worse. It is the authors' belief that traction may benefit the patients by limiting their activity and creating a positive psychologic effect on their expectations for recovery. If traction is used, it is recommended that patients be given a home traction unit rather than be admitted to the hospital.

Manipulation

Spinal manipulation is another popular conservative modality in treating low back pain. In the United States, it is somewhat controversial because it is performed mostly by chiropractors. The principle involved is that any malalignment of the spinal structures can be corrected by manipulation; the assumption here is that the malalignment is the etiology of the patient's pain. Unfortunately, there is no scientific proof for or against either the efficacy of this therapy or its pathophysiological foundation.

The authors' experience is that some patients do have short periods of symptomatic relief after manipulation but must keep returning for repeat sessions to maintain it, substantially increasing the cost of treatment. Some patients, in fact, may be harmed if pathologic bone disease such as a tumor or osteopenia is present when manipulation is performed. At present it is felt that manipulation is not indicated for the routine treatment of chronic low back pain. There is not adequate scientific evidence to justify its routine use.

Braces and Corsets

External support of the lumbar spine with a corset or brace is indicated for only a short period in the average patient's recovery process—and not every patient requires it. As the acute symptoms subside, a properly fitted corset or brace will aid the patient in regaining mobility sooner. As the recovery progresses, the patient usually should abandon the brace in favor of an exercise program. With continued long-term use of a brace, soft-tissue contractures and muscle atrophy will occur. The young patient should rely on a brace only to hasten ambulation. In theory, strong, flexible lumbar and abdominal muscles function as an excellent "internal brace" because they are adjacent to the structures (vertebrae) that they are supporting.

Despite a paucity of clinical data, there are two situations in which the authors believe long-term bracing is a reasonable approach.

One is for the obese patient with weak abdominal muscles. A firm corset with flexible metal stays will reinforce the abdominal muscles. It has been demonstrated that if a lumbosacral corset is properly applied, the intradiscal pressure in the lumbar area will decrease by approximately 30 percent.

The aging patient with multi-level degenerative disease of the lumbar spine is the second type of patient for whom long-term bracing may be beneficial. These older people do not tolerate exercise very well, and in some cases exercise will aggravate their back condition. They can attain significant relief of pain with a well-fitted brace.

Exercises

Some form of exercise is probably the most commonly prescribed therapy for patients recovering from low back pain. There are two regimens commonly advocated: isometric flexion exercises and hyperextension exercises. These programs are purported to reduce the frequency and intensity of low back pain episodes, although there is no scientific evidence to support this contention.

The isometric flexion exercises are the most popular. They are based on the theory that by reducing the lumbar lordosis, back pain is decreased. This goal is achieved by strengthening both the abdominal and lumbar muscles, thereby creating a corset of muscles to support the lumbar spine. Flexion exercises are commonly utilized in patients with spondylolisthesis or spinal stenosis.

Hyperextension exercises are the other form of therapy. They are purported to strengthen the paravertebral muscles. These exercises generally are used after a patient has satisfactorily performed a course of isometric flexion exercises. The goal is to have the paravertebral muscles act as an internal support for the lumbar spine.

The authors believe that an exercise regimen is very important for the rehabilitation of low back patients. This regimen should not be instituted while the patient is experiencing acute pain but may be started after his symptoms have subsided to the point where no list or paravertebral spasm is present. The number of repetitions is increased gradually; if the patient has any recurrence of acute symptoms, the exercises are stopped. The patient is then closely monitored; when his symptoms again decrease, the exercises can be resumed.

Physical Therapy

There are many other treatment modalities used for low back pain. These include hot packs, cold packs, light massage, ultrasound, transcutaneous electrical nerve stimulation, and diathermy. They are all well tolerated and pleasant. Most patients experience some immediate relief of symptoms, but unfortunately, there is not a long-lasting impact on the disease process. There is no evidence that any of these treatment modalities offers any long-term benefit or even adds to the efficacy of decreased physical activity alone.

SUGGESTED READINGS

Boden S, Wiesel SW, Laws E, Rothman RH: The Aging Spine. Philadelphia, WB Saunders Company, 1991.

Borenstein DG, Boden S, Wiesel SW: Low Back Pain: Medical Diagnosis and Comprehensive Management, ed 2. Philadelphia, WB Saunders Company, 1995.

Rothman RH, Simeone FA (eds): The Spine, ed 3. Philadelphia, WB Saunders Company, 1992.

Chapter 9

The Shoulder

Benjamin S. Shaffer

INTRODUCTION

The shoulder is one of the most fascinating and complex joints of the musculoskeletal system. A combination of some four bones, sixteen muscle-tendon units, and four specific articulations, the shoulder is in fact a complex arrangement of multiple structures working interdependently to provide normal shoulder function.

Whether generating the speed and accuracy of a baseball pitch, the strength and endurance of power lifting, or the effortless placement of the hand into nearly any position during daily activity, the shoulder is an extraordinarily versatile joint. Yet there is a price for such versatility, and that is in the ease with which a number of traumatic and atraumatic conditions interfere with its normal functioning. The purpose of this chapter is to describe the shoulder's normal functional anatomy, review techniques of examination, and discuss evaluation and treatment of common shoulder problems.

FUNCTIONAL ANATOMY

The shoulder joint is actually a series of four articulations working in synchrony (Fig. 9–1). The joint we refer to as the "shoulder" is but one of these articulations, the *glenohumeral joint,* composed of the humeral head articulating with the oval-shaped *glenoid.* The *acromioclavicular (AC)* and *sternoclavicular (SC)* joints connect the axial (spine) with the appendicu-

lar (extremity) skeleton. Each is a diarthrodial joint (a joint in which two hyaline cartilage articular surfaces appose each other, surrounded by a synovial lining). The SC joint serves to connect the clavicle to the sternum, while the AC joint connects the distal clavicle to the acromion of the scapula. The *scapulothoracic* articulation involves the scapula upon the posterior thoracic wall.

Each of these articulations variably contribute to normal shoulder motion. In elevation of the arm, for example, motion occurs at the glenohumeral-to-scapulothoracic articulation in a 3 to 2 ratio. To a lesser degree, some joint motion (rotation, elevation) also occurs at the SC and AC joints.

The Glenohumeral Joint

The glenohumeral joint is the most mobile joint in the body, a consequence of its shallow ball-and-socket configuration. Although a rim of surrounding fibrous tissue, known as the *labrum,* enhances the depth of the accommodating socket, the skeletal architecture of the normal shoulder is insufficient to maintain normal stability. The most important design feature in maintaining stability is that of the surrounding soft-tissue envelope, known as the capsule. When viewed from the outside, the shoulder capsule appears to be a fibrous structure similar to that seen in other joints. Yet when viewed from within, either arthroscopically or by histologic examination, we see that the capsule consists of discretely identifiable fibrous bands, each with a specific strategic function.

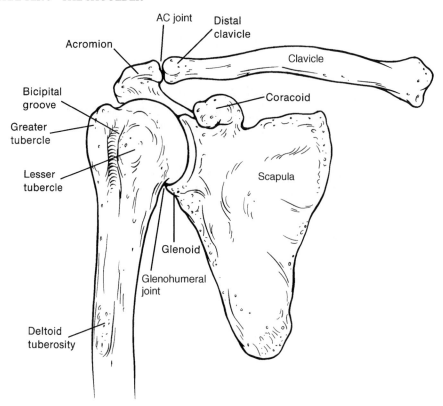

FIGURE 9–1 ■ Anterior view of the shoulder demonstrates the skeletal anatomy and two of the four articulations, the glenohumeral and acromioclavicular joints. (From Essentials in Orthopaedic Surgery, ed 1. p 202; reprinted by permission.)

The anterior capsule is composed of three identifiable ligaments, whose names derive from their glenoid origin: the *superior (SGHL), middle (MGHL)* and *inferior glenohumeral ligaments (IGHL)* (Fig. 9–2).

Of all these structures, the *anterior-inferior glenohumeral ligament (AIGHL) complex* remains the most important and widely studied. This capsular restraint acts like a sling to support the humeral head. As the arm is placed into abduction and external rotation (the "throwing" position), the AIGHL "sling" tightens up, thereby stabilizing the humeral head. Failure to properly tighten, due to laxity (looseness of the tissue) or detachment from the glenoid rim (known as a "Bankart" lesion), is responsible for anterior instability.

The rotator cuff consists of four muscles (the subscapularis, supraspinatus, infraspinatus, and teres minor) that arise from the scapula and coalesce as a tendinous cuff inserting on the lesser and greater tuberosities of the proximal humerus. The long head of the biceps (originating from the supraglenoid tubercle) travels between the subscapularis and supraspinatus and with regard to function is considered with the rotator cuff.

The cuff works with the deltoid as a force couple. Coordinated muscle tension in the cuff (and biceps) exerts a compressive force on the humeral head, centering it within the glenoid fossa, thereby establishing a fulcrum for the deltoid to work effectively during shoulder elevation.

Subacromial Space

The subacromial space provides a frictionless interface between the rotator cuff and the coracoacromial (CA) arch, (consisting of the acromial undersurface, AC joint, and CA ligament). The CA ligament spans the space between the coracoid process and the anterior-inferior acromion.

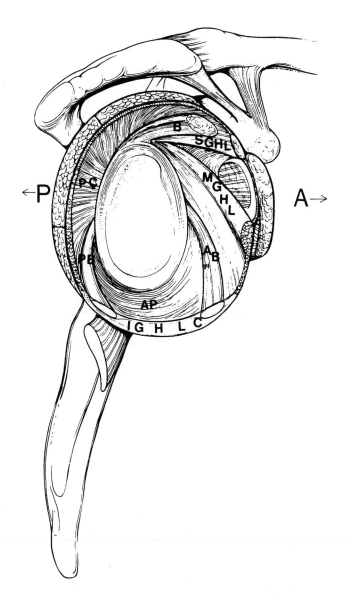

FIGURE 9–2 ■ In this cutaway view of the shoulder joint, the humeral head has been removed, allowing visualization of the interior of the normal glenohumeral anatomy. Notice the discrete ligaments that constitute the anterior shoulder capsule, namely the superior (SGHL), middle (MGHL), and anterior inferior glenohumeral ligaments. In this illustration, the most important anterior restraining structure, the inferior glenohumeral ligament complex (IGHLC), is shown to be further subdivided into having anterior (AB) and posterior (PB) bands and an axillary pouch (AP).

(From Rockwood Jr CA, Matsen III FA (eds): The Shoulder, vol 1. Philadelphia, WB Saunders Company, 1990, p 26; reprinted by permission.)

Acromioclavicular Joint

This diarthrodial joint contains a fibrocartilaginous meniscus and is reinforced by a fibrous capsule. Further stability is provided by the *coracoclavicular (CC) ligaments* (*conoid* and *trapezoid*), which connect the coracoid to the distal clavicle (Fig. 9–3).

Neurovascular Structures

Composed of the anterior nerve roots from C5-T1, the brachial plexus provides motor and sensory function to the upper extremity. Familiarity with the roots, trunks, divisions, cords, and individual branches is crucial to understand peripheral nerve disorders and common shoulder dysfunction. The subclavian artery supplies the upper extremity, becoming the axillary artery as it passes over the first rib. At the inferior border of the latissimus dorsi it becomes the brachial artery.

TECHNIQUES FOR EXAMINATION OF SHOULDER PROBLEMS

Although familiarity with all of the shoulder conditions requires extensive experience on the part of the clinician, most shoulder problems fall into a small number of identifiable conditions. Despite advances in sophisticated imaging studies, the history and physical exam remain the benchmark of diagnostic success.

The most common shoulder complaints are those of pain, stiffness, instability, and weakness. By following an algorithmic ap-

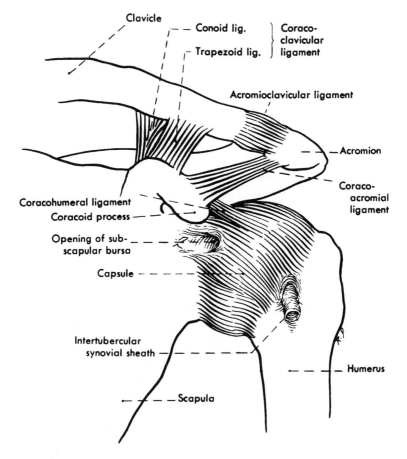

FIGURE 9–3 ■ In this anterior view, note the acromioclavicular joint surrounded by the capsule (acromioclavicular ligament), in addition to the supporting coracoclavicular ligaments, the conoid and trapezoid.

(From Rockwood Jr CA, Matsen III FA (eds): The Shoulder, vol 1. Philadelphia, WB Saunders Company, 1990, p 211; reprinted by permission.)

proach, successful management of most conditions is possible.

History

Determine the nature of the patient's complaint—most commonly pain. When did it begin and how? Was it acute or insidious? What is the nature of the pain? Is it burning in character (think of neurologic causes) or a dull ache over the anterior shoulder (think of rotator cuff pathology)? Does the pain occur during specific activity or with particular positions? For example, pain in the late cocking phase (the shoulder is maximally deducted and externally rotated) of throwing a baseball may be due to mild anterior instability. Alternatively, pain during or after follow-through of the throw may alternatively reflect posterior instability.

The clinician should remember to perform a careful review of systems. Commonly referred patterns of pain are from cervical spine disease or from visceral afferent sources, such as gallstones, peptic ulcer disease, diaphragmatic irritation, cardiac or pulmonary disease.

Several painful conditions, such as rotator cuff impingement or frozen shoulder, may cause pain at night and can lead to nocturnal awakening, usually due to lying on the affected shoulder. Pain at rest may be due to an underlying organic cause, such as tumor or infection.

Stiffness is a common complaint, occurring after trauma, surgery or any period of immobilization. Sometimes, stiffness occurs in the absence of any identifiable cause (i.e., frozen shoulder).

Instability is usually a straightforward complaint, with patients volunteering that they felt their shoulder "go out of place," usually at the time of a traumatic event. Following the first episode, little trauma may be necessary for instability to occur; some patients experience shoulder dislocation when their arm goes over their head while sleeping. Certain types of shoulder instability may present with subluxation (transient incomplete dislocation) rather than dislocation. In the "dead arm syndrome," a feeling of the arm going limp (or "dead") occurs when the shoulder subluxes in the throwing position.

Weakness is the least common shoulder complaint, usually occurring in association with pain, stiffness, or instability. The clinician should inquire about the onset and severity of weakness and the presence of associated symptoms, such as numbness or tingling.

Functional Assessment

Because of the variable severity of shoulder problems as well as differences in handedness, it is important to ascertain arm dominance and in what specific activities the patient is limited. For example, can they perform their daily activities, such as washing under the opposite arm, reaching their perineum, lifting their arm overhead, and sleeping on their affected shoulder? Does their occupation require use of the shoulder?

Physical Examination

A comprehensive and accurate physical examination of the shoulder includes inspection, palpation, range-of-motion assessment, strength testing, and neurovascular examination. Familiarity with some additional tests specific for certain shoulder conditions is diagnostically helpful.

Inspection

Patients should be appropriately gowned to allow inspection of both shoulders and neck. First, perform a quick assessment of the cervical spine, looking for restriction in motion and tenderness to palpation. Have patients raise their arms overhead in order to inspect for pain, referred to as a "painful arc sign," found in patients with impingement. From behind, observe their scapulohumeral rhythm to see if it is smooth and symmetric. Having the patient do a wall push-up may show scapular winging, suggestive of possible serratus anterior weakness (innervation by the long thoracic nerve).

Inspect for evidence of shoulder asymmetry, mass, swelling, erythema, ecchymosis, or muscular atrophy. In AC separation there may be a step-off at the AC joint. In anterior shoulder dislocation, there is anterior shoulder fullness and an abnormally flat contour laterally. In long-standing rotator cuff tears or suprascapular nerve entrapment, the normally full suprascapular and/or infrascapular fossae may be hollow due to muscular atrophy. Ecchymosis may be present in a number of traumatic shoulder conditions, including fracture, dislocations, and acute cuff tears. A globular appearance of the arms' biceps muscle indicates a probable tear of the long head of the biceps.

Palpation

Palpate the shoulder for tenderness, masses, warmth, and crepitus. Begin medially at the SC joint and continue laterally along the clavicle, including the AC joint, coracoid, acromion, and scapular spine. Palpate over the trapezius, deltoid, and spinatae. In acute SC or AC joint sprains, focal tenderness is present. In more chronic conditions, tenderness may be more generalized, with nonspecific trigger points found in the surrounding muscles.

While the patient is actively elevating, palpate directly over the acromion and subacromial space for crepitus. Asymptomatic clicking and/or popping may be normal, but crepitus which is painful and reproduces symptoms, localized to either the AC joint or subacromial bursa, may reflect significant AC joint, rotator cuff, or glenohumeral joint pathology. Crepitus localized to the scapulothoracic bursa may indicate scapulothoracic bursitis, a condition seen in overhand-throwing athletes.

Increased warmth of the shoulder suggests the possibility of infection. Pain on attempted motion is typically present in the septic shoulder. Calcific tendinitis can also present with an acutely painful shoulder mimicking infection, but can be distinguished radiographically by the presence of calcifications near the greater tuberosity.

Range of Motion

In the traumatized or obviously fractured and/or dislocated shoulder, motion assessment should be considered only after obtaining x-rays. In nontraumatized patients, or after ruling out fracture or dislocation, determine patients' active range of motion in forward elevation and external and internal rotation. With the patient seated, forward elevation is determined by having them lift their arm overhead in the plane of the scapula (midway between the coronal and sagittal planes). External rotation is checked with their elbow at their side, rotating their arms out as far as possible. Internal rotation is assessed by having patients put their hand behind them and touch their back as high as they can with their thumb, noting the level of the spinal column reached. As a reference, consider the spine of the scapula T2 and the tip T7.

If there is any discrepancy compared to the opposite side, more careful measurements of passive motion are made with the patient supine, eliminating compensatory spine or trunk motion. Mild restriction is common in a number of conditions, such as following immobilization, trauma, surgery, or with cuff pathology, or arthritis. In moderate-to-severe restriction, consider frozen shoulder as the probable cause.

Strength Testing

Examine for muscular integrity, checking the scapula rotators (ask them to do a wall push-up for the serratus anterior, and a shoulder shrug for the trapezius) and the primary shoulder movers (i.e., pec major and deltoid). The rotator cuff muscles are assessed individually. Integrity of the supraspinatus (the most commonly affected cuff tendon) can be assessed by the *supraspinatus test*. Patients are asked to elevate their arm to a 90-degree position midway between the frontal and coronal plane and hold it, with their thumb pointing downward, against resistance. Weakness and/or a "drop arm" may reflect cuff pathology. The posterior cuff (infraspinatus and teres minor) is examined by having the patient externally rotate against resistance with the elbow at the side.

Neurovascular Assessment

In addition to strength assessment, neurologic exam includes reflex and sensory testing. Biceps (C5), brachioradialis (C6), and triceps (C7) should all be tested. Sensory evaluation relies on the detection of light touch over the thumb web space (radial nerve), the radial aspect of the index finger (median nerve), and the the ulnar aspect of the little finger (ulnar nerve).

Specific Exams

Additional physical examination techniques have been described for specific shoulder conditions, such as rotator cuff impingement, glenohumeral instability, and AC joint arthritis. Impingement signs are useful in identifying rotator cuff pathology (Fig. 9–4). Instability tests attempt to elicit apprehension, pain, or both through provocative shoulder positioning.

Imaging Studies and Other Diagnostic Tests

X-Ray Examination

Standard radiographs include a true anteroposterior (AP) view (AP view of the scapula, not the thorax) (Fig. 9–5) and an axillary lateral view. Additional AP views in internal and external rotation may facilitate identifica-

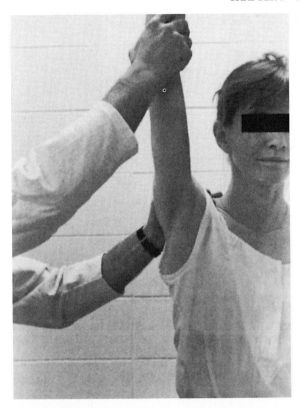

FIGURE 9–4 ■ Impingement of the rotator cuff is demonstrated by passively elevating the shoulder against the fixed scapula. Pain suggests the possibility of mechanical compression of the rotator cuff against the anterior inferior acromion, a process known as impingement.

(From Dele, Jesse C. , Drez, Jr., D. : Orthopaedic Sports Medicine: Principles and Practice, vol 1. Philadelphia, WB Saunders CO, 1994, p 636; reprinted by permission.)

tion of calcific densities that may be otherwise obscured with just a single AP view.

Additional views may sometimes help visualize specific structures. For viewing the AC joint, a "Zanca" view is obtained by tilting the x-ray beam 10 degrees cephalad. The y-outlet lateral view is obtained by shooting the X-ray parallel to the scapular spine, demonstrating the relationship of the humeral head to the glenoid and coracoacromial arch. It is helpful in evaluating calcific deposits, glenohumeral instability, and cuff impingement.

Magnetic Resonance Imaging

Magnetic resonance imaging (MRI) is accurate in identifying full-thickness rotator cuff tears, avascular necrosis, and tumor. In the routine shoulder workup, however, it is an expensive and unnecessary investigative tool.

Arthrogram

This test is performed by injecting radio-opaque contrast into the glenohumeral joint and then looking for the pattern of dye distribution (blunted axillary fold in the frozen shoulder) or abnormal communication of contrast into the subacromial space (indicative of rotator cuff tear).

Bone Scan

Nuclear medicine scans incorporating technetium pyrophosphate have been found to be generally useful in detecting conditions in

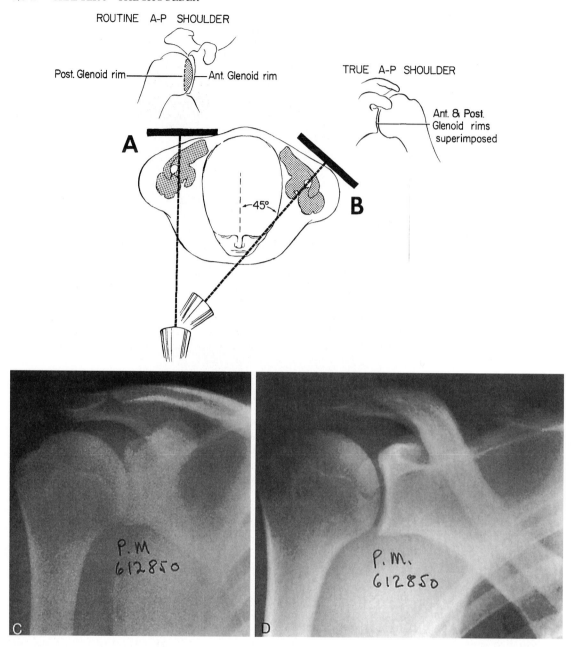

FIGURE 9–5 ■ These illustrations and X-rays demonstrated the importance of obtaining a "true" anteroposterior (AP) perspective of the glenohumeral joint. In X-ray beam (*A*), note that the AP view is actually one of the thorax, yielding an X-ray which shows overlap of the glenohumeral joint. When the beam is angled, however, as in Beam (*B*), a "true" AP view of the glenohumeral joint is obtained. Note the differences in appearance in these views in (*C*) (AP view of the thorax) and (*D*) (true AP view of the glenohumeral joint).

(From Rockwood Jr CA, Matsen III FA (eds): The Shoulder, vol 1. Philadelphia, WB Saunders Company, 1990, p 180; reprinted by permission.)

which there is increased blood supply to an area of the body. Because tumors, infections, fractures, and arthritis can all lead to increased blood flow, bone scans in which certain areas "light up" are not specific. However, when analyzed in the context of the patient's history, physical exam, and x-ray findings, a bone scan can be very useful.

Electrodiagnostic Testing

Electrodiagnostic tests assess the neurologic status of the upper extremity and include electromyography (EMG) and nerve conduction velocity (NCV) testing. In EMG testing, fine wire electrodes are inserted into various muscles and record the resting potential and firing patterns. In NCV testing, the speed with which an electrical impulse is conducted through a specific peripheral nerve is measured, comparing it to the opposite side and reference tables.

Arthroscopy

Diagnostic arthroscopy is the gold standard for evaluation of the shoulder joint. However, it is invasive, expensive, and, in the evaluation of most shoulder problems, unnecessary. Diagnostic arthroscopy is reserved for patients who are refractory to conventional diagnostic evaluation and/or in whom nonoperative treatment has been ineffective.

EVALUATION AND TREATMENT OF COMMON SHOULDER PROBLEMS

The number and variability of different conditions precludes any one treatment approach to the shoulder. An algorithmic approach allows diagnosis and effective management of most problems (Figs. 9–6 and 7).

In principle, initiate treatment immediately after trauma. The application of a sling, ice, and compression decreases bleeding and tissue edema (which often cause greater disability than the injury itself). Rehabilitation, with or without surgery, remains a mainstay of treatment of most shoulder conditions, emphasizing restoration of motion, strength, rhythm, endurance, and function.

The following represents an overview of the basic evaluation and management approach to the most common shoulder problems. For fractures and fracture dislocations of the shoulder, refer to Chapter 3.

AC Joint Sprain (Shoulder Separation)

Sprain of the AC joint is one of the most common traumatic conditions of the shoulder, especially in that segment of the younger population participating in contact sports.

Presentation: Pain directly over the AC joint follows a fall onto the point of the shoulder.

Mechanism of injury: Most commonly this occurs due to direct trauma. The fall applies a significant stress on the AC joint capsule. If the deforming force continues, the stress can injure the supporting CC ligaments.

Relevant anatomy: AC joint stability is rendered by the fibrous AC joint capsule and the CC ligaments (conoid and trapezoid) (Fig. 9–3).

Classification: AC joint injuries are classified according to the amount of damage done to the AC joint and the supporting CC ligaments and are graded type I to VI, based on the degree of injury. Types I and II are inherently stable.

In a type I injury, there is a sprain of the AC joint capsule, without any damage to the underlying CC ligaments. Physical findings are minimal, with focal AC joint tenderness and swelling, but no identifiable deformity on exam or x-ray.

In a type II injury, the AC capsule is completely torn, and the CC ligaments are sprained but still intact. Clinically there may be slight deformity.

In a type III injury, there is "separation" of the shoulder due to complete disruption of both the AC capsule and the CC ligaments, resulting in AC joint instability. There is often an obvious deformity on physical and x-ray examination, showing inferior acromial displacement relative to the relatively prominent distal clavicle.

Types IV, V, and VI are uncommon, unstable AC joint injuries, in which the distal clavicle is markedly displaced posteriorly, superiorly, or inferiorly, respectively, to the acromion.

Physical exam: Findings vary depending on the degree of the sprain, ranging from minimal swelling and tenderness without deformity (type I) to substantial step-off, swelling, and ecchymosis (types III through VI).

X-ray: AC joint radiographs are usually negative in type I, show inferior acromial displacement by up to 50 percent of the clavicle's width in type II, and are ≥100% displaced in type III patients.

Differential diagnosis: Fractures of the distal clavicle are ruled out by x-rays. Osteolysis of the distal clavicle due to repetitive stresses is seen in weight lifters and heavy laborers and causes painful degenerative AC joint changes. Osteoarthritis of the AC joint demonstrates classic radiographic changes (joint space narrowing, sclerosis, osteophyte formation, juxta-articular cysts).

Special tests: Stress views have been recommended to distinguish the stable type II from

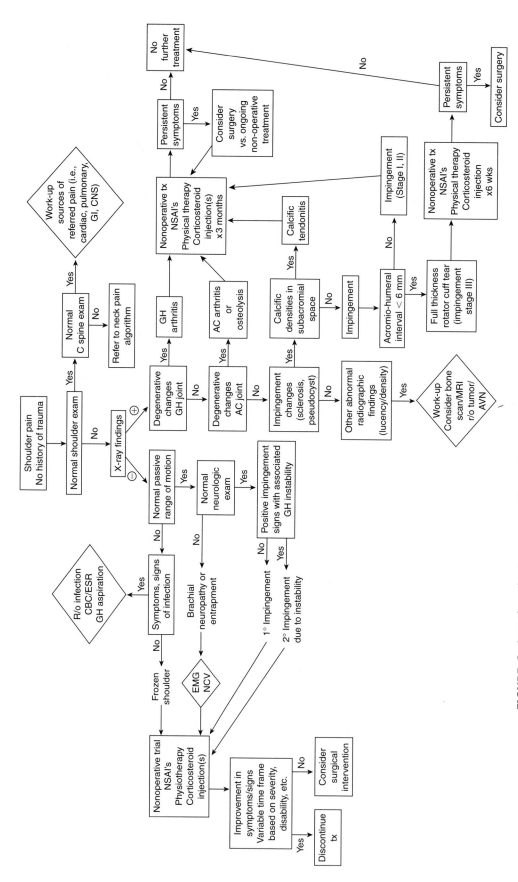

FIGURE 9-6 ■ Algorithmic approach to the diagnosis and treatment of atraumatic shoulder pain.

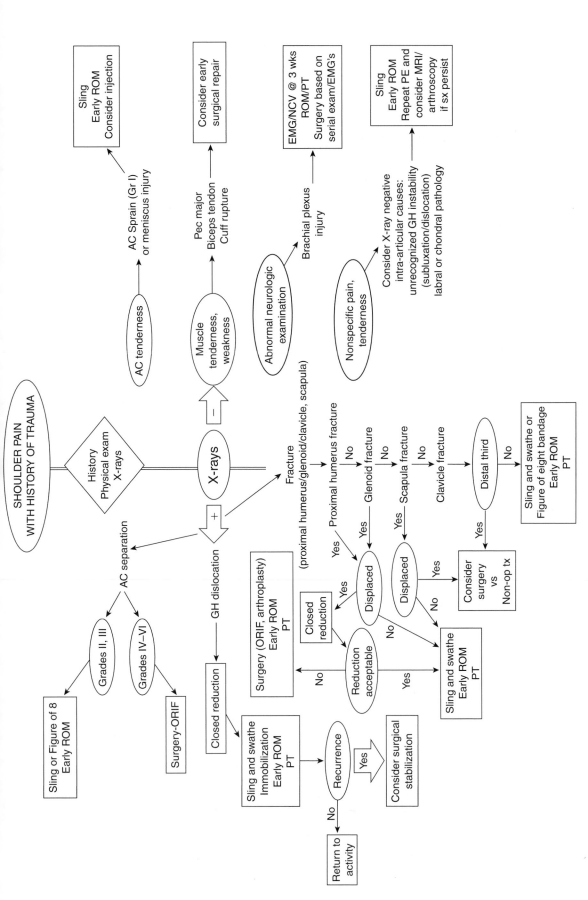

FIGURE 9–7 ■ Algorithmic approach to the diagnosis and treatment of traumatic shoulder pain.

the unstable type III injury. Because the treatment of types II and III is similar, (i.e., nonoperative), however, stress views are probably not only painful, but routinely unindicated. When they are performed, 5 to 15 lbs. of weight should be suspended from the patient's wrists. (If held by the patient, compensatory muscle effort may prevent the detection of instability).

Definitive treatment: Nearly all AC joint injuries are treated symptomatically. All Type I and II injuries are treated nonoperatively with use of a sling or figure-of-eight bandage, ice, and analgesics. Patients are encouraged to use their shoulder as tolerated, with most patients returning to activity within a few weeks. In a small number of cases (<10%), chronic pain may require surgical excision of the distal clavicle (Mumford procedure).

Most Type III injuries are treated nonoperatively as well. The deformity will usually remain noticeable but asymptomatic. In the few patients (10% to 15%) with pain and/or fatigue with overhead activity, surgical reconstruction of the AC joint may be indicated (modified Weaver-Dunn procedure).

Exceptions to nonoperative treatment of type III AC injuries include compromise of the overlying skin, neurovascular injury (rare), or unwillingness to tolerate nonoperative treatment.

Glenohumeral Instability

Of all the joints in the body, the glenohumeral joint is the most commonly dislocated. It is no surprise that the skeletal construct of the shoulder favors mobility at the expense of stability. The large humeral head articulating with the rather flat glenoid fossa makes for an inherently unstable shallow ball and socket design.

Stability is dependent on the surrounding soft-tissue capsular envelope. Injury to this envelope, whether in the form of traumatic capsular disruption or progressive attenuation, leads to subluxation or dislocation.

Instability can be classified according to direction (anterior, posterior, multidirectional); timing (acute, recurrent, chronic); degree (subluxation, dislocation); or cause (traumatic, atraumatic). Anterior dislocation, in which the humeral head dislocates anterior to the glenoid, accounts for the majority of shoulder instability cases.

Presentation: Anterior dislocation most commonly occurs traumatically in teenagers and young adults, usually when the shoulder is abducted and externally rotated. In this position, the humeral head is vulnerable to being levered anteriorly out of its glenoid socket.

Mechanism of injury: Traumatic injury to the shoulder causes tearing and detachment of the anterior soft tissues (the restraint responsible for normal stability—i.e., the AIGHL complex). Detachment of this complex, referred to as a "Bankart lesion," as noted earlier, is thought to be responsible for the instability (Fig. 9–8).

Relevant anatomy: The AIGHL complex (Fig. 9–2) consists of a number of discrete fibrous structures connecting the anterior-inferior glenoid to the proximal humerus. Histologically, discrete identifiable collagen bands have been described, which correspond to visible thickenings in the shoulder capsule. Normally a somewhat loose fold with the arm at the side, this complex has been likened to a hammock, tightening up as the arm is abducted and externally rotated (the "throwing" position), thereby preventing anterior translation. Loss of this normal checkrein—whether due to detachment from the glenoid rim, stretching of its substance, or both—results in anterior instability.

The clinician should be aware of the relationship of the axillary nerve to the proximal humerus, where the nerve is vulnerable to injury. Running along the subscapularis' inferior border, it winds around the humeral neck to emerge posteriorly to supply the teres minor and deltoid. Injury during dislocation or surgical exposure is not uncommon, and familiarity with its location is critical.

Physical exam: In an acute dislocation, the arm is held against the side. The normally rounded lateral shoulder contour is flat, with prominence anteriorly where the humeral head is often palpable. Numbness in the "deltoid patch" due to axillary nerve stretch injury occurs in about 10 percent of patients.

In the patient with a history of suspected or documented recurrent instability, check for anterior instability by provocatively positioning the shoulder in the position of instability. Known as the "anterior apprehension sign," observe the patient as you gently apply an anterior force to the abducted and externally rotated arm. Apprehension or the feeling of impending dislocation ("My arm feels like it's about to come out") confirms the diagnosis.

X-ray: A trauma series must be obtained in any patient with a history of shoulder trauma, including a true AP and an axillary

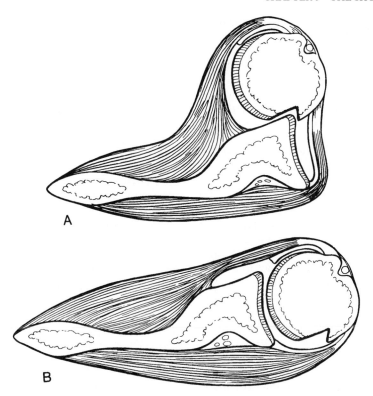

FIGURE 9–8 ■ Viewed from above, the anteriorly dislocated humeral head, the posterolateral articular surface of which is indented against the anterior glenoid, is seen resulting in a so-called "Hill-Sachs" lesion. *(A)* Here the anterior capsule has been detached from the anterior glenoid rim, which is known as a "Bankart lesion." *(B)* At this point the shoulder has reduced, but observe the separation between the anterior glenoid rim and the detached anterior capsule. This illustrates the "Bankart lesion" which is thought responsible for recurrent anterior shoulder instability.

(From Rockwood Jr CA, Matsen III FA (eds): The Shoulder, vol 1. Philadelphia, WB Saunders Company, 1990, p 529; reprinted by permission.)

lateral view. Transthoracic or scapular Y views are acceptable only as additional, not as substitute views, to the axillary lateral.

The Hill-Sachs lesion is a defect in the posterolateral humeral head and has historically been associated with anterior instability (Fig. 9–8). This lesion is thought to occur when the anteriorly dislocated humeral head abuts the anterior glenoid rim during reduction, causing a chondral (cartilage) or osteochondral (bone and cartilage) impression fracture. The presence of this lesion helps confirm previous anterior dislocations, but has otherwise little prognostic value. This fracture can often be seen on x-ray.

Differential diagnosis: Posterior dislocation is ruled out by an axillary lateral x-ray. In patients over the age of 40, associated tearing of the rotator cuff can occur. In the absence of trauma, consider the possibility of multidirectional instability, in which pathologic laxity occurs in more than one direction (most commonly anterior AND inferior).

Special tests: Special tests are unnecessary in most patients. Additional x-ray views may demonstrate a Hill-Sachs (humeral head impression fracture) or a "bony Bankart" lesion. Magnetic resonance imaging and/or an arthrogram are reserved for the patient with suspected rotator cuff injury and are otherwise unreliable and unnecessary in evaluating the soft tissues (labrum and anterior ligaments) after shoulder dislocation. Electrodiagnostic studies are appropriate in the presence of persistent nerve signs and symptoms.

Definitive treatment: Treatment of the first-time dislocator includes appropriate neurovascular and x-ray evaluation, followed by gentle reduction as soon as possible. Reduction is usually achieved more easily when carried out promptly following injury.

Of the numerous described reduction techniques, perhaps the easiest and least traumatic is the Stimson maneuver. Patients are placed prone with their affected arm hanging over the edge of the bed. Secure a small amount of weight (5 to 15 lbs.) to their wrist. Allowing the patient to relax in a dark, quiet area will facilitate reduction. The patient will usually feel the arm slip back into place, with immediate relief. Intravenous sedation and analgesia make this more comfortable, but require observation to avoid respiratory depression and/or emesis and aspiration.

An alternative, more commonly practiced technique is that of traction/counter-traction. During this maneuver, longitudinal traction is applied to the affected arm, while the supine patient is held immobile with a sheet around the torso, either tied or held immobile by an assistant on the patient's opposite side. Gentle sustained traction is almost always rewarded by reduction. Overzealous force can actually hinder reduction efforts and cause more injury. The key to successful reduction is to overcome muscle spasm by steady and sustained effort, rather than abrupt or excessive force.

Following reduction, x-rays are obtained to confirm reduction and rule out any fractures. Physical examination to evaluate axillary nerve function is important. In an older population, manipulation can lead to vascular injury, so be sure to evaluate the patient's radial pulse and look for swelling.

Definitive treatment depends on the patients' age and whether they have had previous instability. In the first-time dislocator, reduction, followed by sling-and-swathe immobilization for a variable period of 1 to 4 weeks, is standard treatment. The risk of recurrent instability is age-related. Under the age of 20, the likelihood of a first-time dislocation becoming a recurrent problem approaches 80 percent. Over the age of 30, the risk is closer to 10 percent. Therefore, most guidelines for treatment, including immobilization, are age-related, with those under 20 subjected to 4 weeks of immobilization, while those over 30 1 to 2 weeks of immobilization. Recent studies question the benefit of immobilization, and some clinicians recommend only minimal sling use.

Progressive motion and strengthening exercises are initiated upon discontinuation of immobilization. The patient is returned to activities when the goals of normal motion, strength, and absence of apprehension are met. Surgery is considered in those patients with recurrent instability, and occasionally in selected elite level athletic patients following a first-time dislocation. Whether performed via conventional open techniques or more recently developed arthroscopic methods, the mainstay of surgical treatment involves reattachment of the detached anterior capsule/labrum (Bankart lesion) to the bony glenoid rim.

Impingement

The most common atraumatic condition affecting the shoulder is *impingement,* also known as rotator cuff tendinitis.

Presentation: The typical presentation is that of insidious onset of anterior shoulder pain sometimes related to overhead activity. The pain is usually a dull ache, which radiates laterally to the region of deltoid insertion.

Mechanism of injury: Conventional theories implicate age-related intrinsic degenerative changes with thinning and weakening of the cuff. Vascular, traumatic, and mechanical processes may each contribute to cuff pathology.

Relevant anatomy: The subscapularis, supraspinatus, infraspinatus, and teres minor coalesce as a tendinous cuff to insert on the proximal humerus. The function of the cuff is primarily that of stabilizing the humeral head, allowing the deltoid to elevate the shoulder.

The subacromial space, immediately above the cuff, provides a frictionless interface between the cuff and the coracoacromial arch. Normal overhead movements result in smooth frictionless gliding of the rotator cuff's bursal surface against the subacromial undersurface, CA ligament, and AC joint. Any process that either (1) interferes with cuff mechanics (resulting in a failure to maintain humeral head/glenoid relationship) or (2) compromises the normal outlet of the coracoacromial arch through which the otherwise normal cuff passes (such as abnormal acromial tilt, shape, or spur) can lead to encroachment on the rotator cuff and is known as "impingement."

Classification: Impingement encompasses a spectrum of pathology, which is classified by clinical criteria into three progressive, overlapping stages. Stage I symptoms are mild, related to overuse or work with the arm overhead, and are seen in younger individuals (<25). Cuff pathology at this early stage is believed to be due to edema and hemorrhage and is reversible with rest.

Stage II impingement occurs in a slightly older patient, between 25 and 40 years of age. Symptoms are often present for weeks or months at the time of presentation. This stage involves less reversible pathologic cuff changes of tendinitis and fibrosis.

In stage III, patients are usually over the age of 45, and symptoms are often chronic. Rotator cuff structural damage is to some degree irreversible, often leading to full-thickness tear of the supraspinatus tendon.

Physical exam: Observation of patients lifting their arm overhead demonstrates the **painful arc sign,** with discomfort from 70 to 120 degrees. Motion is not usually restricted.

The most commonly used physical exam techniques are those described by Neer and Hawkins. In **Neer's impingement sign,** the affected arm is elevated in the sagittal plane against the scapula, compressing the cuff against the unyielding coracoacromial arch. Hawkins emphasized the forcible and internal rotation of the shoulder as a more specific technique. Supraspinatus testing is performed by resisting patients' shoulder elevation midway between the coronal and sagittal plane, with their thumb pointing downward. Pain and/or weakness may indicate cuff involvement. Posterior cuff involvement is assessed through external rotation strength testing.

X-ray: Acromial sclerosis, spurring of the distal clavicle or AC joint, and a "pseudocyst" of the greater tuberosity are common findings. Acromiohumeral interval narrowing is a late finding found in chronic full-thickness cuff tears.

Differential diagnosis: Shoulder pain can be due to a variety of conditions, including frozen shoulder, arthritis (e.g., degenerative, inflammatory), osteonecrosis, infection, traumatic intra-articular injuries, and tumor. In young patients with impingement pain, underlying instability must be considered.

Special tests: In the impingement injection test, symptomatic relief following the injection of a local anesthetic, such as 1 percent lidocaine, into the subacromial bursa indicates the likelihood that pathology within this space is responsible for the symptoms. Imaging tests are ordered only when there is suspicion of a cuff tear, and/or when symptoms fail to respond to treatment. Imaging of the rotator cuff is achieved through arthrography or MRI. In an arthrogram, dye injected into the glenohumeral joint normally outlines the joint and the undersurface of the rotator cuff. The abnormal presence of dye in the subacromial space above the cuff is indicative of a rotator cuff tear.

Magnetic resonance imaging allows direct visualization of the cuff and surrounding soft tissues. It is more sensitive and accurate than arthrography, is noninvasive, and does not involve radiation. It is also considerably more expensive, although the combination of improving technology and managed care is making MRI a more affordable and cost-effective imaging choice.

Definitive treatment: Nonoperative rehabilitation is successful in most patients. The principles of impingement treatment include:

1. eliminating inflammation and pain
2. restoring range of motion
3. improving strength of cuff and scapular rotators
4. optimizing scapulohumeral rhythm and coordination
5. conditioning
6. reinitiating similar biomechanical motion/activity, attending to and correcting activity mechanics as necessary
7. returning the patient to activity.

Corticosteroid preparations injected into the subacromial space have been found to be effective in decreasing pain and inflammation. Because of concern about possible tendon damage, injections are used infrequently and the number of injections limited to no more than three over a 6-month period.

Therapy may last only several weeks for the minimally symptomatic athlete who "overdid it," versus prolonged treatment for the chronically symptomatic individual. The decision to intervene surgically depends on a combination of factors including the patient's stage of involvement, response to treatment, and goals for return to activity.

Surgical treatment is indicated for those patients in whom nonoperative management has been ineffective. Surgery involves either open or arthroscopic decompression of the subacromial space and, when necessary, debridement and/or repair of the rotator cuff.

Calcific Tendinitis

Calcific tendinitis is a common disorder in which calcification occurs within the rotator cuff tendons.

Presentation: Calcific tendinitis presents similarly to impingement, with insidious onset of shoulder pain. Occasionally, the presentation is more acute, with severe pain.

Etiology: Primary degeneration of the fibers of the rotator cuff are thought to be the stimulus for deposition of hydroxyapatite crystals.

Physical exam: Physical findings are similar to those of impingement, with Neer and Hawkins impingement signs. Motion is not usually restricted, although when presenting acutely may be limited due to pain.

X-ray: X-rays establish the diagnosis, with calcific deposits visualized near the cuff's insertion. Because a single AP may miss the deposit due to overlying shadows, additional AP views in internal and external rotation help visualize and localize any calcific densities.

Differential diagnosis: Calcific tendinitis is differentiated from impingement radiographically by the presence of calcific deposits in the former condition. A small number of patients will present with acute calcific tendonitis and clinically present similarly to a septic shoulder. The patient is usually unwilling to allow any passive shoulder movement. Subacromial lidocaine (often with a corticosteroid) injection into the region of the deposit is diagnostically confirmatory and is therapeutic as well. In the patient with suspected septic arthritis, joint aspiration and study of aspirate for cell count, differential, gram stain, and culture is indicated.

Special tests: Radiographs are diagnostic. No further tests are necessary.

Definitive treatment: Most patients respond to simple nonoperative treatment including analgesics, nonsteroidal anti-inflammatory drugs, local modalities, and corticosteroid injections. Some patients benefit from "needling" the deposit percutaneously. For those with symptoms refractory to nonoperative management, open or arthroscopic surgical excision of the calcific deposits is usually effective.

Frozen Shoulder (Adhesive Capsulitis)

Occurring in up to 5 percent of the population, frozen shoulder is a clinical syndrome in which there is restriction in glenohumeral motion for which no specific cause can be determined.

Presentation: The typical presentation is that of a 50-year-old with a several-month history of progressive pain and stiffness in the nondominant shoulder. The pain is generalized, occasionally nocturnal, and accompanied by stiffness. Patients note difficulty reaching behind them or sometimes even washing their hair or raising their arm overhead.

Etiology: The etiology of the frozen shoulder is unknown. The name "adhesive capsulitis" has been used in recognition of the adhesive and restrictive qualities affecting the shoulder capsule.

Classification: There are three overlapping clinical phases in the course of the frozen shoulder: painful, stiffening, and thawing.

Physical exam: The hallmark of the physical exam is restriction in both active and passive motion of variable severity.

X-ray: Except for osteopenia (decreased bone density), there are no specific x-ray findings in the frozen shoulder.

Differential diagnosis: Obtaining an axillary lateral x-ray is paramount before one can rule out posterior shoulder dislocation. Some shoulders are stiff but not truly "frozen." These include patients with other intrinsic shoulder problems in which stiffness is but one component (arthritis, rotator cuff impingement, fracture or dislocation).

Special tests: An arthrogram (injection of contrast agent into the glenohumeral joint) demonstrates <10 cm^3 of contrast fluid (compared to the normal 15 to 20 cm^3) accommodated by the shoulder joint capsule and a blunted (instead of normal) axillary fold.

Definitive treatment: Treatment is nonoperative in most cases. This condition is somewhat frustrating because resolution of tightness is slow, and there is no one predictably effective treatment. The patient is instructed and sometimes supervised in therapy exercises to restore motion, supplemented by corticosteroid injections. Occasionally, the severely or refractory frozen shoulder is manipulated under anesthesia. Surgery to release the extracapsular and capsular adhesions may be necessary, and is effected through either traditional open, or newer arthroscopic methods.

Degenerative Glenohumeral Arthritis

Primary osteoarthritis of the glenohumeral joint is much less common than that of the weight-bearing hip and knee joints.

Presentation: Pain is the most common complaint, often accompanied by stiffness. When secondary to old trauma, avascular necrosis, cuff pathology, or inflammatory arthritis, there is a history of preceding symptoms.

Etiology: A number of diseases and traumatic events can lead to destruction of the normal articular cartilage of the glenohumeral joint.

Physical exam: Pain on active and passive motion is present. Variable restriction in motion may be detected. Crepitus on range of motion is often palpable.

X-ray: Classic features of degenerative arthritis are seen, including joint space narrowing, subchondral sclerosis, osteophyte formation, and the presence of juxta-articular cysts.

Differential diagnosis: The differential is that of the painful, stiff shoulder, which is rather broad. X-rays, however, allow the diagnosis to be readily established by the typical radiographic findings. Septic arthritis, although relatively uncommon, can present similarly, but usually the patient is somewhat debilitated and has constitutional signs (e.g., fever, chills, malaise). Joint aspiration for gram stain, cell count, differential, and culture establish the diagnosis of sepsis. Another sometimes confusing presentation is the neuropathic shoulder, which radiographically shows severe destructive changes which are disproportionate to the patient's mild and occasionally painless presentation. Ossous debris around the joint is a tip-off. Because this condition occurs due to underlying neurologic disease, workup includes a thorough neurologic examination (electrodiagnostic tests, cervical spine x-ray and MRI valuation).

Special tests: For the standard degenerative arthritic shoulder no special tests are necessary.

Definitive treatment: Treatment is symptomatic, with activity modification and analgesics prescribed early in the course, supplemented as necessary with corticosteroid injections. Definitive treatment involves replacing the worn proximal humeral and glenoid articular surfaces with a metal humeral head and a polyethylene glenoid cup.

Other Conditions

A number of other less common conditions afflict the shoulder and should be considered in the differential diagnosis of the patient with shoulder pain. These include inflammatory arthritides, avascular necrosis, reflex-sympathetic dystrophy, intra-articular traumatic disorders (labral tears, chondral lesions), and multidirectional instability. In-depth discussion of each of these less common entities is beyond the scope of this chapter but an understanding of their specific features is important in the management of the patient with shoulder complaints.

CONCLUSION

The shoulder is uniquely designed to provide power and precision through a nearly limitless range of motion. But the price of such mobility is instability, one of the most common problems affecting the shoulder joint. Successful evaluation of most shoulder problems is achieved through a careful history, physical, and radiographic examination. Nonoperative treatment is effective in the management of most shoulder problems.

SUGGESTED READINGS

Rockwood Jr CA, Matsen III FA (eds): The Shoulder. Philadelphia, WB Saunders Company, 1990.

Pettrone FA (ed): Athletic Injuries of the Shoulder. New York, McGraw-Hill, Inc., 1995.

Chapter 10

The Elbow

Benjamin S. Shaffer

INTRODUCTION

Compared to the powerful and mobile shoulder above, and the precise wrist and hand below, the elbow seems functionally outdone. But it is the simple movement and stability of the elbow joint that ensures our ability to perform essential daily activities. The purpose of this chapter is to highlight the elbow's functional anatomy, describe how to evaluate elbow complaints, discuss general principles of treatment and present an overview of common elbow problems.

FUNCTIONAL ANATOMY

Skeletal

The elbow contains two distinct types of joints that allow hinge-like motion in the flexion-extension plane and rotatory motion in the pronation-supination plane. Unlike the shoulder, whose stability is dependent on surrounding soft tissues, the elbow is highly constrained skeletally. The distal humerus contains two articular regions, the trochlea and the capitellum, separated by the trochlear-capitellar groove (Fig. 10–1). Medially, the trochlea articulates precisely, with its mated concave semilunar notch of the proximal ulna of the forearm providing the stable hinge function of the elbow. Laterally, the spherical capitellum articulates against the shallow concavity of the radial head.

Important anatomic skeletal landmarks of the distal humerus are: (1) the medial and lateral epicondyles to which the forearm muscles attach; (2) the olecranon fossa posteriorly, into which the olecranon tip seats in elbow extension; and (3) the coronoid fossa anteriorly, into which the coronoid tip enters during elbow flexion.

The notch of the proximal ulna into which the distal humerus' trochlea of the distal humerus articulates is known as the "semilunar notch." The anterior lip of the notch is known as the "coronoid process," to which the brachialis muscle attaches. The biceps tendon attaches to the bicipital tuberosity of the proximal radius.

Soft Tissue

A number of soft tissues provide additional support to the inherently stable elbow joint. The most important of these is the medial collateral ligament (MCL), composed of anterior, posterior, and transverse bands (Fig. 10–2). The anterior band is the most important structure in providing normal stability. It arises on the anteroinferior surface of the medial epicondyle and attaches to the medial aspect of the coronoid process.

Laterally, there is more variability and less reliance on discrete ligament function. The radial collateral ligament is not as well defined as its medial counterpart. The lateral ulnar collateral ligament originates from the lateral epicondyle and blends with the fibers of the annular ligament to insert on the tubercle of the crest of the supinator on the ulna. This

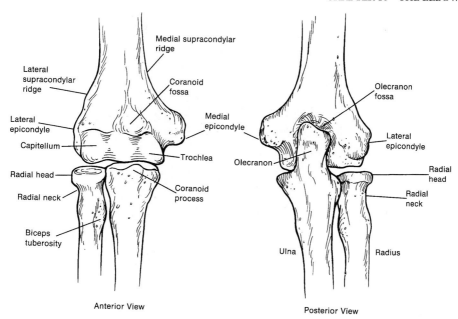

FIGURE 10–1 ■ Anterior and posterior views of the elbow joint demonstrate normal skeletal anatomy, including the three articulations: the ulno trochlear joint, the radio capitellar joint, and the proximal radioulnar joint.

(From Figure 8-1 in The Elbow Chapter 8, in Essentials of Orthopaedic Surgery, First Edition, p 214)

is thought to be the primary lateral stabilizer of the elbow and it is taut throughout flexion and extension. The annular ligament is a circular group of fibers attached to the radial notch of the ulna. This ligament surrounds the radial head and neck, maintaining normal alignment of the proximal radius.

Anteriorly and posteriorly, the elbow joint is lined by a single-cell layer of synovium, which in turn is covered by a relatively thick

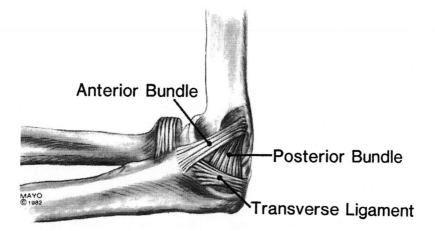

FIGURE 10–2 ■ This sagittal view demonstrates the three bundles or bands of the normal medial collateral ligament. The anterior band is the most important in elbow stability.

(From Morrey BF (ed): The Elbow and Its Disorders, ed 2. Philadelphia, WB Saunders Company, 1993, p 29; reprinted by permission.)

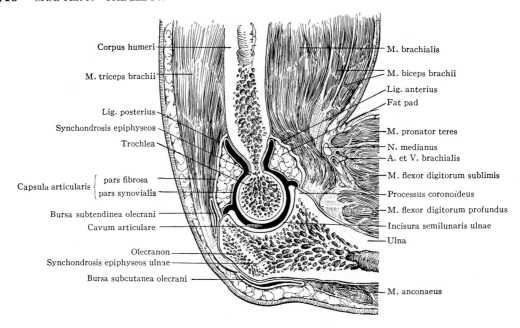

Corpus humeri

M. triceps brachii

Lig. posterius

Synchondrosis epiphyseos

Trochlea

Capsula articularis { pars fibrosa
pars synovialis

Bursa subtendinea olecrani

Cavum articulare

Olecranon

Synchondrosis epiphyseos ulnae

Bursa subcutanea olecrani

M. brachialis

M. biceps brachii

Lig. anterius

Fat pad

M. pronator teres

N. medianus

A. et V. brachialis

M. flexor digitorum sublimis

Processus coronoideus

M. flexor digitorum profundus

Incisura semilunaris ulnae

Ulna

M. anconaeus

FIGURE 10–3 ■ Sagittal illustration of the elbow joint demonstrates the normal skeletal and soft-tissue anatomy. Note the presence of fat pads both anteriorly and posteriorly, directly outside the joint capsule. Intra-articular swelling can lead to displacement out of the olecranon (posterior) or coronoid (anterior) fossa, leading to the appearance of "positive fat pad sign(s)" on lateral x-rays.

(From Morrey BF (ed): The Elbow and Its Disorders, ed 2. Philadelphia, WB Saunders Company, 1993, p 20; reprinted by permission.)

fibrous capsule. In the olecranon and coronoid fossa, a fatty layer of tissue is present between the synovium and the capsule. This layer is of significance in radiographic evaluation of elbow trauma, in which intra-articular (intracapsular) effusion (fluid) or hemarthrosis (bleeding into the joint) causes capsular distension and displacement of these fat pads either anterior or posterior to their usual position (Fig. 10–3). Identification of these usually absent fat pads (particularly the posterior fat pad, which is usually deeply contained within the olecranon fossa) suggests joint injury or fracture.

Muscles

Muscles about the elbow can be divided into four basic groups on the basis of location and function. Anteriorly are the elbow flexors, the strongest of which is the biceps, arising proximally through a long and short head, and inserting through its tendinous attachment to the biceps tuberosity on the proximal radius. The bicipital aponeurosis, or lacertus fibrosis,

is a web-like fascial veil that descends in the antecubital fossa, attaching to the medial and distal deep fascia of the forearm. The other significant elbow flexor, the brachialis muscle, arises from the anterior distal humerus and inserts on the proximal ulna. Both muscles are innervated by the musculocutaneous nerve, a continuation of the lateral cord of the brachial plexus.

Posteriorly lies the triceps, the strongest elbow extensor, arising from three heads (medial, lateral, and long) to insert on the olecranon tip. Innervation is via the radial nerve, a continuation of the posterior cord of the brachial plexus.

Medially lie the "flexor-pronator" muscles, named for their function, including the pronator teres, the flexor carpi radialis, the palmaris longus, and the flexor carpi ulnaris. These muscles arise from the medial epicondyle, and are all innervated by the median nerve. They provide wrist flexion and forearm pronation.

Laterally are the muscles of the "supinator-extensor" group. Including the brachioradialis, the extensor carpi radialis longus and brevis, and the extensor digitorum communis, these muscles arise from the lateral epicondyle and provide wrist extension and forearm supination. All are innervated by branches of the radial nerve.

Neurovascular

In contrast to the deeper-seated peripheral nerves of other extremities, those about the elbow are uniquely vulnerable to both direct and indirect injury. Injuries or symptoms due to nerve involvement around the elbow make familiarization with normal nerve anatomy crucial.

Musculocutaneous Nerve: Continuing from the lateral cord of the brachial plexus, composed of C5-C8 nerve roots, this nerve travels through (and innervates) the biceps and brachialis, terminating as the lateral antebrachial cutaneous nerve of the forearm.

Median Nerve: Arising from C5-T1 nerve roots, combined from the upper and lower cords, the median nerve travels along the anterior brachialis muscle, entering the antecubital fossa and passing medial to the biceps tendon and the brachial artery. It provides motor innervation to the pronator teres, through which it passes, and continues distally in the forearm under the flexor digitorum sublimis. Distally, the median nerve provides sensory innervation of the radial palm and digits.

Radial Nerve: Originating from C6, 7, and 8 nerve roots, the radial nerve is a continuation of the posterior cord that travels in the radial groove of the humerus. It innervates the triceps, brachioradialis, and extensor carpi radialis longus and brevis muscles. In the antecubital fossa the nerve divides into a deep motor branch (posterior interosseous nerve) and a superficial sensory branch. The superficial branch continues underneath the brachioradialis to provide sensation to the middorsal cutaneous forearm.

Ulnar Nerve: Derived from roots C8 and T1, the ulnar nerve continues from the medial cord of the brachial plexus, along the arm, until it passes posteriorly through the inter-

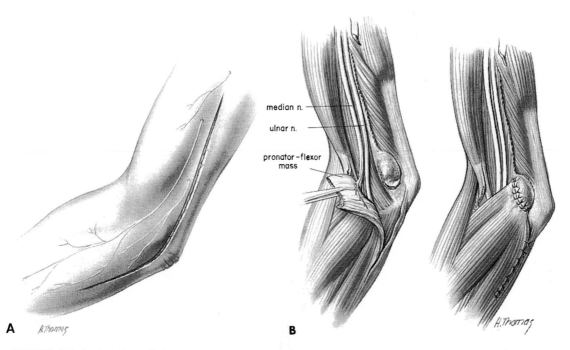

FIGURE 10–4 ■ *A,* A medial incision is made over the elbow, allowing exposure of the ulnar nerve proximal, through, and distal to the cubital tunnel through which it travels. *B,* The ulnar nerve is transposed submuscularly underneath the flexor-pronator muscle mass, after which the muscle origin is reattached to the medial epicondyle.

(From Morrey BF (ed): The Elbow and Its Disorders, ed 2. Philadelphia, WB Saunders Company, 1993, p 823; reprinted by permission.)

muscular septum about 8 cm proximal to the elbow. It then travels through the cubital tunnel, where pathologic compression, traction, or irritation can occur. In the forearm, the ulnar nerve innervates the flexor carpi ulnaris and the ulnar half of the flexor digitorum profundus. Distally, it continues to provide motor to the dorsal interosseous and sensation to the skin of the ulnar wrist and hand.

Brachial Artery: The brachial artery lies anterior to the medial aspect of the brachialis muscle, entering the antecubital space medial to the biceps tendon and lateral to the median nerve. At the level of the radial head, it then divides into its terminal branches, the ulnar and radial arteries.

EVALUATION OF ELBOW PROBLEMS

The evaluation of elbow problems relies on a thorough history, physical, and radiographic examination, supplemented by other pertinent tests when necessary.

History

The most common complaint involving the elbow is pain, although stiffness and occasionally mechanical symptoms such as locking or catching may accompany or overshadow other complaints. How did it start, acutely or insidiously? Characterize the nature of the pain, starting with its location. What is the nature of the pain—is it burning or radiating (nerve) or is it an aching related only to activity (tendinitis)? Does it hurt at rest or at night (tumor, infection)? Is it associated with any other symptoms, such as neck pain (referred pathology from the cervical spine) or wrist pain (distal radioulnar joint problem)?

What is the relationship of the patients' activity to their symptoms? For example, in a throwing athlete, when during the pitch or throw does the pain occur? Medial elbow pain when the arm is in the "cocking position" suggests MCL pathology, whereas medial pain during follow-through suggests involvement of the flexor pronator group.

Determine what treatments, if any, have helped. Have the patients had any cortisone injections? What other type of treatments— e.g., physical therapy, nonsteroidal anti-inflammatory drugs (NSAIDs)—have they had, and with what effect? Have they had previous surgery?

The elbow is commonly involved (and sometimes one of the first joints affected) in inflammatory arthritides, so it is important to elicit a history of other joint complaints, known arthritis, and family history. Is there a history of skin problems (lupus, dermatitis, psoriasis) or gastrointestinal problems (colitis)? Have there been any systemic symptoms of illness (malaise, fevers)?

Numbness, tingling, and weakness may be obvious clues to neurologic involvement, but sometimes nerve entrapment syndromes present with pain only. In addition to inquiring about tingling or numbness, ask about any weakness or clumsiness.

Perhaps the most important part of the history is determining how the symptoms interfere with function. Inability to flex the elbow completely is well tolerated by most patients, because we generally rely on an arc of 30 to 130 degrees for most activities of daily living. But in patients with rheumatoid arthritis, for example, in whom shoulder motion is also compromised, elbow restriction may interfere with their ability to feed or perform simple hygiene themselves.

Physical Examination

Examination of the elbow includes inspection, palpation, range-of-motion assessment, and evaluation for strength and neurovascular integrity. A few special physical exam tests are helpful in evaluating specific conditions. The physical exam must include evaluation of the shoulder and, when relevant, the cervical spine and the wrist/hand.

During inspection, note the presence of swelling, ecchymosis, atrophy, or asymmetry. Note the "carrying angle" formed between the longitudinal axis of the humerus and the forearm, normally 10 to 15 degrees.

With the elbow flexed 90 degrees, note that the normal bony prominence (medial and lateral epicondyles and the olecranon) form an equilateral triangle. In dislocations, this normal relationship is distorted. Look for evidence of joint swelling laterally by inspection of the soft tissue triangle bordered by the radial head, olecranon tip, and lateral epicondyle.

Palpate for tenderness, soft-tissue integrity, and crepitus. Include the anterior, medial, lateral, and posterior structures in an organized systematic fashion. Be specific in trying to identify the exact area of tenderness. For example, lateral epicondylitis (lateral tennis elbow) causes focal tenderness over the lateral epicondyle. Tenderness more distally in the proximal forearm may instead suggest posterior interosseous nerve entrapment. Medial elbow pain may reflect medial epicondylitis (medial tennis elbow), if there is tenderness directly over the epicondyle. When more distal, it may be due to MCL insufficiency. Palpate posteriorly over the olecranon fossa. Notice the presence of any bursae over the olecranon tip, occasionally containing fluid and occasionally palpable fibrous fragments (olecranon bursitis). Palpate over the antecubital fossa for any defect in the biceps tendon attachment (distal biceps tendon rupture).

Check both active and passive motion, noting any difference between them. If passive motion is greater than active motion, consider pain, muscle, or nerve injury as possible causes. Patients tend to splint their elbow between 60 and 90 degrees following trauma because the capsule accommodates the maximum amount of fluid in this position. In the absence of trauma, pain on passive elbow motion suggests infection.

Note the location and timing of pain during motion. Discomfort at terminal extension is common in posterior olecranon impingement. Crepitus over the radiocapitellar joint during pronation/supination may indicate localized synovial or chondral pathology, degenerative changes, or radial neck fracture.

The extent of neurologic evaluation depends on patients' symptoms, but be familiar with sensory, motor, and reflex exam. Check for sensation to light touch in the distribution of the specific peripheral nerves. For the ulnar nerve, check the ulnar border of the little finger. For the median, use the radial border of the index finger. Check radial sensory function over the thumb's dorsal web space. The specific nerve roots have overlapping innervation, but in general, the lateral arm is the C5 dermatome, the lateral forearm C6, the middle finger C7, and the medial forearm and arm C8 and T1.

Strength testing depends on familiarity with the innervation of the various muscle groups. Reflex testing is performed for the biceps (C5), brachioradialis (C6), and triceps (C7).

Vascular assessment includes palpation of the radial and ulnar arteries at the wrist, and the brachial artery at the antecubital fossa.

Additional physical examination tests may be useful depending on the condition suspected. When considering medial epicondylitis, check for pain on wrist flexion or forearm pronation against resistance. Medial collateral ligament sprain or attenuation is determined by applying a valgus stress to the slightly flexed elbow, looking to either reproduce pain or detect abnormal medial joint opening. Lateral epicondylitis can be assessed by reproducing pain by wrist extension and/or forearm supination against resistance.

The Tinel's sign is useful in assessment of nerve problems. Gently tapping over the nerve in the vicinity of suspected entrapment or pathology reproduces the symptoms, causing numbness, tingling, or pain in the nerve's distribution. During flexion and extension, the ulnar nerve may be "unstable," and can be felt subluxing or completely dislocating out of its cubital tunnel.

Imaging Studies and Other Diagnostic Tests

X-Ray Examination

Anteroposterior (AP) and lateral x-rays are the minimum views necessary to evaluate the elbow joint. Following trauma, additional views are sometimes helpful, including oblique, radial head, and axillary views.

Stress X-rays

Stress views may be helpful in evaluating the patient with a suspected tear of the MCL. This is achieved through manual stress, during which the clinician applies a valgus stress to the elbow in an effort to open up the medial side. Difference between the affected and normal elbow of >2mm is probably significant.

Computerized Tomography/Magnetic Resonance Imaging Examination

Computerized tomography scans are effective in preoperative planning of complex elbow trauma and may be useful in evaluating for loose bodies of the elbow.

Magnetic resonance imaging provides superior soft tissue imaging. Its current utility about the elbow is in helping to image tumors, demonstrate joint effusion, and evaluate osteochondritis dissecans. It is unnecessary and unreliable in evaluating medial or lateral epicondylitis or MCL injury, and it is rarely helpful in nerve entrapment syndrome workup.

Technetium-99 Bone Scan

Technetium-99 injected intravenously is taken up in areas of increased vascularity. Although it is very sensitive, this test is not very specific, because increased blood flow can occur in a variety of conditions, such as fracture, infection, tumor, or arthritis. In patients with heterotopic ossification, serial bone scans over time may help determine when the process has become quiescent enough to permit safe bone mass excision.

Electrodiagnostic Tests

Electromyography and nerve conduction velocity testing have definite indications in the patient with suspected nerve entrapment or injury. Such testing may indicate the site of the compression or injury. However, failure to demonstrate specific neurologic findings by electrodiagnostic testing does not rule out their presence. This is commonly the problem in working up the patient with early ulnar nerve symptoms or the patient with suspected posterior interosseous nerve entrapment syndrome, in whom such even electrodiagnostic tests are commonly negative.

Arthroscopy

Although generally reserved for therapeutic use, arthroscopy provides a minimally invasive means with which to visually inspect, and when necessary, palpate and/or treat the intra-articular structures. The indications for diagnostic arthroscopy include persistent symptoms unresponsive to nonoperative treatment, and/or symptoms undiagnosed by other noninvasive means.

TREATMENT OF ELBOW PROBLEMS

Treatment of elbow problems is algorithmic, dividing conditions into those resulting from either a traumatic or an atraumatic cause (Figs. 10–5 and 10–6). In traumatic conditions, treatment is divided into immediate and definitive strategies. Immediate treatment for elbow trauma is similar to that of traumatic injury elsewhere, and includes the principles of RICE: rest, ice, compression and elevation. The combination of vascular vulnerability and relatively confining soft-tissue envelope of the forearm renders elbow trauma at risk of leading to compartment syndromes.

Nonoperative Treatment

Rehabilitation

The goals of rehabilitation include (1) decrease pain and inflammation, (2) restore motion, (3) optimize strength, and (4) return to normal function and activity.

Inflammation and pain are treated with activity modification, analgesics, NSAIDs, and local modalities, including ice, heat, electrical stimulation, and ultrasound.

Elbow stiffness is best treated by prevention. Do not immobilize or use a sling any longer than absolutely necessary. Motion loss is usually in extension (inability to completely straighten the elbow), and takes much longer to regain than to lose. Once lost, motion return is best achieved through active exercise by the patient, rather than passive stretching by the therapist. A unique characteristic of the elbow is its propensity to develop heterotopic ossification—that is, bone formation within the soft tissues. This is particularly common anteriorly because of the presence of the brachialis muscle immediately anterior to the elbow capsule. The risk of ossification is increased with passive stretching, and for this reason, aggressive passive motion is discouraged. Specially designed splints that exert a dynamic force across the elbow are sometimes effective in restoring motion.

Corticosteroid Injections

The use of corticosteroids about the elbow facilitates treatment of a number of conditions, including medial and lateral epicondylitis, olecranon bursitis, and, less commonly, inflammatory or degenerative arthritis.

Because corticosteroid injections can lead to tendon damage, dermal depigmentation, and infection, they should not be used arbitrarily or excessively. Generally, their use is reserved for conditions that fail initial activity modification, NSAIDs and therapy. The exact timing and number of injections is controversial, but in general no more than three injections should be given over a 6-month time period.

Operative Treatment

Surgery is reserved for those patients whose symptoms are refractory to or inappropriately treated by nonoperative means. Surgery can

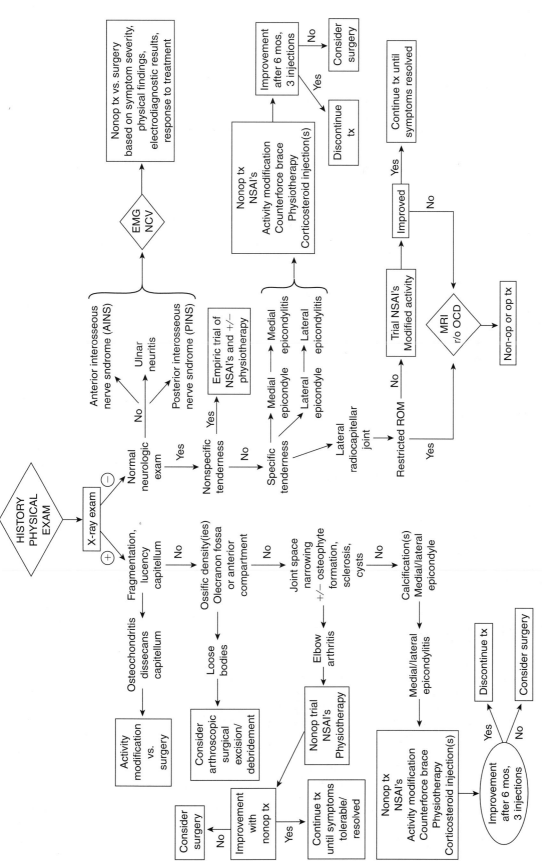

FIGURE 10–5 ■ Algorithmic approach to the diagnosis and treatment of atraumatic elbow pain.

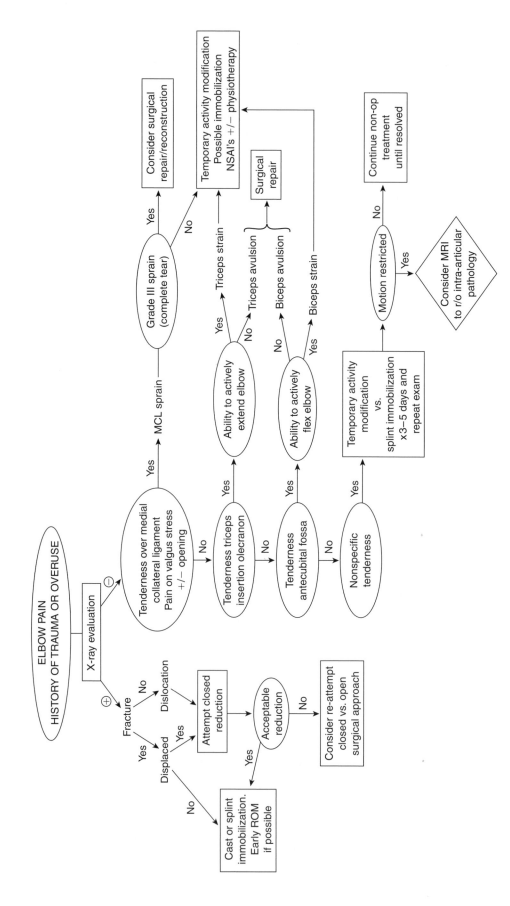

FIGURE 10-6 ■ Algorithmic approach to the diagnosis and treatment of traumatic elbow pain.

be performed via open or arthroscopic technique. Arthroscopy is an effective technique for removal of loose bodies, synovial biopsy, and osteochondral debridement (osteochondritis dissecans, trauma, arthritis).

EVALUATION AND TREATMENT OF COMMON ELBOW PROBLEMS

The following discussion highlights selected examples of common elbow problems. For more specific discussion of fracture evaluation and management, the reader is referred to Chapter 3 on fractures.

Elbow Dislocation

The elbow is the second most commonly dislocated major joint of the body, and is the most common dislocation seen in children under the age of 10. By far the most common type is posterior, in which the olecranon dislocates posteriorly relative to the humerus.

Presentation: A fall on the outstretched upper extremity accounts for most dislocations.

Relevant anatomy: Posterior dislocation results in complete tearing of the MCL. Associated injuries are common, such as radial head and neck fractures (5 to 10%), avulsion fractures from the medial or lateral epicondyle (12%), and fractures of the coronoid process (10%).

Classification: The most common type is posterior, followed by anterior, and rarely, divergent.

Physical exam: There is visible deformity, with loss of the normal bony equilateral triangle. Swelling is common. The ulnar nerve is the most commonly injured nerve. Significant swelling anteriorly can lead to compartment syndrome of the forearm.

X-ray: An AP and lateral x-ray are sufficient to make the diagnosis. The radial head should line up with the capitellum on both views. Failure to do so suggests residual subluxation.

Differential diagnosis: X-rays rule out fractures and establish the diagnosis.

Special tests: None are necessary. In the patient with median nerve injuries, think of arterial injury because of the median nerve's proximity to the brachial artery. If there is any question, arteriographic evaluation is appropriate.

Definitive treatment: Initial neurovascular and radiographic assessment is followed by prompt reduction. Reduction is effected through manual forearm traction and brachial countertraction. The elbow is assessed for stability following reduction. If it is stable throughout the range of motion, application of a splint and sling, followed by early range of motion exercises is indicated. If the elbow starts to sublux or dislocate, immobilization at 90 degrees is appropriate for a longer period, but usually no more than 3 weeks to minimize the risk of permanent stiffness.

Medial Collateral Ligament Sprain

Medial collateral ligament sprain can occur due to a single traumatic or, more commonly, to repetitive stresses. It is particularly common among baseball pitchers.

Presentation: The athlete will usually complain of pain on throwing. Pain typically occurs when the arm is in the "cocking position" of throwing—that is, with the shoulder abducted and externally rotated. Occasionally the patient has sudden onset of symptoms with one particular event such as in javelin throwing, but more commonly, prodromal symptoms precede the "final event" when the ligament completely tears.

Etiology: Either acute or repetitive stresses compromise the integrity of the ligament, resulting in either permanent stretch or outright ligament tear.

Relevant anatomy: The anterior band of the MCL is responsible for stability to valgus stress.

Classification: As in any sprain, injury to the MCL can be classified as grade I, II, or III, depending on the severity. In a grade I there is microscopic hemorrhage, but little ligament damage. In a grade II, there is stretching out, but the ligament is intact. A grade III indicates complete tear of the MCL, with elbow instability to valgus stress.

Physical exam: Physical examination shows focal tenderness over the MCL or its coronoid insertion. On valgus stress there may be pain, tenderness, or the subtle sensation of medial joint opening. Look for signs of ulnar nerve irritability, which commonly accompanies MCL pathology.

X-ray: X-rays may show ossification or the "spur" sign at the ulnar insertion of the ligament.

Differential diagnosis: The most difficult

differential is that of medial epicondylitis. Valgus stress may cause pain in this condition as well because of stress on the medial epicondylar tendinous origin. However, in the isolated MCL sprain, forearm pronation or wrist flexion against resistance (common in epicondylitis) should not cause pain.

Special tests: Special stress x-rays may be helpful to document this subtle instability. By flexing the elbow 30 degrees, thereby unlocking the olecranon from its fossa, either gravity or manual force can apply a valgus stress. Probably any opening is of some significance, although it is appropriate to compare with the other side. When positive, these stress views are confirmatory. When negative however, they do not necessarily exclude MCL insufficiency.

Definitive treatment: In almost all grade I and II injuries, symptomatic treatment, including rest, ice, compression, and strengthening allow return to activity. Grade III tears often require surgical reconstruction in which the palmaris longus is used to reconstruct the MCL.

Little League Elbow

In the skeletally immature athlete, injury to the medial epicondylar structures is known as "Little League" elbow because of its relative incidence in this population.

Presentation: Most commonly, these kids present with medial elbow pain, diminished throwing effectiveness, and decreased throwing distance.

Etiology: Repetitive stresses to the vulnerable epicondylar origin of the flexor-pronator group and MCL, during both acceleration and follow-through, results in abnormalities in secondary ossification and physeal plate structures.

Physical exam: On examination there is focal tenderness over the medial epicondyle and pain on attempting active wrist flexion or forearm pronation, especially against resistance.

X-ray: X-ray findings vary, and include apophyseal fragmentation, irregularity or enlargement, abnormality of the physis, or avulsion of the medial epicondyle.

Differential diagnosis: Medial epicondylitis is seen in the older, usually skeletally mature, population.

Special tests: In contrast, medial epicondyle avulsion stress views are useful; even

an innocent-appearing minimally displaced, fracture may be unstable.

Definitive treatment: Fortunately, treatment is rarely operative, and includes rest, ice, and gradual return to activity as pain resolves. Restricting the number of innings pitched in Little League has led to a reduction in the incidence of elbow complaints. Surgery is reserved for those with displaced or unstable avulsion injuries, or symptomatic nonunions.

Medial Epicondylitis (Medial Tennis Elbow)

In skeletally mature individuals, repetitive stresses on the medial epicondyle result in medial epicondylitis. Although more common in athletic endeavors (tennis, baseball, golf), it can occur with any repetitive stress.

Presentation: Patients complain of pain on activity over the medial elbow.

Etiology: The flexor pronator group arising from the medial epicondyle is subjected to repetitive stresses. The tendon origin is thought to undergo microtears, degeneration, replacement with abnormal scar and granulation tissue (so-called "angiofibroblastic hyperplasia" due to its microscopic appearance) within the pronator teres and flexor carpi radialis.

Physical exam: The key finding is focal tenderness over the medial epicondyle. Wrist flexion and forearm pronation against resistance reproduce the symptoms.

X-ray: X-rays are usually unremarkable although calcifications near the medial epicondyle may be seen in up to 25 percent of patients.

Differential diagnosis: Differentiate from Little League elbow (skeletally immature athlete) and MCL injury (pain and/or opening on valgus stress, stress X-ray).

Special tests: None are necessary.

Definitive treatment: Treatment is almost always conservative, emphasizing rest, ice, avoidance of provocative activities and NSAIDs. In addition, physical therapy (PT) modalities such as ice, heat, or contrast therapy are helpful. Identification and correction of faulty technique, use of a counterforce brace, and a structured PT program can be helpful. Cortisone injections are used in those unresponsive to conservative management. Surgery may be indicated in patients unresponsive to an appropriate conservative trial, usually considered to be at least 6 months' duration and up to three injections of cortisone. Successful surgery involves identification and debridement of the pathologic tissue, usually located within the substance of the flexor carpi radialis and PT.

Ulnar Neuritis

Presentation: Symptoms are those of numbness and tingling in the distribution of the ulnar nerve. There may be elbow pain with or without radiation. Patients may feel clumsy or weak in grasping or throwing. They may note actual "snapping" in cases in which the ulnar nerve is unstable.

Etiology and relevant anatomy: The ulnar nerve's confined position within the cubital tunnel renders it susceptible to both direct and indirect trauma. Any entrapment (whether due to adhesions, scar, or mild fixation) can result in traction with motion in the relatively fixed cubital tunnel. Up to 16 percent of patients are further predisposed to symptoms by having "instability," with either subluxation or frank dislocation out of the groove.

Physical exam: There is usually no sensory or motor deficit, although Tinel's sign over the cubital tunnel may be positive. Check for nerve mobility by flexing and extending elbow while feeling the ulnar nerve.

X-ray: X-rays are almost always negative.

Special tests: Electrodiagnostic tests are usually unrewarding.

Differential diagnosis: Remember to rule out other similarly presenting compressive neuropathies (cervical rib or disc, or compression at Guyon's canal at the wrist).

Definitive treatment: Treatment is initially nonoperative, with rest, ice, NSAIDs, and occasionally splint or cast immobilization for 2 to 3 weeks. In some patients and most athletes, conservative management fails, and surgery is necessary. Surgery usually involves nerve decompression combined with nerve transposition (Fig. 10–4).

Lateral Epicondylitis (Tennis Elbow)

Although more frequently afflicting the non–tennis-playing population, pain over the lateral elbow has become synonymous with "tennis elbow." Only about 5 percent of patients with lateral epicondylitis actually play tennis.

Among tennis players, however, the incidence is about 50 percent over the course of their playing.

Presentation: Symptoms include pain over the lateral elbow, often radiating into the forearm.

Etiology: Repetitive stresses to the lateral epicondylar origin of the extensor-supinator tendons are thought to lead to microtears, degeneration, and abnormal scar formation. This tissue has been termed "angiofibroblastic hyperplasia," and is found most commonly within the ECRB tendon origin.

Physical exam: There is focal tenderness over the lateral epicondyle, with pain on active wrist extension and forearm supination against resistance.

X-ray: X-rays show calcification in the region of the epicondyle about 25 percent of the time.

Differential diagnosis: Differential diagnosis includes radiocapitellar joint arthritis, synovitis, and posterior interosseous nerve (PIN) entrapment, quoted to occur in about 5 percent of "resistant" tennis elbow cases. In skeletally immature athletes, lateral elbow pain may be due to osteochondritis dissecans of the capitellum.

Special tests: None.

Definitive treatment: Treatment of lateral epicondylitis involves the same as for other overuse injuries—rest, ice, NSAIDs, and physiotherapy. Use of a counterforce brace, in which tension on the extensor-supinator origin is relieved, can be helpful.

Identification and correction of errors in athletic technique are important and usually require the expertise of a coach or trainer. Equipment modification includes the use of a larger racquet head (decreasing the incidence of off-center hits). In addition, appropriate string tension, grip size, and the use of graphite or epoxies to absorb vibratory stress may all be helpful.

Surgery is necessary in fewer than 10 percent of all cases. Surgery involves identification and excision of the grayish homogenous abnormal tissue, usually located on the undersurface of the ECRB.

Osteochondritis Dissecans (Panner's Disease)

This condition is particularly common amongst adolescent throwing and gymnastic athletes. It has been described as the leading cause of permanent disability in the young, throwing athlete.

Presentation: The most common symptom is that of lateral elbow pain, related to activity. There may be associated swelling, limitation of motion, catching, or locking episodes.

Etiology: In throwing, enormous valgus stresses are imparted to the elbow joint. Absorbed primarily by the MCL, the second line of defense is the radiocapitellar buttress, which is subjected to significant compression and shear. This also occurs in gymnastics, particularly during vaulting, balance beam, uneven parallel bars, and floor exercises. In skeletally immature individuals, such repetitive stresses are thought to compromise the vascularity to the vulnerable epiphysis, with consequent avascular necrosis of the capitellum.

Classification: Classification is from I–III, based on articular involvement. Type I lesions have no articular involvement. In types II and III, there is articular involvement. In type II, there is no fragment separation, and in III there is separation with loose body formation.

Physical exam: There may be restriction in motion, crepitus on supination/pronation, and tenderness over the radiocapitellar joint.

X-ray: Initially, x-rays are often normal, although there may be lucency and/or irregular ossification. In later stages, there may be a crescent sign, fragmentation or loose-body formation.

Differential diagnosis: Synovitis can occur in post-traumatic or inflammatory elbow disorders.

Special tests: Magnetic resonance imaging or CT-arthrogram is probably the best method of establishing the diagnosis and assessing the degree of articular involvement. Magnetic resonance imaging is also useful in assessing subchondral involvement and the extent and status of healing of the lesion.

Definitive treatment: Treatment depends on clinical and radiographic findings. Nonoperative treatment for type I includes rest, ice, NSAIDs, and PT modalities. Resumption of activities is usually contraindicated because of the time required for healing. Because the healing process is slow, the area must be protected against overzealous activity (i.e., hard throwing or weight-bearing) for a long time. Treatment of type II and III (articular involvement) lesions is usually operative, arthroscopically removing loose bodies, curetting, and/or drilling the lesion's base.

Arthritis

Arthritis of the elbow is much less common than that of the hip or knee. Yet among patients with inflammatory (rheumatoid) arthritis, 20 to 50 percent have elbow involvement.

Presentation: Insidious pain, swelling, stiffness, and disability mark the development of elbow arthritis. Progressive limitation in movement can seriously affect patients with concomitant shoulder and/or wrist involvement. Patients may be unable to reach their mouth or perform usual hygiene functions.

Etiology: Inflammatory arthritis involves progressive joint destruction mediated through synovial proliferation, articular and subchondral erosion, and loss of joint congruity.

Physical exam: Swelling, restriction, and pain on attempted motion are common.

X-ray: Inflammatory changes are variable, ranging from osteopenia, subchondral erosions, destructive-appearing joint collapse, and ultimately bony ankylosis.

Differential diagnosis: In the acutely painful elbow, consider pyogenic (septic) arthritis and crystalline-induced (gout, pseudogout) arthritis, differentiated by joint aspiration and cell count, differential, gram stain, and crystal examination. Degenerative arthritis shows typical radiographic appearance of joint narrowing, sclerosis, and osteophyte formation.

Special tests: Appropriate lab tests for evaluation of systemic arthritis include erythrocyte sedimentation rate, anti-nuclear antibody test, rheumatoid factor test, and complete blood count. Additional rheumatologic tests should be determined in consultation with a rheumatologist.

Definitive treatment: Treatment varies with the stage of presentation. Early in the course, anti-inflammatory medication, analgesics, and activity modification may be sufficient. Initial goals are to decrease pain and inflammation, maintain motion, and avoid further destructive changes. Later, efforts to relieve pain and improve function may rely on surgical treatment, and, in end-stage disease, joint replacement.

CONCLUSION

The elbow is the critical link between the mobile positioning shoulder joint, and the precisely coordinated wrist/hand complex. Conditions that interfere with the elbow's normal motion can significantly compromise patients' ability to feed, dress, and clean themselves. In the athlete, compromise in function precludes the ability to participate. Fortunately, most conditions affecting the elbow do not result in significant limitations. Most elbow problems are readily diagnosable with a thorough history, physical, and basic radiographic examination. An algorithmic approach to treatment facilitates resolution of most problems of the elbow.

SUGGESTED READING

Morrey BF (ed): The Elbow and Its Disorders, ed 2. Philadelphia, WB Saunders Company, 1993.

11

The Hand

George P. Bogumill

Surgery of the hand is a subspecialty practiced by surgeons who have a special interest in the hand and who usually have undergone a year or more of study and experience beyond their primary specialty training in orthopaedic, plastic, or general surgery. Since most hand problems are seen initially by individuals with minimal experience in hand surgery, it is very important for <u>all</u> physicians to have a rudimentary knowledge of the field so the patient with a hand problem can be referred where and when appropriate.

HISTORY

As in all fields of medicine, the history starts with a chief complaint, followed by a detailed history of the present illness. The usual questions of what, when, where, how, how much, and the like are asked.

When one is presented with a congenital deformity, information about any problems that might have occurred during pregnancy or whether similar problems are present in other family members must be sought. Specific details of any accident should be requested and <u>recorded,</u> since the initial history taken is often the most accurate and less likely to be influenced by medicolegal or workman's compensation considerations. Also, the site of occurrence of open injuries might have a major influence on the treatment (a barnyard crush laceration would be treated differently than a clean cut occurring while the patient was washing dishes).

What are the patient's age, occupation, and hobbies? Has there been any previous injury or hand impairment? Which hand is dominant? How long since injury took place, where and how did it occur, and has there been any prior treatment? These are all important considerations in an injury.

For noninjury situations, one should determine when the problem began, how it has progressed, how function is impaired for usual activities, whether other areas of the body are involved, and what makes the situation worse or better. A history of any medical problems such as diabetes or heart disease is important, as is information regarding any medications the patient may be taking, such as nonsteroidal anti-inflammatory drugs (NSAIDs) or anticoagulants, that could influence the treatment plan.

PHYSICAL EXAMINATION

A thorough examination of the upper limb begins at the shoulder or, occasionally, at the cervical spine. After the patient is made comfortable, the upper limb must be undressed and evaluated. Active and passive range of motion of the shoulder and elbow as well as rotation of the forearm should be noted. Skin color, texture, and temperature are important to note. Any visible atrophy, enlargement, swellings, or masses should be noted and, in many cases, measured and compared to the opposite side. Range of motion of fingers, wrist, and thumb should be recorded for comparison with later evaluations. This is quite tedious but important, particularly in cases of injury or progressive diseases such as rheumatoid arthritis and Dupuytren's contracture.

A careful systematic check must be made during the examination of skin, vascular system, tendon excursion and position at rest, and obvious deformities from fractures or dislocations. A discrepancy in active range of motion when compared to passive range of motion might indicate tendon laceration or adherence. In fresh wounds, delving into the wound itself is seldom indicated, even if there is significant bleeding.

It is much more appropriate to cover the wound with a dry, sterile dressing and evaluate the parts distal to the site of the open wound. A decision can then be made regarding the need for early surgery. Nerve injury can be adequately evaluated by checking for sweating of the parts distal to the laceration or by muscle function when the patient is asked to move a part. Sweating is a function of the autonomic nervous system and ceases as soon as a peripheral nerve is cut.

PATHOPHYSIOLOGY

Hand problems can be grouped into the same seven major categories of disease common to most of medicine: congenital, developmental, inflammatory, traumatic, metabolic, circulatory, and neoplastic. It may be difficult to decide the specific category of disease in which any given patient's problem belongs, but by eliminating categories that are obviously not concerned, the appropriate diagnosis and treatment choices become easier to ascertain. A discussion of some of the most common hand problems in each category provides a place to start in evaluating a hand problem.

Congenital Disease

Failure of Formation of Parts (Arrest of Development)

The limb bud appears during the fourth week after fertilization and develops in a proximal-to-distal sequence. Any insult to the limb bud during this time period can damage the terminal epithelium of the bud and stop all subsequent development (transverse failure or congenital amputation). This will be manifested by failure of terminal limb parts to appear, varying from absence of one or more fingertips to absence of the entire upper limb (Fig. 11–1B).

If the intrauterine insult spares the terminal epithelium but damages other structures that are still in a state of early development, a partially normal hand may be attached to an abnormal forearm (longitudinal failure). This is often seen in genetic situations such as radial (Fig. 11–1A) or ulnar clubhand, in which the major deficiency is partial or complete absence of one of the forearm bones. Rarely, one sees a hand attached in the region of the shoulder without intervening humerus or forearm (phocomelia, seal flipper limb).

Failure of Differentiation (Separation) of Parts

Failure of differentiation can vary from the simple skin bridging seen in simpler forms of syndactyly (Fig. 11–1C) to the complex fusion of parts seen in Apert's syndrome. Bony fusions occur in the proximal forearm as congenital synostosis, which prevents forearm rotation. Often this deformity is not noted by parents until children are in school because the children compensate so well functionally. Fusion of carpal bones, especially lunate to triquetrum, is quite common. Symphalangism, the fusion of proximal interphalangeal (PIP) joints, interferes in the individual's ability to grasp with force.

Duplication

Polydactyly can be radial, ulnar, or central. Splitting of the early embryonic part is seen as duplication. It is most common on the thumb (Fig. 11–2A) or little finger and less common in the central three rays. Removal of the extra partial digit must be carefully planned, particularly when the attachment is at a joint, since each phalanx will have one of the collateral ligaments attached and an unstable joint may result if the ligament is not reattached.

Other Congenital Anomalies

Overgrowth (gigantism) may affect a single digit or the entire limb. Most cases show overgrowth of the soft tissues (fat, vessels, fibrous tissue), with or without overgrowth of the skeletal elements (Fig. 11–2B). Undergrowth (hypoplasia) is incomplete or defective development of the entire limb or any part. Congenital constriction band syndrome produces a deep indentation in a circular fashion around the limb or a part. It may lead to amputation. Generalized skeletal abnormali-

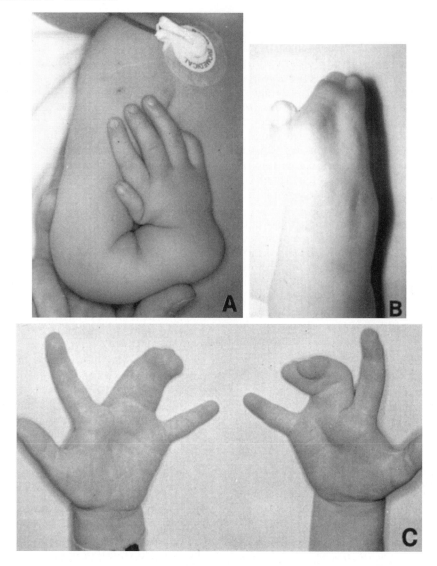

FIGURE 11–1 ■ Congenital malformations. *A,* Radial clubhand produced by longitudinal absence of radius. *B,* Failure of formation of parts combined with failure of separation. *C,* Simple syndactyly of middle and ring fingers.

ties (enchondromatosis, osteochondromatosis, osteogenesis imperfecta, osteopetrosis, etc.) will be manifested in the hand to a smaller extent than in larger bones. Growth-plate anomalies will often show well because of the large number of growth plates in the digits.

Developmental or Acquired Disease

Dupuytren's Contracture

This common affliction, primarily of older men, causes contracture of the fascia of the palm and/or fingers. It begins as a nodule that may be tender at onset and progresses unpredictably and somewhat relentlessly to fibrous bands that cause contractures in the fingers. There is often a strong familial history, particularly when the onset is in younger men and the deformity progresses rapidly.

The contractures are seldom painful; they cause restriction of extension (Fig. 11–2C) but not of flexion since they do not involve the flexor tendons. Treatment is surgical.

Arthritides

Rheumatoid arthritis in the hand ordinarily is part of a generalized process with manifestations in other joints. Patients should be under the care of a rheumatologist for their generalized synovitis before they are referred to a surgeon. In the hand, the synovitis may involve the synovial sheaths of the extensor tendons at the wrist or the flexor tendons in the carpal tunnel or digital sheath, as well as the digital and wrist joints (Fig. 11–3A). Progression of the disease often presents the hand surgeon with ruptured tendons (Fig. 11–3B), dislocated joints with marked instability or contractures, ulnar drift of the fingers, and the like (Fig. 11–3C). Swelling and morning stiffness are helpful findings in the early diagnosis.

The early treatment is medical, but eventually many patients require surgery. Synovectomy is often helpful in isolated joints that have failed to respond to medical treatment or in tendon sheaths that are so full of hypertrophic synovium they cannot function properly. Repair or transfer to replace tendons that have ruptured (usually extensors) is common. Arthrodesis or arthroplasty of destroyed joints leads to improved function (Fig. 11–3D).

Osteoarthritis usually begins in the distal interphalangeal (DIP) joints and is more common in women than men. Hard nodular enlargement of the edges of the joints resulting

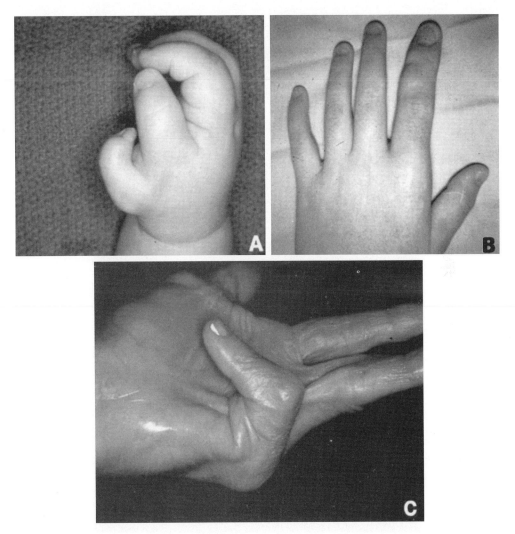

FIGURE 11–2 ■ Congenital and developmental anomalies. *A*, Duplication of thumb. *B*, Gigantism of index finger with enlarged soft tissues as well as skeleton. *C*, Dupuytren's contracture. Bands extending from proximal palm into middle segment of finger have caused near 90-degree contractures of MCP and PIP joints with dimpling and shortening of skin.

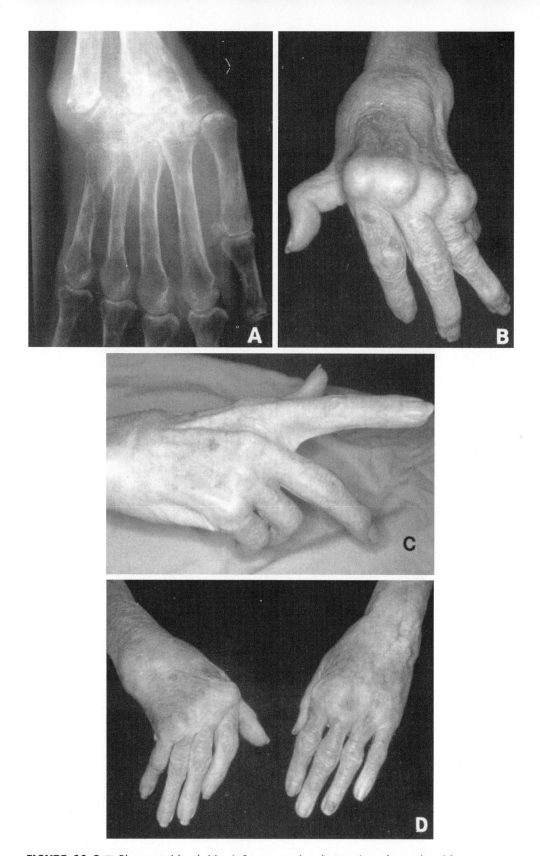

FIGURE 11–3 ■ Rheumatoid arthritis. *A,* Severe erosive destruction of carpal and forearm bones with dislocation of distal radioulnar joint and moderate osteoporosis of all bones. *B,* Clinical picture of advanced rheumatoid changes with tenosynovitis at wrist, dislocations of MCP joints of fingers resulting in ulnar drift, and typical deformities of the thumb. *C,* Rupture of extensors of ulnar three digits as a result of tenosynovitis at wrist with dislocation of distal radioulnar joint. *D,* Results of surgery with relocation of MCP joints of fingers by prosthetic insertion, fusion of thumb joints, and synovectomy of wrist joint and extensor tendons.

from osteophyte formation are referred to as Heberden's nodes. They may be red and painful as they develop. Similar nodules may develop at the PIP joint but seldom at the metacarpophalangeal (MCP) joint. The base of the thumb is a common location of "wear and tear" arthritis, with subluxation of the metacarpal on the trapezium during strong pinch. Compressing the thumb in its long axis and rotating the metacarpal ("compression/grind test") usually elicits pain and crepitation in involved joints. Arthroplasty, with or without tissue or silicone interposition, is often helpful for trapezial-metacarpal or PIP joints. Arthrodesis of the wrist or finger joints, especially the DIP joints, can give pain relief and provide stability—thereby increasing the power of grip and pinch.

Nerve Compression Syndromes

Carpal tunnel syndrome is a common affliction of median nerve compression beneath the transverse carpal ligament. It is being recognized more and more often in industrial workers who perform repetitive hand movements. Patients are often awakened at night with pain in the hand that may extend up the forearm beyond the elbow. The hand "goes to sleep," with numbness and tingling primarily in the middle and ring fingers, although the index finger and thumb are usually involved as well. Patients often do not realize the little finger is spared until asked specifically.

Symptoms are often initiated by such activities as driving a car or holding a phone, book, or hair dryer in the affected hand. The entity is more common in women and is seldom seen in children or adolescents. It occurs whenever a situation is present that will cause impingement on the volume of the carpal tunnel. Thus it is commonly seen in Colles' fractures, rheumatoid arthritis, pregnancy, hypothyroidism, and the like. Most cases, however, have no systemic component.

Physical examination combined with appropriate history will often make the diagnosis. Tapping the nerve from midpalm proximally to the distal forearm may elicit electric shock sensations extending into the fingers or proximally into the forearm. The wrist flexion test or thumb pressure over the canal may also elicit the numbness and paresthesias of which the patient complains. Providing a patient with a simple night splint may cause abatement of the symptoms for prolonged periods. Steroid injections into the carpal tunnel and surgical

release of the transverse carpal ligament are other treatment modalities. When the history and findings are not clear-cut, as is often the situation in workman's compensation cases, electrical testing can be helpful.

Cubital tunnel syndrome refers to compression of the ulnar nerve at the elbow. Clumsiness of hand function and numbness in the little finger are common complaints. Electrical testing may be required (electromyogram and nerve conduction velocity) to determine whether the compression is at the elbow or wrist or even at the root of the neck, where the lower trunk, which gives rise to the ulnar nerve, may be stretched by a cervical rib or by a Pancoast tumor of the lung apex.

Tendon Compression Syndromes

Trigger finger or thumb is a form of stenosing tenosynovitis. An enlargement of the flexor tendon or inflammation of the sheath can lead to a discrepancy in the size of the tendon and the pulley, particularly the first annular pulley over the volar plate of the MCP joint. The tendon can be pulled through by the flexor muscle, but difficulty and a painful snap are experienced when trying to extend the digit. Congenital trigger thumb is fairly common in infants and young children and is manifested by the inability to extend the terminal thumb joint.

De Quervain's stenosing tenosynovitis presents with painful wrist and thumb motion. Resisted extension of the thumb, or grasping the thumb and abruptly deviating the wrist toward the ulna (the Finklestein test) causes pain over the radial styloid and first extensor compartment housing the abductor pollicis longus and extensor pollicis brevis tendons. Treatment by splinting and administration of NSAIDs such as indomethacin or ibuprofen may be quite helpful in the early acute phase of a case. Steroid injections are often employed.

Inflammation

Paronychia is an infection of the soft tissues overlying the base of the nail. It is usually caused by staphylococcus, and presents as a red, swollen, and painful abscess overlying the root of the nail (Fig. 11–4A). Surgical drainage is often required.

Felon is a deep infection of the pulp at the end of the digit. The pulp is very tense and

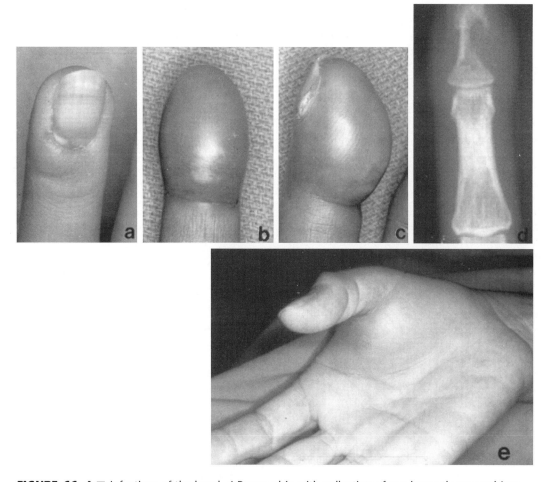

FIGURE 11–4 ■ Infections of the hand. *A,*Paronychia with collection of pus beneath eponychium and base of nail. *B–D,* Felon with marked distention of pulp of finger, impending necrosis of skin on palmar surface, and dissolution of bone of distal phalanx. *E,* Thenar space abscess.

painful, leading the patient to seek early medical attention. If not drained early, it can spread into tendon sheath or bone (Fig. 11–4B–D). Purulent tenosynovitis is a very serious infection that can result in loss of a finger if not treated aggressively. The patient presents with tender swelling along the palmar surface of the entire digit, which is held in a slightly flexed position. Attempts to extend the digit are quite painful and are resisted by the patient. There is usually moderate-to-marked swelling over the dorsum of the hand, but there is no pus present there. Palmar space infections can result from untreated tenosynovitis, with rupture of the tendon sheath abscess into the thenar or mid-palmar spaces (Fig. 11–4E). Death occasionally resulted from these infections in the preantibiotic era, before it was realized that surgical drainage was imperative.

Granulomatous infections of the hand are uncommon but potentially serious. Tuberculosis is seldom seen in this day and age, but atypical mycobacterial infections are being recognized more often and can be very destructive.

Human bite infections can cause extensive damage before treatment is begun. The injury often occurs in a fight; the metacarpal head strikes a tooth and is seeded with a mixture of potent bacteria. Such wounds should never be closed primarily.

Trauma

Lacerations

Lacerations can be trivial or serious, and the decision as to the category a specific laceration fits requires careful examination. Seldom do lacerations present with life-threatening bleeding. Even major vessels will retract and clot when completely severed. However, they can bleed profusely if partially severed and not able to retract. Vessels should not be clamped blindly because they often are in close proximity to nerves or other important structures that can be injured by such clamping. Direct pressure is the best method for controlling heavy bleeding.

A clean, dry dressing should be placed over the wound and a systematic examination done of the parts distal to the laceration. Nowhere is a thorough knowledge of anatomy more important than in examination of the injured hand, because the initial treatment so often determines the eventual outcome. One must consider what structures might have been injured, then carefully test each tendon or nerve for loss of function. The posture of the hand or lack of sweating of a part will often make the diagnosis and allow a determination that this injury must be treated in the operating room and not the emergency room. A partially lacerated tendon may allow movement of a part against no resistance, but pain and/or weakness are disclosed when the movement is resisted. Lack of sweating can be detected immediately after nerve laceration and does not require cooperation by the patient (useful in children or unconscious patients).

Fractures and Dislocations

Fractures can often be diagnosed by physical examination alone but must be confirmed by radiographs for appropriate treatment as well as for the record. They may be open (simple) or closed (compound) and relatively clean or heavily contaminated. Tendon, nerve, or vessel injury may be associated and affect the treatment.

Phalanges may present shaft fractures of various configurations. They usually heal within 4 weeks (sooner if spiral rather than transverse). The presence of angular or rotatory deformity must be carefully corrected and monitored frequently during the healing process to avoid recurrence with healing in a position of deformity. Intra-articular fractures are particularly troublesome and often require open reduction and internal fixation because of their tendency to slip and cause deformity during splinting.

Metacarpal fractures are managed in much the same way as phalangeal fractures.

Control of rotation is particularly important, shortening less so. "Boxer's fracture" usually involves angulation of the end of the metacarpal into the palm. It is not much of a problem for the fifth metacarpal because of mobility at its base, but can be a moderate problem when the second or third metacarpal is involved. Bennett's fracture of the base of the first metacarpal is an intra-articular fracture that results in displacement of the metacarpal by pull of the abductor tendons attached to its base. It is difficult to maintain reduction in a cast and often internal fixation is required after reduction.

Carpal bone fractures are common. The most frequently fractured carpal is the scaphoid (Fig. 11–5). Even if the initial radiographs fail to show a fracture, it should be suspected any time there is a history of injury associated with tenderness in the anatomic snuffbox—including when the initial radiographs fail to show a fracture.

Casting the injury for 2 to 3 weeks would be good treatment if the diagnosis turns out to be a "sprain" and would also be good initial treatment if immobilization allows enough resorption to occur at the fracture line to make the fracture visible on radiograph. Many wrist sprains will show a small chip of bone overlying the dorsum of the wrist on the lateral view. These avulsion fractures can be treated adequately with 3 weeks of cast immobilization.

Dislocations of the interphalangeal and MCP joints are often simple to reduce and quite stable when reduced. If the collateral ligaments are intact when tested after reduction, 10 days of immobilization is adequate. If laxity is present on one side, 3 weeks will be needed. "Gamekeeper's thumb" is common in skiers and other athletes and involves rupture of the ulnar collateral ligament of the thumb MCP joint. These often require skilled and experienced evaluation to determine the need for open repair. Sprains and strains (so-called "jamming injuries") are very common in weekend athletes, are often presented rather late for treatment, and result in swelling and limited motion for a surprisingly long time (6 to 12 months is not unusual).

Severe or Complex Injuries

Amputations of portions of the upper limb, especially the fingertips, are very common because of the exposure of the hand to multiple injuring forces during work and play. Modern microvascular surgery often provides

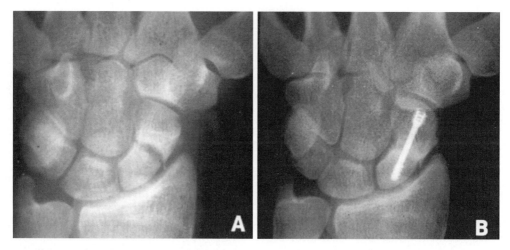

FIGURE 11–5 ■ Fracture with nonunion of carpal scaphoid. *A,* Established nonunion with sclerosis and cyst formation 6 months after untreated "wrist sprain." *B,* Operative treatment with screw resulted in union.

the opportunity for reimplantation of the amputated part with restoration of cosmesis, and of function that is superior to a prosthesis. The decision concerning reimplantation must be made by an experienced hand surgeon as soon as possible to diminish avascular time. The severed part should be wrapped in a moist, sterile wrapping, placed in a container that can then be immersed in ice, and transported with the patient to the treatment facility. Dry ice should never be used.

Extensive mangling injuries must be treated by an experienced hand surgeon as soon as possible. The initial care rendered often determines the final outcome and therefore must be carefully planned with the long-term outcome firmly in mind. Inadequate debridement, primary closure, improper splinting, and the like all too often result unnecessarily in significant disability.

Crush injuries should always be carefully evaluated for the development of compartment syndrome. The early symptoms may be very subtle, the history of crushing may be vague (e.g., a drugged patient sleeping on the arm for a long period), and the damage may take a long time to develop. Iatrogenic causes may include tight casts or dressings and subfascial fluid injections. A high degree of suspicion and careful observation of the patient for increasing pain, loss of sensation or motor function, and distal discoloration will lead to diagnosis before irreversible damage has been done to muscles and nerves.

The condition occurs from increased pressure in the forearm or hand muscle compartments with backup pressure closing down the veins, the capillaries, and finally the arteries (a pulse may persist distal to the compartment for some time after the muscle has closed down its functional capillary bed).

These cases are surgical emergencies! Physical examination is the best method of diagnosis, although a number of devices are available for measuring the compartment pressures.

Thermal, chemical, or electrical injuries cause tissue injury of varying depth. The skin is the initial point of contact and may show first-degree (red), second-degree (blister), or third-degree (charred) injury, particularly in burns. Early care of the second-degree injury can minimize the chance of an infection converting it to third-degree injury. Early referral to a hand therapist for exercise and splinting may avoid extensive late contracture. Third-degree burns should be treated by early surgical excision of the eschar and skin grafting. Cold injury varies from minor frostbite to extensive freezing of tissues in peripheral parts. Early amputation is not necessary in the absence of infection. Electrical burns are deceptive as to the extent of damage and require repeated evaluation.

Other Injuries

Mallet finger may occur from rupture of the terminal extensor tendon, often with trivial injury. Fracture of the dorsal lip of the terminal phalanx may be seen on radiograph; a laceration of the tendon may also cause the drooping of the terminal phalanx and hyperextension of the PIP joint. Passive full extension is present but active extension is not. Treatment is usually splinting in extension for 6 or more weeks.

Boutonnière deformity occurs from disruption of the central slip of the extensor tendon over the PIP joint by blunt trauma or laceration. The lateral bands slip progressively anteriorly with time and lose their capacity to extend the PIP joint. Thus, one sees flexion of the PIP joint (which may be passively correctable early) and hyperextension of the DIP joint. The lesion must be suspected early and treated by appropriate splinting. If seen late, surgery is often required.

Metabolic Disease

Storage diseases, hyperparathyroidism, diabetes mellitus, and the like can cause changes in the hand but seldom require treatment by a surgeon. The destructive action of urate crystal deposition in articular cartilage in patients with tophaceous gout is no longer common since medical treatment of the metabolic defect is more effective in preventing the large deposits. Surgical treatment may be needed to treat skin breakdown or joint destruction.

Circulatory

Arteriovenous malformations may be either congenital or acquired and may or may not present with gigantism. Excision of the lesion may be required; occasionally, amputation is necessary. Raynaud's syndrome or phenomenon is a common circulatory disturbance of the terminal portions of the digits that can lead to dry gangrene of the fingertips, requiring amputation.

Neoplasms

Tumors of Soft Parts

Tumors of soft parts can be either benign (common) or malignant (rare in the hand). They can arise in any of the tissues making up the hand, such as nerves, vessels, fat, and fascia. Lesions of the synovium comprise the most common "tumors" of the hand (i.e., ganglion, mucous cyst, and giant cell tumor of the ten-

don sheath). Ganglia occur in four locations: on the dorsum of the wrist, volarly beneath the radial artery, from the flexor sheath at the base of a finger, and over the dorsum of the DIP joint (mucous cyst), usually associated with osteoarthritis and osteophyte formation of that joint. Larger ganglia can be aspirated; seldom is surgery required except for cosmetic reasons. A giant cell tumor of the tendon sheath is a solid lesion arising from the synovium of the sheath or one of the digital joints. Simple excision is usually curative, although occasional recurrence does occur.

Skin Cancers

Skin cancers (squamous cell and basal cell carcinomas and melanoma) are relatively common, especially in the elderly or in those with predisposing factors. These factors include prolonged sun exposure in farmers and sailors and excessive exposure to x-rays, arsenicals, or other chemicals (Fig. 11–6A). Squamous and basal cell carcinomas can usually be cured by wide excision if they have not already spread. Melanomas are much more unpredictable in their behavior (Fig. 11–6B).

Tumors of Bone

Benign tumors of the hand skeleton are often diagnosed on radiographic examination for trauma. The most common is the enchondroma (Fig. 11–6C). Treatment is not often required unless pathologic fracture has occurred through the lesion. Simple curettage with or without bone grafting often suffices. Osteochondromas, fibrous dysplasia, and giant cell tumor of bone can also present in the small hand bones and may require surgery for diagnosis or treatment.

Malignant tumors of the hand skeleton are very rare. Partial or total hand amputation may be required along with adjuvant radiotherapy or chemotherapy. Metastatic tumors of the hand seldom occur as isolated metastases but are not uncommon during widespread metastatic disease, particularly from lung or breast lesions.

MANAGEMENT PROTOCOLS

When a patient presents with hand or wrist pain, the physician is usually faced with a specific complaint but seldom an established diagnosis. The physician must obtain a good

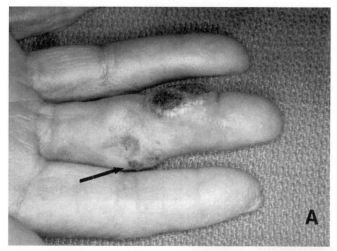

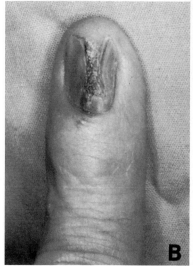

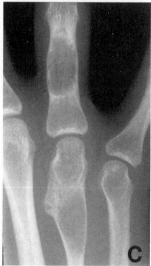

FIGURE 11–6 ■ Neoplasms of the hand. *A,* Squamous cell carcinoma of finger in patient with 30-year history of holding children being radiographed. Note atrophic skin changes *(arrow)* from the radiation exposure. *B,* Subungual melanoma with splitting of the nail from involvement of nail bed. *C,* Enchondroma of proximal phalanx with expansion of the diaphysis. Note the enchondroma of the metacarpal with callus from a healed pathologic fracture.

history, examine the patient, and obtain appropriate studies, particularly radiographs. Use of a standardized approach will save time and expense in arriving at a diagnosis and treatment plan. Such a standardized approach is presented in the form of an algorithm. The algorithm is an organized pattern of decision making and thought processes that allows the

patient to receive the most helpful diagnostic and therapeutic measures at the optimal time and at reasonable expense.

The management protocol begins with the universe of patients who are initially evaluated for hand and wrist pain. After a medical history is first taken and physical examination performed and assessed under the assumption that the symptoms are originating from the hand and wrist, the patient is placed into one of two major groups: those with acute hand injuries and those with symptoms but no history of a specific injury. Regardless of which group, however, the patient needs a set of radiographs. An algorithm has been developed for each group to present a standardized approach through a series of easy-to-follow and clearly defined decision-making processes.

The first algorithm pertains to individuals with hand and wrist pain following an injury (Fig. 11–7). A radiograph is taken but may show no derangement. This would lead the examiner to search for ligament damage or tendon disruption. Localizing the tenderness and loss of function should lead to the correct diagnosis and treatment. When the radiograph is positive for fracture or dislocation, reduction is usually done closed and the situation evaluated for stability to determine whether surgery with or without internal fixation is necessary.

The second algorithm should assist in evaluating a patient who has hand or wrist pain but no history of injury (Fig. 11–8). Again, radiographs are necessary in most cases. Localizing signs of heat, redness, and limitation of motion resulting from swelling or pain should make one think of inflammation. If only one digit is involved, particularly around the base of the nail or in the finger pulp, an infection should be suspected. Various arthritides have some of the same findings but usually involve more than one area of the hand or body. Localized snapping of a digit of the thumb may mean trigger finger or other forms of stenosing tenosynovitis. Numbness, tingling, or pain leads one to consider nerve compression syndromes. Masses, with or without pain, are fairly common about the hand and wrist. The common ganglion is by far the most common tumor and can be diagnosed with a degree of confidence by its location and by transillumination with a penlight. Masses that do not transilluminate should not be neglected; the amount of preoperative workup needed depends on the characteristics of the mass and how it presents.

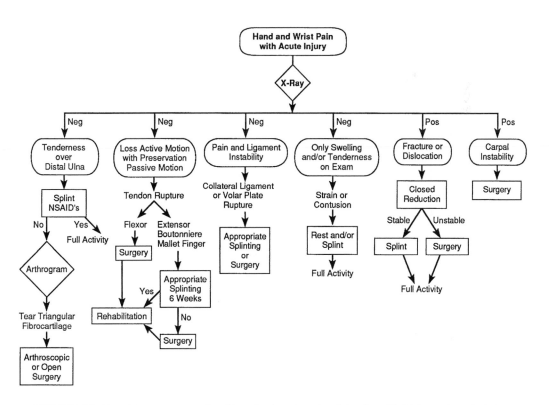

FIGURE 11–7 ■ Management algorithm for hand and wrist pain with history of acute injury.

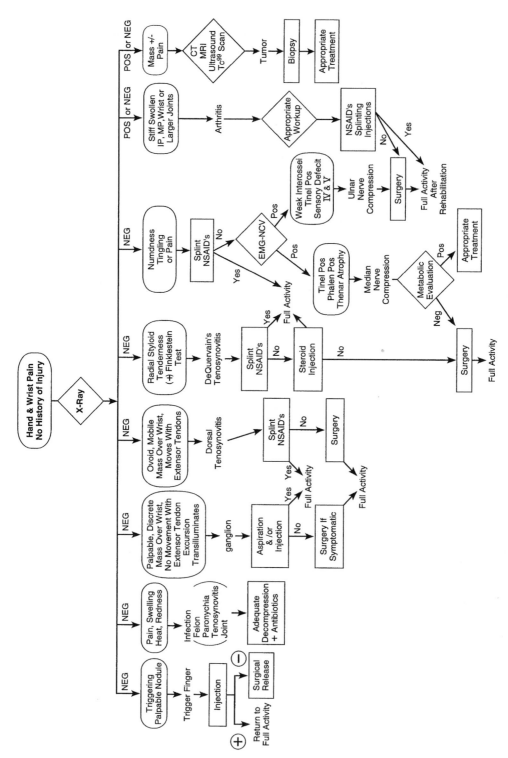

FIGURE 11-8 ■ Management algorithm for hand and wrist pain with no history of injury.

SUGGESTED READINGS

American Society for Surgery of the Hand: The Hand: Examination and Diagnosis. Edinburgh, Churchill Livingstone, 1983.

American Society for Surgery of the Hand: The Hand: Primary Care of Common Problems. Edinburgh, Churchill Livingstone, 1985.

Bogumill GP, Fleegler EJ: Tumours of the Hand and Upper Limb. Edinburgh, Churchill Livingstone, 1993.

Lichtman DM: The Wrist and Its Disorders. Philadelphia, WB Saunders Company, 1988.

Lister G: The Hand: Diagnosis and Indications, ed 2. Edinburgh, Churchill Livingstone, 1984.

The Hip

Brian G. Evans

The primary function of the lower extremities is locomotion. Injuries or disease in the lower extremities will therefore be manifested through alteration in the ability to ambulate. The hip is the most proximal joint in the lower extremity. Alteration in the hip due to disease will effect the biomechanics of gait and place abnormal stress on the joints above and below the hip.

This chapter will briefly review the anatomy of the hip and its relationship to normal and pathologic gait. The important history and physical examination findings of hip pathology will be discussed. Several of the common disorders of the hip will be presented and the appropriate treatment outlined. Surgical management of end-stage disease of the hip is commonly treated by one of several options and these will be discussed, with the indications and outcome for each treatment option outlined.

ANATOMY

Development

The hip joint is a ball and socket joint with the round femoral head articulating within the round acetabular socket. The acetabulum is formed from three structures: the ischium, the ilium, and the pubis. In skeletally immature patients these three bones are joined in the medial acetabulum by the triradiate cartilage, which is a growth plate for the medial acetabulum (Fig. 12–1). There is also appositional growth from the edges of the acetabulum resulting in increased depth of the acetabulum. Optimal development of the acetabulum requires the femoral head to articulate with the acetabular cartilage. If the femoral head is dislocated or subluxed, then the acetabular socket will not develop normally. This will result in developmental dysplasia of the hip.

Osteology and Musculature

The innominate bone consists of the ilium, the ischium, and the pubis, which, as noted above, are joined in the area of the acetabulum. The ilium is a large flat bone providing broad surfaces for muscular attachment. The ischium extends posteriorly and forms the posterior aspect of the acetabulum. The ischium joins the ilium superiorly and the pubis inferiorly through the inferior pubic ramus. The ischium also serves as the origin of the hamstring and short external rotator muscles of the hip. The pubis consists of the superior pubic ramus, inferior pubic ramus, and the pubic symphysis. The superior pubic ramus connects the pubic symphisis with the ilium and the inferior pubic ramus connects the pubic symphisis with the ischium. The pubis serves as the site of insertion of the musculature of the abdominal wall as well as the site of origin for the adductor muscles of the thigh.

Where these three bones meet is the acetabulum: the ilium forms the superior dome of the acetabulum, the ischium forms the posterior acetabulum, and the pubis forms the anterior acetabulum. The lateral opening of the acetabulum forms a horseshoe

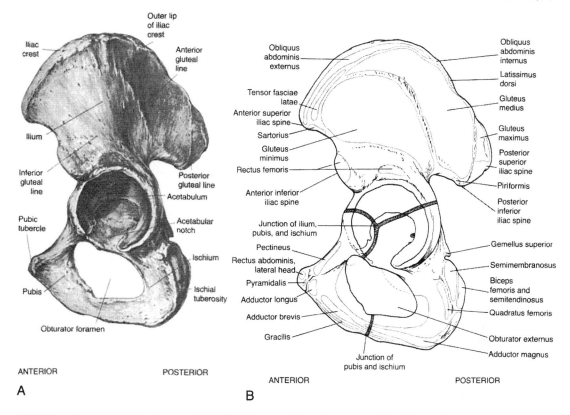

FIGURE 12–1 ■ *A,* Lateral aspect of left hip bone. *B,* Attachments and epiphyseal lines are shown.
(From Williams PL, Warwick R: Gray's Anatomy, ed 36.•••, Churchill Livingstone, 1980, pp 378-379; reprinted by permission.) (From Steinberg M (ed): The Hip and Its Disorders. Philadelphia, WB Saunders Company, 1991, P 32; reprinted by permission.)

with the open end directed inferiorly. The medial base of the acetabulum contains a depression called the *acetabular fovea.* This is filled with a fatty tissue called the *pulvinar* and with the ligamentum teres.

The fovea of the femur is a depression on the femoral head. This depression and the fovea of the acetabulum are the sites of attachment for the ligamentum teres. This ligament links the femoral head to the acetabulum. It also contains the foveal artery, which supplies a small portion of the femoral head. Attached to the rim of the horseshoe is a fibrocartilagenous labrum, which is similar to the meniscus in the knee. This serves to improve stability and to cushion the femoral neck when the femur is rotated and impinges upon the acetabular rim at the extremes of motion. The hip joint capsule is a dense fibrous structure extending from the base of the intertrochanteric region of the femur to the acetabular rim. Thickenings within the capsule are the iliofemoral and pubofemoral ligaments anteriorly and the ischiofemoral

ligament posteriorly. These ligaments as well as the ligamentum teres and the labrum augment the stability of the hip joint.

The femoral head is essentially spherical in geometry (Figs. 12–2 and 12–3). The spherical portion of the femoral head is covered by articular cartilage. The sphere is altered in two areas. Laterally, where the femoral neck begins and medially, at the fovea of the femoral head. The femoral neck joins the femur at approximately a 125-degree angle. The neck is also rotated anteriorly 12 to 14 degrees relative to the axis represented by the posterior femoral condyles (Fig. 12–4). The femoral neck flares laterally to join the proximal femur in between the greater and lesser trochanters. The greater trochanter is continuous with a ridge anteriorly and posteriorly that allows for the attachment of various muscles.

The muscles of the hip form several distinct groups. The anterior muscles are the hip flexors. These consist of the iliopsoas and rectus femorus and sartorius muscles. The rectus and sartorius are innervated by the

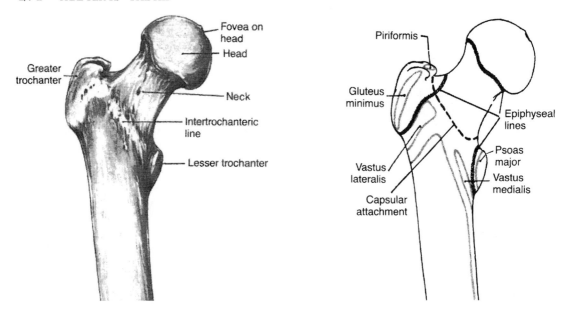

FIGURE 12–2 ■ *A,* Anterior aspect of proximal right femur. *B,* Attachments and epiphyseal lines.
(From Williams PL, Warwick R: Gray's Anatomy, ed 36.•••, Churchill Livingstone, 1980, pp 392–393; reprinted by permission.) (From Steinberg M (ed): The Hip and Its Disorders. Philadelphia, WB Saunders Company, 1991, p 28; reprinted by permission.)

femoral nerve. The iliopsosas is innervated by motor branches from spinal roots L2, 3, and 4.

The lateral group consists of the abductors—the gluteus medius, minimus, and tensor fascia lata. These muscles are essential for normal gait. The anterior one third of the gluteus medius muscle is the principal internal rotator of the hip. The lateral muscles are

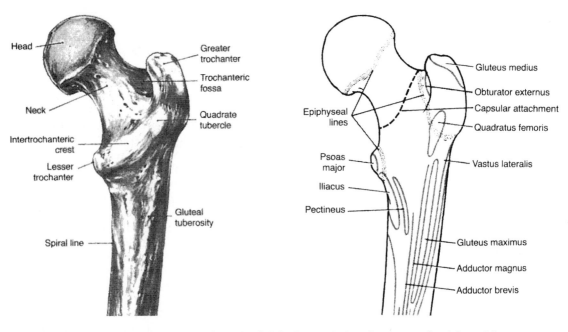

FIGURE 12–3 ■ *A,* Posterior aspect of proximal right femur. *B,* Attachments and epiphyseal lines.
(From Williams PL, Warwick R: Gray's Anatomy, ed 36.•••, Churchill Livingstone, 1980, p 394, reprinted by permission.)(From Steinberg M (ed): The Hip and Its Disorders. Philadelphia, WB Saunders Company, 1991, p 28; reprinted by permission.)

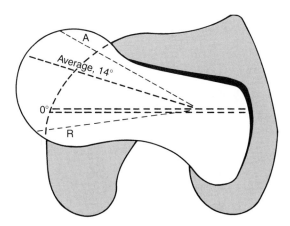

FIGURE 12–4 ■ Average rotary, or torsion, angle of the femur. It may be anteverted (A) or retroverted (R).

(From Steinberg M (ed): The Hip and Its Disorders. Philadelphia, WB Saunders Company, 1991, p 29; reprinted by permission.)

innervated by the superior gluteal nerve. The posterior muscles are in two layers. The superficial layer consists of the gluteus maximus, the primary extensor of the hip. This is innervated by the inferior gluteal nerve. The deep layer consists of the short external rotators of the hip: the piriformis, superior gemellus, obturator internus, inferior gemellus, obturator externus, and quadratus femoris. These muscles externally rotate the femur, and the upper four provide some abduction force. They are innervated by small branches from the sacral plexus. The medial muscle group consists of the pectineus, the adductor brevis, longus, and magnus, and the gracillus. The adductors and gracillis are supplied by the obturator nerve, with the posterior portion of the adductor magnus also receiving innervation from the tibial division of the sciatic nerve. The pectintus is innervated by the femoral nerve.

The sciatic nerve crosses the hip joint posteriorly. It exits the pelvis under the piriformis muscle and lies superficial to the short external rotators. The nerve has two distinct divisions within the single nerve sheath—the tibial and the peroneal. Of the two, the peroneal division is more susceptible to injury, at all levels along the course of the sciatic nerve. Therefore a partial injury to the sciatic nerve will commonly result in a foot drop, clinically similar to the deficits seen in an isolated injury to the common peroneal nerve injury at the level of the fibular neck. One anatomic point with important clinical relevance is that the

peroneal division of the sciatic nerve has only one motor branch in the posterior thigh—the short head of the biceps. Determining if the short head of the biceps is normally innervated can assist in determining the level of sciatic nerve injury clinically (i.e., in the hip or knee).

Vascular Anatomy of the Proximal Femur and Femoral Head

The medial and lateral femoral circumflex vessels, in conjunction with the artery of the ligamentum teres, provide the vascular supply to the proximal femur and femoral head (Fig. 12–5). The medial femoral circumflex artery extends posteriorly and ascends proximally deep to the quadratus femorus muscle. At the level of the hip it joins an arterial ring at the base of the femoral neck. The lateral femoral circumflex artery extends anteriorly and gives off an ascending branch that also joins the arterial ring at the base of the femoral neck. This vascular ring gives rise to a group of vessels that run in the retinacular tissue inside the capsule to enter the femoral head at the base of the articular surface. These vessels provide 80 to 90 percent of the blood supply to the femoral head. The artery of the ligamentum teres, a branch of the obturator artery, travels within the ligamentum teres and supplies only 10 to 20 percent of the vascularity to the femoral head.

Biomechanics

The joint reaction force is the force that is placed across a joint and includes components from gravity, body weight, and muscle forces acting upon the joint. In a two-legged stance with both feet on the ground and static conditions, a joint reaction force of approximately 1.3 to 1.5 times body weight will cross each hip joint. However, in a single-limb stance this force will increase to 2.5 to 3 times body weight across the hip joint. The primary contribution to the increase is the force generated by the abductor muscles to maintain balance and to keep the pelvis level. If the system is in motion, such as with walking, the joint reaction forces can be as high as 4 times body weight.

Several studies have measured the actual joint reaction forces during rehabilitation using actual inserted, instrumented prostheses. The greatest joint reaction force was noted when patients arose from a low chair or during stair climbing. However, even non-weight-

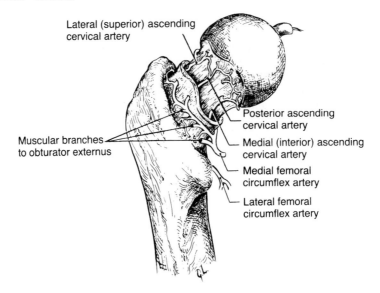

FIGURE 12–5 ■ Arterial supply to the head and neck of the posterior aspect of the left proximal femur. Note the extracapsular arterial ring on the surface of the capsule, the ascending cervical arteries on the neck of the femur, and the intra-articular sub-synovial arterial ring at the articular cartilage margin.
(From Steinberg M (ed): The Hip and Its Disorders. Philadelphia, WB Saunders Company, 1991, p 19; reprinted by permission.)

bearing activities such as getting onto a bed pan were found to have a joint reaction force of 1.5 to 1.8 times body weight. The lowest joint reaction forces with ambulation were recorded when patients used touch-down weight-bearing. Touch-down weight-bearing allows the patient to rest the foot on the ground to balance the weight of the leg but not to step down or bear weight on the involved lower extremity.

Gait

As mentioned previously the principal function of the lower extremities is ambulation. In gait analysis, a gait cycle examines one leg, beginning with heel strike and continues until the next heel strike of the same leg. Gait can be divided into two principal phases—stance and swing. The stance phase is defined as that portion of the gait cycle when the foot is in contact with the ground. The swing phase is, therefore, the portion of each step when the foot is not in contact with the ground. The stance phase makes up 60 percent of each step with the remainder being made up by the swing phase. Therefore, during 20 percent of

the gait cycle both feet are in contact with the ground. Normal gait requires a stable pelvis, which is provided by the hip abductor muscles. Normal gait also requires 40 degrees of hip flexion and 10 degrees of internal rotation and external rotation.

PATIENT EVALUATION

History

The evaluation of a patient with hip pain requires careful attention to the history, physical examination, and radiographic studies. The character, nature, and duration of the patient's pain should be documented. Acute or recent onset pain will be associated more commonly with trauma or infection. Chronic and gradually progressive pain is associated with arthritic conditions. Intra-articular pain is usually described as a deep aching pain. Pain from the hip joint will commonly be noted anteriorly in the groin or in the region of the greater trochanter. Hip pain can radiate down the inner thigh to the knee with little or no pain in the area of the hip. This is particularly true in adolescent patients. Posterior pain and buttock pain is more commonly associated with lumbar spine pathology. Spine pain will also commonly radiate down the posterior thigh and below the knee. The insidious onset of a deep boring pain or a pain that awakens the patient at night suggest either infection or neoplastic disease.

Hip pain is commonly aggravated by activity and relieved by rest. Patients will report difficulty donning and doffing their shoes and socks and difficulty with nail care on the involved extremity. As it progresses, the pain will begin to be felt on prolonged sitting and at night as patients try to go to sleep. Those with hip arthritis will report that if they sit for a prolonged period of time when they get up to walk the hip will feel out of place or painful for the first few steps. This feeling will resolve quickly after a few minutes of walking.

The use of a cane, walking stick, or crutch should be documented. The patient may also have begun to take over-the-counter anti-inflammatories or pain relievers. The medication and the amount the patient is taking, as well as the level of relief provided, needs to be recorded. Walking tolerance can be measured in terms of blocks the patient can walk or in terms of how many minutes the patient can be ambulatory doing grocery shopping or in a mall. The above data will give a detailed picture of the degree of pain and the patient's functional limitations.

Patients should also be questioned about past problems with the hip such as hip dislocation at birth, delays in ambulation as an infant, and any bracing as a child. If previous surgery or trauma to the hips has occurred, this should be explored in detail. The past medical history and any medications the patient is taking should be noted. This information can have implications for the patient's hip problems and may have an impact upon what treatment may be instituted.

Physical Examination

The most important aspect of the physical examination in patients with hip disease is to evaluate their gait pattern. This will reveal important information about patients' ambulatory status and their pain. Patients with significant hip pain will manifest a coxalgic gait. This gait pattern is represented by a reduced stance phase on the painful leg, with the shoulders lurching over the affected hip. Patients

with mild pain or weakness in the abductor muscles may have a stance phase equal to the opposite leg but the shoulders will continue to lurch over the affected leg. This lurch results in moving the center of gravity closer to the center of rotation of the hip. This, in turn, reduces the force necessary to stabilize the pelvis in stance phase. This gait is referred to as a "Trendelenburg gait" (equal stance phase, with the shoulders lurching over the affected hip). The hip should be inspected for previous scars, swelling, bruises, or abrasions. The region then should be palpated to identify areas of focal tenderness such as over the greater trochanter, sciatic nerve, or anterior hip capsule. The range of motion of the hip should then be determined. Normal range of motion of the hip is flexion to 130 degrees, extension to 0 degrees, adduction to 30 degrees, abduction to 40 degrees, internal rotation to 30 degrees, and external rotation to 60 degrees. When assessing the range of motion of the hip it is important to stabilize the lumbar spine. Motion in the lumbar spine may be attributed to the hip if the examiner is not careful. The Thomas test will stabilize the lumbar spine to measure for a flexion contracture of the hip (Fig. 12–6). Movement of the pelvis with abduction and adduction can be accurately assessed by placing a hand on the opposite anterior superior iliac spine and recording the patient's motion as the amount of motion prior to pelvic abduction.

To assess the function of the hip abductor muscles the patient should be standing, and the involved leg should be lifted off the floor. The patient should now be standing on the uninvolved leg, and the pelvis should remain level. The patient then stands on the involved leg and lifts the uninvolved leg off the floor. If the pelvis is level, then the patient has normal strength of the abductor muscles. If the pelvis is noted to lower on the elevated leg, then the abductor muscles are weak or the hip is one in which weight-bearing is painful. This is referred to as the "Trendelenburg sign."

In addition to assessing the hip, a careful neurologic exam and lumbar spine exam are essential to assessing the possibility of spine pathology producing pain radiating to the hip. Patients with significant arthritic disease in the hip will also commonly have spine pathology as well. The distal pulses should also be palpated. If a significant reduction in pulse is noted, a vascular noninvasive evaluation should be obtained.

Radiographic Evaluation

Routine radiography of the pelvis and hips is the most useful study in evaluating hip pathology. Standard anterioposterior (AP) radiography of the pelvis will reveal the lower lumbar spine, sacroiliac joints, innominate bone, pubic symphysis, hip joint and proximal femurs. Frequently, in unilateral disease the normal side can be used for comparison (Fig. 12–7). Lateral views of the proximal femurs can also be helpful in defining pathology and in determining the location of a pathologic lesion.

Computerized tomography of the pelvis is most helpful in evaluating trauma—particularly fractures in the posterior pelvis and sacrum, which is usually poorly visualized in routine radiography. Fractures to the ac-

A.

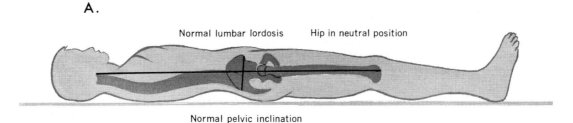

Normal lumbar lordosis   Hip in neutral position

Normal pelvic inclination

B.

Note increased pelvic inclination

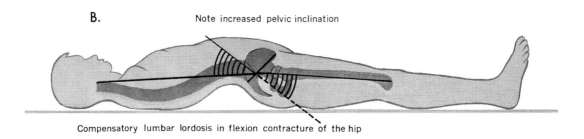

Compensatory lumbar lordosis in flexion contracture of the hip

C.

Opposite hip and knee
are maximally flexed

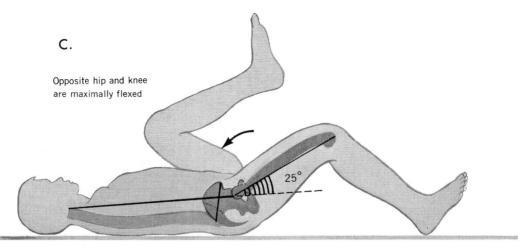

25°

Lumbar spine flattens   Note flexion contracture of hip

FIGURE 12–6 ■ Diagrammatic representation of the Thomas test to assess hip flexion contracture. (Adapted from von Lanz T, Wachsmith W: Praktische Anatomic. Berlin, Julius Springer, 1938, p 157.) (From Tachdjian MO: Pediatric Orthopaedics, ed 2. Philadelphia, WB Saunders Company, 1990, p 28; reprinted by permission.)

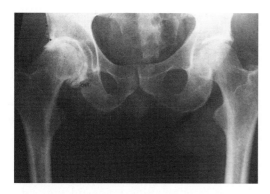

FIGURE 12–7 ■ Anteroposterior pelvic radiograph of a 65-year-old male with osteoarthritis of the right hip. The contralateral left hip is normal.

etabulum are also well visualized on computerized axial tomography scan images. Magnetic resonance imaging of the hips is indicated in patients where a periarticular lesion is suspected or to evaluate for the presence of avascular necrosis (AVN) of the femoral heads.

The bone scan can be helpful in identifying occult fracture of the femoral neck in elderly patients who are osteopenic. The bone scan is also helpful for identifying neoplastic disease in the region of the hip.

Aspiration of the hip should be performed under fluoroscopic guidance. Aspiration is essential in the evaluation of a possibly septic joint in a child or an adult. Aspiration of the hip and intra-articular injection with a local anesthetic agent can be helpful in differentiating hip from spine pathology. If the intra-articular local anesthetic results in near complete relief of pain, the pain is most likely intra-articular in origin. If the pain is not altered by the local anesthetic agent, extra-articular pathology or spine disease should be investigated.

The use of these radiographic techniques is directed by the patient's history and physical examination. The appropriate use of these diagnostic tests can result in a cost-effective and accurate diagnosis and properly directed treatment.

HIP PATHOLOGY

Fractures, infection, metabolic bone disease, and neoplastic disease have been reviewed in

previous chapters of this text. This review will focus on arthritic conditions affecting the hip and AVN. Avascular necrosis is a condition that most commonly affects the femoral head. However, this condition can also affect the proximal humerus, knee, and talus.

The specific mechanism causing AVN is unclear. Several factors have been associated with increased risk of developing this condition. The most common factors are trauma to the proximal femur, excessive alcohol intake, and systemic corticosteroid administration (Fig. 12–8). In addition to these factors, there is a long list of less common causative factors such as hemoglobinopathies, metabolic conditions, and inflammatory conditions. However, in as many as one third of patients with nontraumatic AVN, no specific etiology can be identified.

In all cases there is compromise of the blood supply of the femoral head, which leads to necrosis of a portion of the femoral head. If the avascular segment is large and in a weight-bearing area as the necrotic trabeculae weaken, the support of the subchondral bone is compromised, the round femoral head will collapse, and the joint will progressively degenerate.

In early cases, prior to collapse of the femoral head, attempts can be made to save the femoral head and restore vascularity. These techniques are surgical and involve drilling a core tract into the avascular portion of the

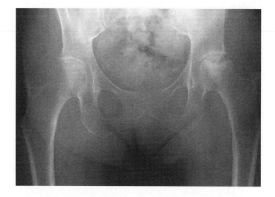

FIGURE 12–8 ■ Anteroposterior radiograph of a 57-year-old female who was treated with systemic corticosteroids to prevent rejection of a cardiac transplant. She presented with left hip pain, and the radiograph demonstrates avascular necrosis of the femoral head on the right side. The outer contour of the femoral head remains round.

femoral head in an attempt to restore vascularity and possibly heal the lesion. Several techniques have been described to augment this procedure—from cancellous bone grafting to using one of the patient's fibulae on a vascular pedicle to place vascularized bone into the lesion.

In patients who undergo no treatment of their AVN, 70 percent will require a total hip replacement within 5 years. Patients who have had a core decompression-type procedure will require a total hip replacement (THR) in 30 to 35 percent of cases within 5 years. Although such results are an improvement over no treatment, the success rate is less than we would prefer. As the AVN progresses and the hip becomes severely degenerated, hip replacement offers the most reliable means of restoring function and relieving pain.

A wide variety of arthritidies can affect the hip joint. While the medical therapy can vary based upon the specific diagnosis, the operative treatments fall into several broad categories and will be discussed as such.

Hip Arthritis

Arthritis is defined as any condition which results in cartilage damage with resulting pain and limitation of the motion of a joint. Hip arthritis can be divided into several broad categories (Table 12–1). The nonoperative treatment will vary based upon the specific diagnosis. Osteoarthritis (OA), whether primary or secondary, is treated in a similar fashion.

The treatment for the majority of patients with osteoarthritis is nonoperative. There are five primary interventions in the nonoperative management of the patient with osteoarthritis (Table 12–2).

These five interventions should be used in combination as indicated. Non-steroidal anti-inflammatory drugs (NSAIDs) can be very effective in eliminating pain and improving function. However, there is a large individual variation in the efficacy of these agents. Patients should be tried on several NSAIDs from different chemical classes before this arm of therapy is abandoned.

Intra-articular corticosteroid injections are helpful for acute exacerbations in pain. Intra-articular injections are beneficial in the treatment of shoulder and knee pathology. They have not been as widely utilized for arthritis of the hip. Injection of the hip with local anesthetic can be helpful in differentiating referred back pain from intra-articular pathology. However, injections are limited in their ability to provide long-term relief of symptoms. Corticosteroid injection for arthritis should not be done more than 3 times per year. If the patient requires more frequent injections for pain control, other therapeutic measures or surgery should be considered.

TABLE 12–1 ■ *Classification of Hip Arthritis*

CATEGORY	EXAMPLES	ETIOLOGY
Osteoarthritis	Primary osteoarthritis	Idiopathic
	Secondary osteoarthritis	Congenital
		Developmental
		Avascular necrosis
		Posttraumatic
Inflammatory arthritis	Rheumatoid arthritis	Immunogenic
	Ankylosing spondylitis	
	Psoriatic arthritis	
	Systemic lupus	
Infectious	Pyogenic	*S. aureus,*
		S. epidermidis,
		Gonococcal
	Lyme Disease	*Borrellia*
	Nonpyogenic	Mycobacterium
Other	Crystals	Gout, Pseudogout
	Hemophilia	Hemosiderin
		Deposition

TABLE 12–2 ■ *Primary Interventions in the Nonoperative Management of Osteoarthritis*

Nonsteroidal anti-inflammatory drugs (NSAIDs)
Physical Therapy
Intra-articular injection of corticosteroids
Assistive devices
Modification of activities

Repeated injection of the joint is not indicated. This will result in acceleration of the articular cartilage degeneration and increases the risks of complications such as infection.

Physical therapy can be beneficial in reducing pain and improving range of motion for OA involving the knee or shoulder, although limited benefit has been found for the treatment of OA involving the hip. However, all patients should be encouraged to strive for aerobic fitness to maintain their joint function as well as their general health.

Assistive devices including crutches, cane, and a walker can be quite effective in the relief of stress across the joint surface with ambulation in patients with OA involving the lower extremities. A cane used in the contralateral hand of a patient with isolated hip arthritis can reduce the joint reaction force by as much as 30 percent. However, the use of these devices is associated with a significant change in patients' perception of themselves and their global health status.

Modification of activities is one of the most significant aspects in the non-operative management of arthritis. This includes modification in a patient's activities of daily living and self care. The reduction of certain activities, such as running or racquet sports, can improve the patient's joint symptoms. However, this will result in a gradual progressive decrease in the patient's quality of life. The level of social interaction and activities in which the patient can comfortably participate thus may become markedly reduced.

Modification of activities should also address patients who are overweight. Reduction in weight can significantly improve patients' symptoms, increase their mobility, and improve their global health status. In addition, reduction in weight will lessen the stress placed upon the joint replacement implants if they require surgery.

The nonoperative management of a patient with OA involves all of the above therapies. However, as the arthritis progresses, pain and limitation of activities will continue to increase. When the patient fails to achieve acceptable symptomatic relief with the nonoperative regimen, joint replacement should be discussed. No significant change in the complexity of the surgery or outcome will be noted in patients with hip arthritis who delay having an operative intervention in favor of nonoperative treatment.

SURGICAL MANAGEMENT

Osteotomy

Osteotomy involves redirecting the joint forces by realigning the bone of the pelvis or proximal femur. The bone is transected, redirected, and then fixed rigidly in some fashion. If there is arthritis in only one portion of a joint, by having the patient undergo an osteotomy, the damaged cartilage can be moved away from the weight-bearing area and undamaged articular surfaces transferred into the high-stress area. This will result in reduced pain and prolong the functional life of the patient's native joint. Prerequisites for an osteotomy are that the patient have an adequate range of motion of the joint, that the joint be stable, and that the articular damage is only in a limited area of the joint. If extensive arthritis is present, then the osteotomy will not be successful.

In properly selected patients, hip osteotomies can have a success rate of 80 percent at 8 to 10 years follow-up. For young patients with focal articular damage, osteotomy can provide an acceptable option, retaining their own hip joint without the need for replacement with artificial materials that can wear or become loose (Fig. 12–9). Osteotomy of the proximal femur can make a future hip replacement more difficult by altering the anatomy of the proximal femur.

Arthrodesis

Arthrodesis involves the fusion of the proximal femur to the pelvis. This procedure can result in a strong, stable, painless lower extremity. The patient can even return to heavy labor without the risk of loosening or doing damage to the arthrodesis. However, the hip will be stiff, and over a period of 15 to 20 years the arthrodesis can result in low back pain and pain in the ipsilateral knee. Several reports have noted between 50 to 60 percent of pa-

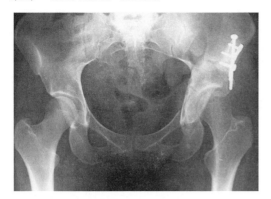

FIGURE 12–9 ■ Anteroposterior radiograph of a 26-year-old female 6 months after a left pelvic osteotomy was performed to deepen her acetabulum and improve coverage of the femoral head. Her primary diagnosis was developmental dysplasia of the hip, which left her with a shallow left acetabulum.

goes inside the canal of the femur. Two principal types of implants are used today. Those inserted with bone cement and those inserted without cement and designed to allow bone to grow onto or into a porous metal surface (Fig. 12–10). The principal advantage of utilizing bone cement is that immediate rigid fixation is obtained. The bone does not need to respond to the implant to obtain fixation. In patients with an average age of 65 years, excellent survival of 20 years or greater has been noted. Non-cemented fixation requires the bone to respond to the implant to provide rigid, long-term fixation. However, if the bone does stabilize the implant as the bone remodels over time, rigid fixation should be maintained over the long term. Postoperatively, the patient is mobilized to a chair the day after surgery and begins physical therapy on the second postoperative day. If the femoral component is cemented, the patient may fully bear weight on

tients complaining of pain in the back or knee at 25 to 50 years follow-up. If the pain is severe, the fusion can be taken down surgically and a total hip replacement performed. The outcome of this surgery depends upon the functional status of the hip abductor muscles. However, the return to a mobile hip can relieve the patient's low back pain.

The indications for arthrodesis are patients with significant hip arthritis who are relatively young, may be heavy laborers, have no preexisting back or ipsilateral knee pain, and have unilateral hip involvement. Patients with bilateral disease or an inflammatory arthritis are not appropriate candidates for arthrodesis.

Hip Replacement Surgery

Total hip replacement is a common operation today. Approximately 200,000 replacements are performed each year. The primary goal of hip replacement surgery is to relieve pain. This can be accomplished in >95 percent of patients. The results of THR can last approximately 15 years. In fact, one study found that 80 percent of patients with THRs survived a minimum of 20 years.

In THR both the socket and the ball are replaced with metal and plastic parts. The socket is replaced with either a plastic cup cemented onto the bone or by a metal shell with a removable plastic liner. The ball is replaced by a metal ball attached to a stem that

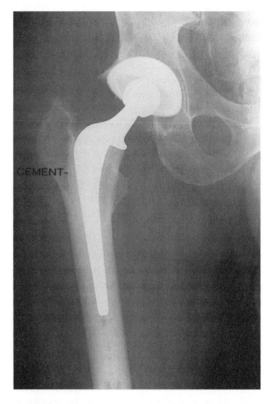

FIGURE 12–10 ■ Anteroposterior view of the right hip after "hybrid" total hip replacement in the 65-year-old male pictured in Fig. 12–7. In the "hybrid" replacement, the femoral component is cemented in place and the acetabular component is inserted in a noncemented fashion.

the operative leg immediately. If porous ingrowth fixation is utilized some surgeons will allow restricted weight-bearing for 6 weeks to allow for bone ingrowth. Patients need to be careful not to flex the hip beyond 90 degrees and to keep their legs abducted for the first 6 weeks to prevent the ball from dislocating out of the socket.

Aseptic loosening of the implant from bone occurs at a low rate with modern techniques. A recent study reviewing the minimum 20-year follow-up of patients after cemented THR revealed approximately 90 percent of patients had retained their original implant until they had died or until their minimum 20-year follow-up evaluation. Revision surgery had been performed on 15 percent of the surviving patients. Eleven percent of the revisions were for aseptic loosening. The rate of loosening of the femoral component was found to be 3 percent and 10 percent for the acetabular component in the surviving patients. Eighty-five percent of the patients who survived a minimum of 20 years had retained their initial implant. One study demonstrated that the rate of femoral loosening is greater in the first 5 years and decreases after 5 years. Acetabular loosening however, was noted to increase over time when cemented components were used. The use of modern cementing techniques has decreased the rate of early failure of cemented stems. Modern techniques, however, have not resulted in any significant change in the rate of acetabular loosening.

The survival of cemented implants in patients <50 years of age is a lower rate than that noted in older patients. This is most likely related to the higher demands and higher activity level in this younger group of patients.

In an attempt to reduce the rate of aseptic loosening after THR, surgeons have tried to achieve implant fixation directly to bone. This can be accomplished through the use of porous surfaces made of small beads or wires sintered onto the base stem. If this surface is closely approximated to bone and essentially no motion occurs at the interface, bone trabeculae will interdigitate into the porous surface and secure the implant. Little long-term data exist to support the use of porous ingrowth devices. However, the early data are encouraging. The rate of early loosening of the porous ingrowth femoral implants is slightly greater in most series compared to cemented stems. The rate of loosening appears to vary with the stem design for the porous ingrowth devices. There-

fore data should be analyzed for each implant. Porous ingrowth hemispherical acetabular components, however, appear to have a lower rate of loosening compared to cemented acetabular components.

An additional disadvantage of the porous ingrowth femoral devices is the presence of thigh pain. This is a mechanical type of pain, increasing with weight-bearing and relieved by rest. The rate of thigh pain varies with the individual implant design and ranges from 5 to 20 percent. The etiology of thigh pain is unclear at present. However, it may be related to the stiffness of the noncemented implants in direct contact with bone.

At the present time a "hybrid" total hip arthroplasty is recommended for the majority of patients receiving THR. This includes the use of a cemented femoral stem and a porous ingrowth acetabular component. This arthroplasty takes advantage of the excellent long-term results with the use of cemented femoral stems and the improved fixation with modern cementing as well as the very encouraging results with the use of porous ingrowth acetabular components.

Complications

The most frequent complication after THR is thromboembolic disease. This includes deep venous thrombosis and pulmonary embolism. Early in the history of THR, the rate of fatal pulmonary embolism was 1 to 2 percent. However, at that time patients were kept at bed rest for as long as 2 to 3 weeks and up to 6 weeks in the hospital. Early mobilization of patients has undoubtedly contributed to the significant reduction in the rate of fatal pulmonary embolism.

However, significant reduction has also occurred through the use of regional anesthesia, shorter operating times, and lower blood loss. In the United States, THR is considered a significant risk factor for thromboembolic disease, and therefore routine use of medical and/or mechanical prophylaxis has been recommended. At present the rate of thromboembolic disease ranges between 5 and 15 percent. The rate of fatal pulmonary embolism is low, approximately 0.01 percent. The principal methods of prophylaxis are low-dose Coumadin, aspirin, and pneumatic compression stockings. Interest is now focusing upon low molecular-weight heparin for routine prophylaxis.

Dislocation of the prosthetic femoral head from the acetabular component occurs in 2 to 5 percent of patients after THR. Postoperatively, patients are instructed to not bend their replaced hip beyond 80 degrees and to keep their legs abducted. These restrictions should be followed closely for the first 6 to 8 weeks following surgery. After this time, the patient should have formed a sufficient pseudocapsule to protect against dislocation. However, a replaced hip is always at greater risk for dislocation compared to a native hip joint. The majority of patients who dislocate their hip in the early postoperative period can be reduced without additional surgery and protected with a hip abduction brace for 6 weeks to allow healing of the pseudocapsule. In addition to patient compliance, the other etiologies for dislocation are component malposition, excessive soft-tissue laxity, and impingement of the prosthetic or osseous structures resulting in levering of the femoral head out of the acetabulum. If a patient recurrently dislocates, revision surgery may be indicated.

The most devastating complication after THR is deep sepsis. Early post-operative infection occurs in approximately 0.3 to 0.5 percent of cases after primary THR. If detected within the first 2 weeks postoperatively, open debridement and synovectomy combined with intravenous antibiotics may be successful. However, if the infection recurs after debridement or is detected beyond 2 weeks, treatment must include removal of the prosthetic components and all cement. The prosthesis is left out for at least 6 weeks. If the pathologic organisms are highly virulent and resistant to antibiotic therapy, reimplantation may be delayed for more than 12 months. Serum bactericidal titers (SBT) should be determined and a titer of at least 1 to 8 maintained during the 6-week course of therapy. During the antibiotic therapy, patients may be mobilized to the extent that they can tolerate with the use of a walker. Reimplantation can proceed when the wound is sterile if sufficient bone stock and soft-tissue integrity remain. The use of antibiotic-impregnated cement for the femoral component is recommended. If the SBT was maintained at 1 to 8 for 6 weeks, reimplantation of a new prosthesis will be successful in 90 percent of cases. Recent data has demonstrated a higher rate of recurrence in patients reimplanted without cement.

Heterotopic ossification (HO) can form around a THR in 5 to 25 percent of cases. Frequently, the presence of HO will not compromise the clinical result. Associated risk factors are patients with hypertrophic osteoarthritis, males over the age of 65, previous HO formation after surgery, and ankylosing spondylitis. Patients who are at high risk for this complication can receive prophylaxis using indomethacin for 6 weeks or low-dose radiation therapy.

CONCLUSION

The accurate diagnosis and treatment of hip disease requires a careful analysis of the patient's history, a thorough physical examination, and a review of the appropriate radiographic studies. While there are many conditions leading to degeneration and pain in the hip joint, the treatment options are similar. Many patients, particularly those who are older, will benefit from hip replacement; however, in properly selected patients, osteotomy or arthrodesis may offer good results without implants.

SUGGESTED READINGS

Evans BG, Salvati EA: Total Hip Arthroplasty in the Elderly: Cost Effective Alternatives. Instructional Course Lectures, vol 43. Chicago, American Academy of Orthopaedic Surgery, 1994.

Evans BG, Salvati EA: The Case for Cemented Total Hip Arthroplasty. Orthopaedic Clinics in North America. Philadelphia, WB Saunders Company, 24(2), 1993.

Schulte KR, Callaghan JJ, Kelley SS, Johnston RC: The outcome of Charnley total hip arthroplasty with cement after a minimum twenty-year follow-up: The results of one surgeon. J Bone and Joint Surg. 75-A:961–971, 1993.

Wedge JH, Cummiskey DJ: Primary arthroplasty of the hip in patients who are less than twenty-one years old. J Bone and Joint Surg 76-A:1732–1742, 1994.

13

The Knee

Brian G. Evans

This chapter will discuss the anatomy, evaluation, and pathology of the knee. The function of the knee is provided primarily by the soft tissue. Therefore, injury to these soft-tissue structures will have significant impact upon the stability of the knee.

ANATOMY

The osseous anatomy of the knee consists of the proximal tibia, distal femur, and the patella (Fig. 13–1). The distal femur consists of the medial and lateral condyles, the medial and lateral epicondyles, femoral trochlear groove, and the intercondylar notch. The medial condyle is larger and extends slightly distal compared to the lateral condyle. Both condyles are covered with articular cartilage. The trochlear groove lies on the anterior aspect of the distal femur between the medial and lateral femoral condyles. This surface is also covered by articular cartilage and serves as the site of articulation of the patella. The lateral rim of the trochlear groove is frequently more prominent than the medial side to allow for proper patellar tracking along the femur.

The epicondyles serve as the site of insertion of several important structures. The deep and superficial medial collateral ligament (MCL) attaches to the medial epicondyle. The proximal margin of the medial epicondyle is enlarged and serves as the site of insertion of the adductor magnus (the adductor tubercle). The lateral, or fibular, collateral ligament (LCL) attaches to the lateral epicondyle. Infe-

rior to the attachment of the LCL is the insertion of the popliteus muscle at the junction of the lateral condyle and epicondyle. The medial and lateral heads of the gastrocnemius muscle originate from the medial and lateral posterior femoral condyles. The intercondylar notch is the site of the femoral attachment of the cruciate ligaments. The anterior cruciate ligament (ACL) attaches in the posterior lateral aspect of the notch, while the posterior cruciate ligament (PCL) attaches in the anterior medial aspect of the notch.

The proximal tibial surface is composed of the medial and lateral plateaus and the intercondylar eminence. The medial plateau is larger and extends further posterior compared to the lateral plateau. The surface of the medial plateau is relatively flat. The lateral tibial plateau is, in fact, slightly convex. Both of the tibial plateaus are covered with articular cartilage. The intercondylar eminence is the site of attachment between the menisci and the cruciate ligaments.

The patella is a sesamoid bone within the tendon of the quadriceps mechanism. There are two major facets on the patella—the medial and lateral facets. There is significant variability in the size and orientation of these facets. However, normally the lateral facet is broader and the medial facet is more acutely oriented to the femoral trochlea.

The osseous anatomy of the knee provides little to the stability of the knee. Stability and function are therefore provided by the complex soft-tissue envelope around and in the knee (Figs. 13–2 and 3). The soft-tissue components of the knee can be divided into

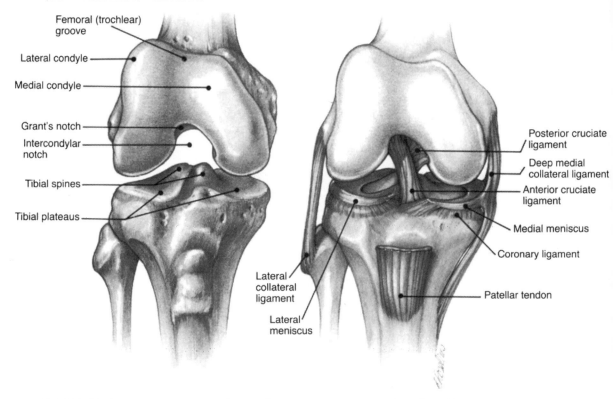

FIGURE 13–1 ■ Bony anatomy and major ligamentous structures of the flexed knee joint (anterior view).

(From Wiesel S, Delahay J, Connell M (eds): Essentials of Orthopaedic Surgery. Philadelphia, WB Saunders Co, 1993, p 252.)

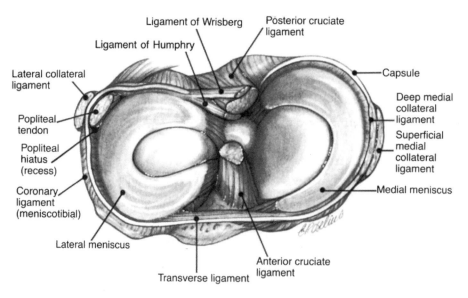

FIGURE 13–2 ■ Cross-section of the knee demonstrating the menisci and associated ligaments.

(From Wiesel S, Delahay J, Connell M (eds): Essentials of Orthopaedic Surgery. Philadelphia, WB Saunders Co, 1993, p 253.)

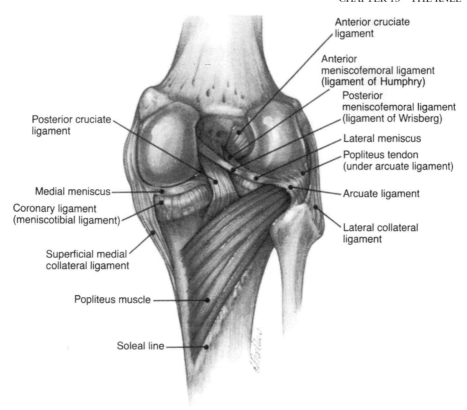

Posterior cruciate ligament

Medial meniscus

Coronary ligament (meniscotibial ligament)

Superficial medial collateral ligament

Popliteus muscle

Soleal line

Anterior cruciate ligament

Anterior meniscofemoral ligament (ligament of Humphry)

Posterior meniscofemoral ligament (ligament of Wrisberg)

Lateral meniscus

Popliteus tendon (under arcuate ligament)

Arcuate ligament

Lateral collateral ligament

FIGURE 13–3 ■ Posterior aspect of the knee joint.

(From Wiesel S, Delahay J, Connell M (eds): Essentials of Orthopaedic Surgery. Philadelphia, WB Saunders Co, 1993, p 254.)

several components: static restraints (ligaments), dynamic restraints (muscles and tendons), and the menisci. The static restraints are represented by the MCL, LCL, ACL, and PCL. These structures also resist valgus and varus stress and anterior and posterior translation of the tibial relative to the femur. The MCL consists of two layers. The deep MCL spans from the medial epicondyle of the femur to the proximal tibial border just below the medial tibial plateau. The superficial MCL has the same femoral origin; however, the ligament has a broad tibial insertion extending 6 to 10 cm below the tibial plateau along the posterior medial border of the tibia. The LCL is a more discrete band along the lateral aspect of the knee. It spans from the lateral epicondyle to the fibular head.

The ACL resists the anterior translation of the tibia relative to the femur. The ligament runs from the anterior aspect of the tibial eminence to the posterior lateral aspect of the femoral notch. The PCL resists posterior translation of the tibia relative to the femur and resists hyperextension of the knee. The ligament extends from the posterior aspect of the intercondylar eminence and proximal tibia in the midline to the anterior medial aspect of the femoral intercondylar notch.

The dynamic restraints in the knee are the muscles and tendons that cross the knee joint. These are broadly divided into muscles that act to extend and those that act to flex the knee. The extensor muscles are the quadriceps femoris and the tensor facia lata. The quadriceps make up a group of four muscles all inserting onto the patella and the patellar tendon, which in turn, inserts upon the anterior tibial tubercle. The muscles that make up the quadriceps are the rectus femoris, vastus lateralis, vastus medialis, and vastus intermedius. These are all supplied by the femoral nerve. The tensor fascia lata originates upon the pelvic brim and inserts at Gerdy's tubercle on the proximal anterior lateral tibia. The tensor fascia lata is innervated by the superior gluteal nerve.

The primary flexors of the knee are the

hamstring muscles: the semimembranosis, the semitendonosis and biceps femoris, and the sartorius, and gracillis. The hamstring muscles originate on the ischium and insert on the posterior medial and lateral proximal tibia. They receive their innervation from the sciatic nerve; all are innervated by the tibial division of the sciatic nerve except the short head of the biceps, which is innervated by the peroneal division of the sciatic nerve. The sartorius originates from the anterior superior iliac spine, and the gracillis originates from the pubis. Both of these muscles with the semitendonosis insert into the proximal medial tibia in the pes anserine (goose's foot, relating to the appearance of the three tendons inserting together). The sartorius is innervated by the femoral nerve and the gracillis by the obturator nerve.

The other muscles that serve to flex the knee are the gastrocnemius and popliteus, which extend from the posterior aspect of the femoral condyles to the calcaneous and proximal tibia, respectively.

The menisci are two crescent-shaped cartilaginous structures attached to the proximal tibial surface. These structures serve two purposes in the knee. They increase the surface area for weight-bearing, therefore, reducing the peak stress in the articular cartilage. They also provide a small degree of stability to the knee by changing the flat tibial articular surface to a cupped surface. The menisci are composed of dense, organized cartilage tissue.

Biomechanics of the Knee

The mechanical axis of the lower extremity extends from the center of rotation of the hip to the center of the ankle joint. This normally crosses the knee joint in the lateral third of the medial tibial plateau. The normal anatomic alignment of the knee is in 7 degrees of valgus. When the knee is loaded, the medial compartment sees 60 percent of the weight-bearing stress and the lateral compartment sees 40 percent of the weight-bearing stress. This difference in the applied load in the normal knee is why the medial tibial plateau and medial femoral condyle are larger than the lateral side. Patients with significant angular deformity in the knee will have altered weight-bearing, and this will result in increased stress in the medial (with varus or bow-legged deformity) or lateral (with valgus or knock-knee deformity) compartment. The increased stress

will frequently result in early arthritis in the overused compartment of the knee.

The highest joint forces, however, are found in the patello-femoral articulation. Forces as high as 5 to 8 times body weight can be noted for activities such as stair climbing and jumping. The function of the patella has been controversial, however, most now recognize the patella's role in providing a mechanical advantage to the quadriceps tendon. The patella moves the line of pull of the quadriceps further away from the center of rotation, therefore acting as a lever and reducing the force required to extend the knee. Patients who have had the patella removed because of arthritis or trauma are noted to have approximately 30 percent reduction in the force in the quadriceps compared to patients with a patella.

EVALUATION OF THE PAINFUL KNEE

History

The history should begin with the chief complaint and how long the patient noticed the problem. The specific location of pain, any radiation, the nature of the pain (ache, burning, stabbing, etc.), and any exacerbating or ameliorating factors. In particular, the relationship of the pain with activity and rest are important to note. Commonly, pain in the musculoskeletal system will be relieved with rest. Severe pain, which is present at rest, suggests a septic process or neoplasm, which may be primary or metastatic.

Frequently, knee problems begin with an injury. Detailed history describing the injury can be very helpful in determining the structures that are injured. The nature of any external force contacting the knee, as well as the position of the knee at the time of injury, should be elicited. Did an audible or palpable pop occur at the time of the injury? Shifting or abnormal movement of the knee may also have been noted at the time of injury. The degree and nature of any swelling around the knee is important to record. In addition to a description of the injury, it is helpful to inquire about the patient's ability to use the knee after the injury. Was the patient able to bear weight? Was the onset of pain or swelling immediate or delayed? Could the patient flex or extend the knee after injury? These are all important questions to ask the patient after knee injury.

In addition to pain, patients with knee problems will complain of mechanical problems in the knee. Patients may note an inability to fully bend or straighten the knee. This is referred to as locking of the knee. Locking can be a result of a loose body in the knee becoming lodged between the femoral condyle and tibial plateau similar to a wedge "door stop." The patients who note intermittent locking of the knee will usually be able to relieve the locked knee by gently moving the knee without weight bearing. This maneuver allows the loose fragment to be released from between the femur and tibia and motion will be restored. However, inability to fully flex and extend the knee can also be noted in patients with large effusions and in patients with ligament injuries.

Instability is another frequent complaint of patients with knee injuries. Patients will observe that their knee will shift or buckle with particular activities. Instability can result from two general etiologies. The first are ligamentous injuries. As noted previously, the stability of the knee is a result of the ligaments that cross from the tibia to the femur. Disruption of the ligaments will result in alteration of knee function; the knee may shift or sublux with activity. The second common cause of a knee buckling or giving way are problems in the patella-femoral joint. Instability of the patella in the trochlear groove will result in a giving way sensation as the patella subluxes. Damage to the articular surfaces of the patella or the trochlear groove will result in pain as the patella tracks over the trochlea. This can occasionally lead to a sharp acute pain that will lead to the quadriceps releasing its contraction while the patient is weight-bearing on the leg as a result of a primitive reflex arc. The patient will note a giving way or buckling sensation in the knee, and a few patients may actually fall as a result.

The majority of knee complaints are aggravated by activities. The specific problems the patient has encountered are important to note. Patients will commonly have difficulty ascending and descending stairs. Frequently, descending stairs will be the most symptomatic as this places high stress across the patella-femoral joint. Bicycling can also aggravate the patella-femoral joint. Activities that involve quadriceps contraction with the knee in flexion may result in subluxation in patients with patellar instability. Patients with meniscal tears will have difficulty squatting and may notice snapping or pain when rising from a chair or ascending stairs. Activities that involve stopping and turning or cutting will result in the knee shifting or giving way if there is insufficiency in the collateral or cruciate ligaments.

Physical Examination

Physical examination of the patient with a knee complaint begins inspection. Observation of the alignment of the lower extremity should demonstrate a normal 7-degree valgus (knock-knee) angle at the knee when a patient is standing. Deformity of the leg in varus or valgus beyond 7 degrees can be associated with either a ligamentous or osseous deficiency. Any swelling, bruising, or ecchymosis should be recorded.

Next, the evaluation should focus upon the patient's gait. Normal gait involves range of motion from 0 to 65 degrees of flexion. The gait should have a smooth cadence, with the length of each step being equal on the left and right sides. The knee should not demonstrate any sudden shift to either the lateral or medial sides. If abnormal lateral motion is noted, this is recorded as a medial or lateral thrust.

The knee should then be examined with patients sitting with their legs over the edge of the examining table. The position of the patella should be anterior and symmetric. The patellar tracking can then be followed by asking the patient to flex and extend the knee, with the examiner palpating the patella. There should be little lateral movement. Crepitus may also be noted as a grinding sensation between the patella and the femoral trochlear groove.

The knee should then be examined with the patient supine. For all aspects of the examination, the contralateral knee can be used as a normal control. Effusion or fluid within the knee can be assessed by placing both hands on the knee with one below the patella and one above the patella. Any fluid in the knee can then be displaced and palpated proximally and distally. The knee can be palpated to determine the specific site of maximum tenderness. The range of motion of the knee is measured with the knee in straight extension at 0 degrees of flexion; normal full flexion is approximately 135 degrees.

The collateral ligaments are then assessed by stabilizing the thigh with one hand and placing a varus or valgus stress on the knee with the other hand. A normal knee will have a small amount of medial and lateral laxity in the collateral ligaments. However, if any laxity is excessive or if pain is elicited, it should be noted. The cruciate ligaments can also be assessed. The ACL is best assessed using the Lachman test. The examiner should stand by the patient's feet. The femur is stabilized with one hand holding the distal medial thigh. The tibia is held with a thumb at the lateral joint line. The examiner then attempts to displace the tibia forward in relation to the femur. Translation <5 mm should be noted, and the ACL should be felt to "snap taut." Injury to the PCL can be demonstrated by noting the degree of recurvatum (back-knee) that can be obtained passively compared to the contralateral knee. Also, with both knees flexed 60 to 90 degrees and the patient supine, the tibia on the deficient side will be noted to sag posteriorly compared to the uninjured leg when viewed from the side. Comparison to the contralateral knee is very important for examination of the collateral and cruciate ligaments.

The menisci are examined by palpation of their outer margin along the joint line at the proximal tibial articular surface. In addition meniscal tears can be detected by the McMurray maneuver. This is done by flexing the knee internally and externally rotating the tibia and then extending the knee with a valgus force applied. If a reproducible snap is palpated or pain elicited at the joint line, this is suggestive of a tear. Patients with meniscal tears will also report pain when asked to squat down with the knees flexed.

Imaging

All of the available imaging techniques have been utilized in the evaluation of patients with knee problems. Plain radiographs are the most commonly obtained studies (Fig. 13–4). Plain radiographs are helpful in the evaluation of fractures and subluxation of the joint; in addition, the condition of the articular surfaces can be investigated. The standard series of routine x-rays of the knee should include a standing anteroposterior (AP) radiograph of both knees, a lateral view and a "Merchant" or "sunrise" view. The sunrise view is a view taken with the knee in 45 degrees of flexion with the beam directed inferiorly and parallel to the patellar articular surface. There should be a space of 5 to 10 mm between the end of the femoral condyles and the tibial surface and beneath the patellar surface and the femoral trochlea. This "clear space" is, in fact, occupied by articular cartilage.

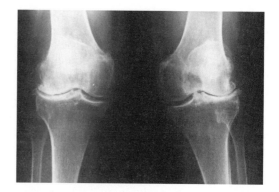

FIGURE 13–4 ■ Standing anteroposterior radiograph of the knees in a 70-year-old female with osteoarthritis of both knees with a valgus (knock-knee deformity). Note the asymmetric space between the medial and lateral femoral condyles and the tibial surface.

Routine radiography is an excellent tool for the evaluation of the knee for trauma, arthritis, and alignment. Plain radiographs, however, only demonstrate the osseous structures. As mentioned earlier the soft tissues provide the stability and allow the knee to function. Arthrography has been used in the past to evaluate the knee for meniscal pathology. However, this technique was inaccurate and invasive. The development of arthroscopy, a technique that allows the direct visualization of the structures within the knee with a minor surgical procedure. However, this technique is also invasive and while arthroscopy is accurate, the procedure is relatively expensive compared to an imaging modality alone. Nuclear medicine studies are of limited use in the knee. These studies are sensitive, however, the specificity of these studies is limited. Magnetic resonance imaging (MRI) represents a dramatic step forward in our ability to diagnose soft-tissue injury to the knee. Providing accurate and noninvasive evaluation of all of the soft-tissue structures within the knee (Fig. 13–5), MRI is currently the study of choice for the evaluation of intra-articular pathology within the knee.

KNEE PATHOLOGY

Soft-tissue injury is common in the knee. A knee with a bloody effusion after an injury has an incidence as high as 80 percent of significant soft-tissue injury. The differential diagnosis of a posttraumatic bloody effusion in the absence of an intra-articular fracture is meniscal tear, ACL tear, or a patellar dislocation.

Meniscal Tears

Tears of the meniscus can occur in two settings. One is as the result of a specific injury. This usually involves a twisting injury with the knee in some flexion. Swelling and pain are noted immediately after the injury. There is increased pain with attempts at movement, and there is a limitation in the range of motion. Pain with squatting down or arising from a chair are commonly reported. The torn meniscus can block motion. Occasionally, the knee can be gently manipulated to reduce the torn meniscal fragment and motion will be restored. However, the fragment will fre-

quently redisplace and intermittent locking may occur. This form of a tear is usually in younger patients with stout meniscal tissue.

In older individuals, the meniscal tissues soften and the edge becomes frayed. As this occurs, the frayed edges can become entrapped between the edges of the bone initiating a tear which can extend into the meniscal substance. This tear can occur with little or no trauma, minimal swelling, and pain initially. The diagnosis is made by joint line pain, effusion, and rarely locking. Patients with locking will frequently require arthroscopic surgery to debride the torn portion of the meniscus. In older patients with meniscal tears, if the tear does not cause locking, frequently, these can be treated with nonsteroidal anti-inflammatory drugs (NSAIDs) and an intra-articular corticosteroid injection. These treatments will reduce the effusion and pain. With continued activity the soft meniscal tis-

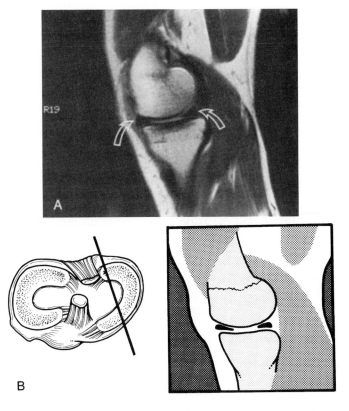

FIGURE 13–5 ■ *A,* Normal T1-weighted MRI sagittal image of the medial meniscus. *B,* Schematic illustration showing the section cut of *A.* (MRI indicates magnetic resonance imaging).

(From Wiesel S, Delahay J, Connell M (eds): Essentials of Orthopaedic Surgery. Philadelphia, WB Saunders Co, 1993, p 257.)

sue can be worn down and a stable edge reestablished.

Ligament Injuries

Injury to the ligamentous structures are manifested by instability in the knee. In addition to pain and swelling, patients will report a sense of the knee shifting or giving way. This may be with only specific activities such as descending stairs or when turning on the loaded extremity. The initial management of these injuries is rest, ice, and elevation. A splint or knee immobilizer can also be helpful to protect the knee. As the initial pain subsides it is important to begin to work on restoring the range of motion using a brace to protect the injured ligament. As the pain further decreases strengthening is begun. If, after the strengthening program is completed, the knee remains unstable the patient may be a candidate for surgical reconstruction.

Patella-femoral Pathology

The patella-femoral joint is one of the most common areas of pain in the knee. Common complaints are anterior knee pain which is aggravated by activities involving high loads on a flexed knee such as stair climbing or bicycling. This pain can be the result of degenerative changes in the patella-femoral articulation or a result of mal-tracking of the patella within the trochlear groove. A grinding or snapping sensation may also be noted. Pain is usually relieved by rest; however, if the patient is sitting for a prolonged period of time with the knee flexed, such as in a theater, on a plane, or during a long car ride, anterior knee pain will result. Frequently, patients will try to change the position of the knee to relieve their discomfort. This phenomenon is known as "movie sign" and is indicative of degenerative changes in the patella-femoral joint. Softening of the articular surface is referred to as "chondromalacia patella." This can be a primary problem or it may be secondary to excessive trauma to the joint due to mal-tracking of the patella within the trochlear groove.

The treatment of these conditions is primarily nonoperative. Improving the patellar tracking can be done through a series of exercises to retrain the quadriceps and through patellar mobilization exercises. The exercise program needs to be maintained for a minimum of 6 to 8 weeks to demonstrate benefit.

The symptoms can frequently be recurrent. If the symptoms are recurrent, do not respond to the nonoperative regimen, and patellar mal-tracking is evident, operative intervention may be indicated. Operative intervention is directed at correcting the patellar tracking and maximizing the quadriceps function with postoperative physical therapy.

Arthritis

The management of arthritic symptoms within the knee are similar to management elsewhere. The nonoperative management of arthritis within the knee consists of a five-modality approach. The first line of therapy is the use of NSAIDs. These medications will reduce the pain and swelling associated with the knee. Although all NSAIDs function in a similar fashion, there is a wide variation in individual patient response. Therefore, a minimum of two or three different NSAIDs should be tried. The most common side effect of this course of treatment is dyspepsia.

The second line of treatment of arthritis is the selected use of intra-articular corticosteroid medication. This can be effective in patients who have an acute exacerbation of the arthritic pain. The injection can quiet their pain and restore them to a baseline level of discomfort. The injection should not be utilized for the control of baseline pain. If the injection is required at a frequency of greater than one every 6 to 8 weeks some other course of treatment should be initiated, such as surgery.

Physical therapy can be very helpful in the treatment of arthritis of the knee. Because the soft-tissue sleeve is very important to the function of the knee, by optimizing the function of the soft tissues the symptoms of arthritis can be reduced. The physical therapy should be directed at maintaining the range of motion of the knee and optimizing the strength of the quadriceps and the hamstring muscles. In the late stages of degenerative arthritis, physical therapy may worsen the patient's symptoms and should be limited to the patient's tolerance.

Assistive devices such as a cane or crutch may be of assistance in the management of arthritis of the knee. This can limit the stress across the painful knee and improve the patient's walking tolerance. The final approach to the management of arthritis of the knee is modification of activities. This includes alterations in the patient's activities such as sports, work environment, and possibly even assisting in arranging special parking for the patient. Frequently, patients with significant knee arthritis are also overweight. Weight loss in these patients can significantly reduce symptoms and the need for other treatment modalities.

Surgical Reconstruction for Arthritis

When all of the nonoperative measures have failed to relieve the symptoms of knee arthritis, surgical intervention should be contemplated. The surgical correction of knee arthritis can be separated into treatments which retain the patient's articular surfaces and knee replacement. Non-replacement options include the use of arthroscopy to "clean out" the knee; this procedure can remove the small cartilage fragments that accumulate in arthritic joints and debride any loose articular fragments. The pain relief from this procedure, however, is short lived, lasting only 3 to 6 months.

Patients with osteoarthritis of the knee will frequently develop angular deformities. The most common deformity is varus angulation of the knee. This results from erosion of the medial compartment of the knee. As the deformity progresses, a greater portion of the weight-bearing stress is concentrated in the medial compartment of the knee. Osteotomy is a procedure to realign the articulation. The proximal tibia is transected and a wedge of bone is removed from the lateral aspect. When the two new surfaces are brought together the varus deformity is corrected. This redistributes some of the weight-bearing stress to the lateral compartment and can result in improved symptoms in the knee. The result is generally successful for 5 to 10 years. Osteotomy is contraindicated in knees that are stiff or unstable. When the symptoms return, knee replacement surgery is indicated.

Arthrodesis or fusion of the knee is an option for the management of young, active patients, particularly physical laborers. This will result in a stiff, straight knee that will allow the patient to ambulate and stand for long periods of time without difficulty. However, significant limitations also exist. The gait pattern is significantly abnormal. Also patients will have difficulty sitting, particularly in confined spaces such as public transportation and theaters. Resection arthroplasty is a procedure where the articular surfaces are resected and a fibrous pseudoarthrosis forms within the joint space. Pain may be decreased; however, the knee is significantly unstable, requiring a brace for ambulation. Arthrodesis and resection arthroplasty are not commonly performed. Currently, these procedures are reserved for the management of a failed total knee replacement (TKR).

Total Knee Replacement is commonly utilized to relieve the symptoms of knee arthritis and restore function (Fig. 13–6). Approximately 200,000 arthroplasties are performed annually in the United States, with an average age of patients receiving a TKR being 70 to 74 years. Successful results can be obtained in over 95 percent of patients with survivorship at 10 to 15 years of 90 to 92 percent. All components are currently fixed with polymethyl methacrylate bone cement. Noncemented components, those used with porous ingrowth surfaces for bone ingrowth, have been associated with a higher incidence of loosening and pain.

The proximal tibia is cut perpendicular to the long axis of the shaft, and the femoral articular surface is cut using specific guides to remove the femoral trochlea, distal, and posterior femoral condyles. The anterior cruciate ligament is removed; however, the posterior cruciate ligament can be resected or retained depending on the design of implant chosen. For proper function of the arthroplasty the MCL, LCL, and (if retained) PCL must be carefully balanced. The components are then fixed to the surfaces of the tibia and femur with bone cement. The patella is normally resurfaced as well, after resecting the articular surface parallel to the anterior surface.

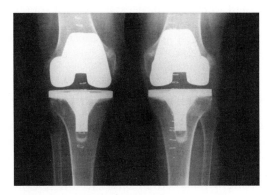

FIGURE 13–6 ■ Standing anteroposterior radiograph of both knees 2 weeks after one-stage bilateral knee replacements in the 70-year-old female whose preoperative radiograph is shown in Fig. 13–4.

The patient is mobilized into a chair on the first postoperative day, and full weight-bearing may be allowed immediately. However, a knee immobilizer should be utilized to protect the knee from acute flexion while walking. This is continued until the quadriceps function returns. The critical element of the postoperative therapy is the restoration of motion. If the motion is not restored within the first 3 to 6 weeks, maturation of the scar tissue will prevent major gains in motion after that point. Many patients can be safely discharged at 4 to 6 days after surgery.

Frequently, however, these patients will require home physical therapy to continue to work on range of motion and ambulation in the first few weeks after surgery. While the total rehabilitation period after TKR is between 3 and 6 months, patients are functionally mobile after 2 to 3 weeks. Knee replacement can be performed bilaterally in one stage in medically healthy patients (Fig. 13–6). The initial increase in debilitation post-operatively is offset by a reduction in the overall period of rehabilitation after sequential unilateral TKR.

Aseptic loosening of the implants after TKR occurs at a low rate. Several studies have documented a 10-year survivorship of >90 percent and <0.5 percent per-year rate of aseptic loosening after cemented THR. Young age, marked obesity, and high demand will negatively impact upon the long-term survival of the replacement. To date, the best data for noncemented TKR is equal to the cemented replacement. Several studies suggest poorer results when cement is not used particularly for fixation of the tibial component. Increased tibial loosening and pain have been noted with these devices. At present, due to the generally increased cost for the noncemented, porous-coated implants and poorer clinical results, the use of these devices is difficult to justify.

The majority of the complaints after cemented TKR are related to patella-femoral joint. This can be the result of poor soft-tissue alignment at the time of arthroplasty. This may lead to painful subluxation or dislocation of the patellar component. If inadequate bone is resected from the patella at the time of resurfacing, a marked increase in the patella-femoral stress can be noted which may become painful. Several authors have advocated not resurfacing the patella. However, several studies now demonstrate a higher rate of patella-femoral complaints after TKR without patellar resurfacing. If significant patella-femoral arthritis exists at the time of arthroplasty, weight >60 kg, height >160 cm, patients will have more pain postoperatively if the patella is not resurfaced.

The most common complication after TKR is thromboembolic disease. The rate of deep venous thrombosis ranges from 25 to 50 percent of cases in patients evaluated with venography or duplex Doppler analysis. As with patients receiving total hip replacement (THR) it is currently recommended that all patients receive some form of prophylaxis against thromboembolic disease. Mechanical methods such as the pneumatic compression stockings appear to have a greater benefit after TKR compared to THR. Low-dose Coumadin and aspirin are currently the most commonly utilized medications. The efficacy of low molecular-weight heparin is currently under investigation.

Deep infection occurs at a rate of approximately 1 percent after TKR for osteoarthritis over the life of the implant. The most common organisms are skin flora, primarily *Staphylococcus aureus* and *S. epidermidis*. In knee replacement in particular, the relatively thin soft-tissue envelope at the inferior aspect of the skin incision can lead to breakdown and allow entry of the flora into the joint. Any area of skin breakdown after TKR should be treated aggressively to prevent deep infection. This is particularly true in patients with prior incisions and in those with diabetes of significant vascular disease.

If a deep infection is established the only way to eradicate the infection is to remove the implants and then cement and thoroughly debride the joint. A cement spacer is then placed into the joint space, and the patient should receive 6 weeks of intravenous antibiotics. The Serum Bactericidal Titer (SBT) should exceed a ratio of 1 to 8. After 6 weeks, the knee can be reimplanted if adequate soft tissue and bone remains. However, due to the inevitable scarring, the clinical result is compromised.

Occasionally after TKR, range of motion of the knee does not progress well after surgery. If it is being seen less than 2 to 6 weeks since surgery, a return trip to the operating room for gentle manipulation of the knee, with the patient under anesthesia, may be beneficial. If the motion cannot be restored, particularly if the patient is beyond 6 weeks after replacement, additional surgery may be necessary to restore functional range of motion.

soft-tissue envelope with directed physical therapy is essential to an optimal outcome.

CONCLUSION

The knee is a complex joint with function provided by the combination of osseous and soft-tissue structures. The soft-tissue envelope plays a significant role in the pathology of the knee and in the management of these conditions. With careful history, physical examination, and appropriate use of the available diagnostic modalities, knee pathology can be accurately determined and successful treatment instituted. Successful management of knee pathology includes treatment of the specific etiology, but optimal management of the

SUGGESTED READINGS

Heck DA, Murray DG: Biomechanics in the Knee. In: Evarts CM (ed): Surgery of the Musculoskeletal System, ed 2. New York, Churchill Livingston, 1990, pp 3243-3254.

Stern SH, Insall JN: Posterior stabilized prosthesis: Results after follow-up of nine to twelve years. J Bone and Joint Surg 74-A:980-986, 1992.

Rand JA, Ilstrup DM: Survivorship analysis of total knee arthroplasty: Cumulative rates of survival of 9200 total knee arthroplasties. J Bone and Joint Surg. 73-A:397-409, 1991.

The Foot and Ankle

John N. Delahay

Always discussed at the end of every textbook about the musculoskeletal system, this anatomic segment still remains in many ways an orphan. Its anatomy is complex when compared to the hip; its afflictions are not nearly as glamorous as those that affect the knee; its surgical treatment is not as impressive as the extensive procedures used on the spine. Nevertheless, this seemingly boring anatomic region should be familiar territory for all physicians, if for no other reason than the fact that its afflictions are so commonplace.

Most adults at some time or another have painful feet. Many athletes will almost certainly sprain their ankle during the course of their endeavors. Most grandmothers will have corns, calluses, hammer toes, or bunions. Most children will start their walking career with apparent flat feet and toes pointing in. Thus, problems of the foot and ankle are important to both sexes and all age groups.

It is safe to assume that all physicians, despite their specialty, will at sometime during their career be asked to evaluate a patient with a painful foot. It is hoped that this chapter will allow that physician to be somewhat more conversant with the relevant anatomy of the region, the diagnostic evaluation of the painful foot, the broad categories of disease that impact on the foot and ankle, and a number of specific entities that might be considered. The final summary presents an algorithm that can be used as a logical guide in the diagnosis and treatment of afflictions of the foot and ankle.

STRUCTURAL ANATOMY

Osteology

The foot itself is generally divided for descriptive purposes into three anatomic regions: forefoot, midfoot, and hindfoot (Fig. 14–1). The forefoot is composed of the five metatarsals and 14 phalanges. The midfoot consists of five tarsal bones—the cuboid, the navicular, and three cuneiforms, which together form a trapezoid, larger base medial. The hindfoot contains the calcaneus (os calcis), which is the bone of the heel, providing a surface for ground contact; and the talus, which is at the apex of the foot, where it articulates in the ankle joint. The talus in many ways is indeed the "keystone" of the foot-ankle relationship. It is somewhat unique in that about 60 to 70 percent of its surface is covered with articular cartilage and it has *no* musculotendinous attachments.

The Joints

The ankle is for all intents and purposes a hinge joint (Figs. 14–2 and 14–3). The talus, which has a head, neck, body, and dome, is held firmly between two malleoli, tibial and fibular, to create a "mortise joint." The dome of the talus is a trapezoid when viewed from above; the wider base is anterior. Hence, when the foot is plantar flexed, the narrower posterior base is held between the malleoli, allowing some medial-lateral "play" in the ankle,

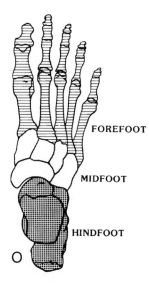

FIGURE 14–1 ■ Anatomic regions of the foot.
(From Weissman BNW, Sledge CB: Orthopedic
Radiology. Philadelphia, WB Saunders Company, 1986,
p 628; reprinted by permission.)

whereas, with the foot dorsiflexed, the wider
base is articulating and the "play" is reduced,
resulting in a more stable configuration.

The medial (tibial) malleolus covers
about one third of the medial side of the talus,
whereas the lateral (fibular) malleolus extends
to cover the entire lateral surface. In addition,
the medial malleolus is located slightly anterior to the lateral in the normal anatomic
position. This relationship places the transmalleolar axis out of the coronal plane, externally
rotated about 30 degrees. Thus, when standing, the foot is normally externally rotated
relative to the knee.

The subtalar joint is the talocalcaneal
joint (Fig. 14–4). It consists of three facets that
lie in different planes and create a complex
situation for simultaneous motion in different
planes. Essentially, this joint permits inversion
(elevating the medial border of the heel) and
eversion (elevating the lateral border of the
heel). In addition to the three facets, there are
two synovial-lined cavities with a canal between them. This canal is trumpet shaped,
opening laterally just anterior to the lateral
malleolus as the sinus tarsi. The canal contains
a dense ligament and a small neurovascular
bundle.

Chopart's joint is actually two articulations (Fig. 14–5)—the talonavicular joint and
the calcaneocuboid joint. Chopart's joint geo-

graphically is the junction of the hindfoot and
midfoot, and is named for the French surgeon
who popularized an amputation at this level.

Lisfranc's joint (Fig. 14–6) is also a misnomer since it really is a composite of all
metatarsal-tarsal articulations that mark the
junction of the forefoot and midfoot. Named
for Napoleon's surgeon, this "joint" allows for
a portion of forefoot supination (raising of the
medial border) and pronation (raising of the
lateral border) and is the site of a classic
fracture-dislocation.

The metatarsophalangeal joints are
simple condylar joints. Most significant is the
fact that their distal projection varies because
of the differential lengths of their metatarsals.
Normally, the second metatarsal is the longest,
followed by the third, first, fourth, and fifth.
Alterations in these lengths resulting from
numerous causes are a frequent source of static
foot deformities and pain.

Musculature

The muscles that move the foot and ankle
classically are divided into two groups: extrinsic and intrinsic. The extrinsic muscles (Fig.
14–7) are those that originate outside the foot
but act on it. They are subdivided into four
groups:

1. *Posterior group*—the muscles of the "triceps surae" group. The gastrocnemius-
   soleus complex and plantaris act as a
   group to plantar flex the foot. If the foot
   is bearing weight, they elevate the heel
   from the floor.

2. *Anterior group*—the pretibial muscles.
   The anterior tibial, extensor digitorum
   longus, and extensor hallucis longus act
   in concert to dorsiflex the ankle, and the
   latter two also extend the toes. The anterior tibial muscle also tends to invert the
   hindfoot.

3. *Medial group*—muscles of the lower leg.
   The tibialis posterior, flexor digitorum
   communis, and flexor hallucis longus all
   distribute their tendons behind and below the medial malleolus. As a group they
   plantar flex the foot and invert the hindfoot; the latter two flex the toes.

4. *Lateral group.* The tendons of the peroneus longus and brevis pass behind the
   lateral malleolus and are the major ever-
   tors of the hindfoot. In this role they are
   the antagonists of the two major in-

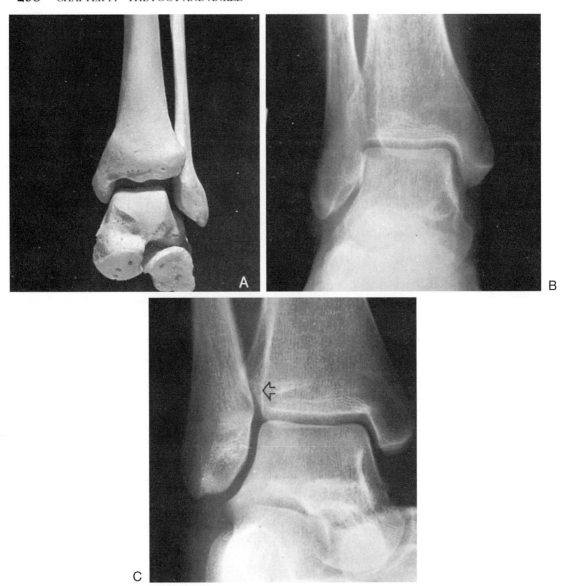

FIGURE 14–2 ■ Photographic diagrammatic, and radiologic anatomy of the normal ankle in anteroposterior (*A* and *B*). Note equal width of cartilage spaces and alignment of lateral talus with posterior cortex *(arrow)* on mortise view.

(From Weissman BNW, Sledge CB: Orthopedic Radiology. Philadelphia, WB Saunders Company, 1986, p 590; reprinted by permission.)

vertors—the tibialis anterior and tibialis posterior.

The intrinsic muscles originate and act within the foot. With the exception of the extensor digitorum brevis, they are all found in the sole of the foot. Many believe that their major role is to curl the plantar surface of the foot, essentially acting in concert with the ligaments and extrinsic musculature in maintenance of the longitudinal arch.

Ligaments

Most important are the ligamentous medial and lateral ankle stabilizers. Medially the deltoid ligament is a fan-shaped structure of four different ligaments—the tibionavicular, anterior talotibial, posterior talotibial, and calcaneotibial. The deltoid, considered as a composite, has two layers, superficial and deep. This structure is a key stabilizer of the ankle mortise and as such its compromise allows pathologic "play" to occur in the ankle.

The lateral side, in contrast, is stabilized by three ligamentous bands—the anterior talofibular, posterior talofibular, and calcaneofibular. This composite is less dense and less critical for lateral stability, considering that the lateral malleolus extends further distally, hence providing increased bony stability.

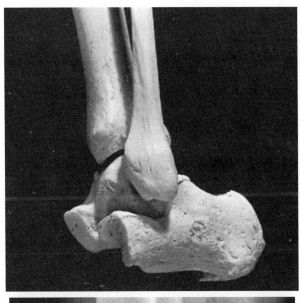

A

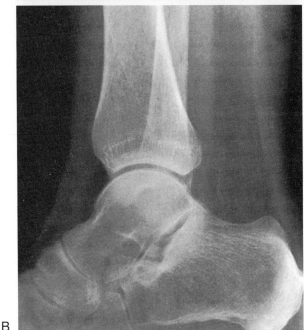

B

FIGURE 14–3 ■ Photographic *(A)* and radiologic *(B)* anatomy of the normal ankle in lateral projection.
(From Weissman BNW, Sledge CB: Orthopedic Radiology. Philadelphia, WB Saunders Company, 1986, p 591; reprinted by permission.)

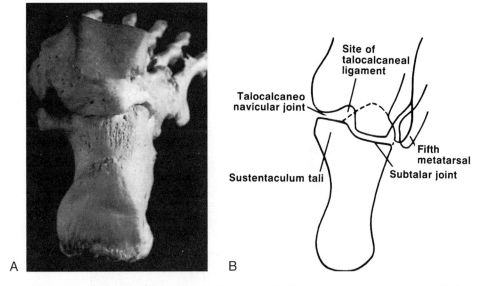

FIGURE 14–4 ■ Photographic *(A)* and diagrammatic *(B)* anatomy of the normal ankle in tangential calcaneal (Harris) projection.
(From Weissman BNW, Sledge CB: Orthopedic Radiology. Philadelphia, WB Saunders Company, 1986, p 628; reprinted by permission.)

Interosseous ligaments exist between the tibia and fibula distally and play an adjunctive role in maintaining the mortise. Together they are referred to as the distal tibiofibular syndesmosis (Fig. 14–8).

There are numerous ligamentous structures in the foot, some named and some unnamed, that span the many small articulations within the foot. Their role, however, is critical. In concert with the confining bony architecture and muscles, they maintain the arches of the foot.

The classic arches of the foot are the transverse arch and the longitudinal arch. The *transverse arch* is a rigid arch at the midfoot level established by the integral relationship of the five tarsals of the midfoot maintained by interosseous ligaments and supported by musculature. The middle cuneiform functions as the keystone of this arch. The typical *longitudinal* arch is reflected primarily on the medial border of the foot. It is created by the configuration of portions of the forefoot, midfoot, and hindfoot and maintained by the plantar fascia and the intrinsic musculature. To some degree this arch is genetically determined. The longitudinal arch has sweeping significance in many pathologic states, but it should be remembered that there is a wide variation of "normal."

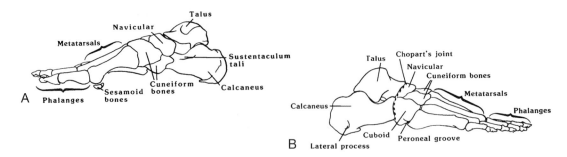

FIGURE 14–5 ■ Diagrammatic *(A* and *B)* anatomy of the normal foot in lateral projections.
(From Weissman BNW, Sledge CB: Orthopedic Radiology. Philadelphia, WB Saunders Company, 1986, p 627; reprinted by permission.)

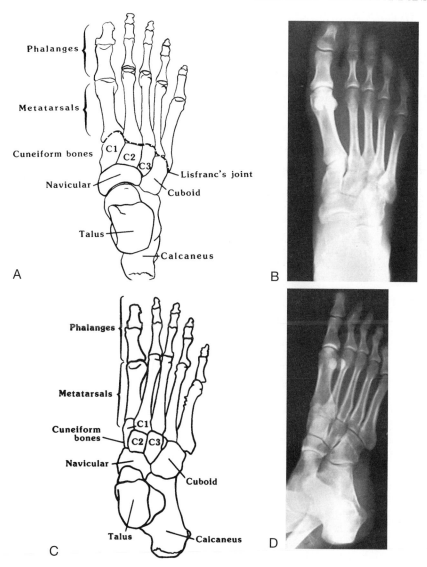

FIGURE 14–6 ■ Photographic, diagrammatic, and radiologic anatomy of the normal foot in posteroanterior *(A–B)* and internal oblique *(C–D)* projections.

(From Weissman BNW, Sledge CB: Orthopedic Radiology. Philadelphia, WB Saunders Company, 1986, p 626; reprinted by permission.)

Nerves

The sciatic nerve ends at the upper extent of the popliteal fossa behind the knee. Here it splits into the tibial nerve and the common peroneal nerve.

The tibial nerve enters the leg in the posterior compartment and supplies the muscles of the posterior and medial groups. These, it will be remembered, plantar flex and invert the foot. Its terminal branches, the medial and lateral plantar nerves, supply the intrinsic muscles and skin of the foot.

The common peroneal nerve itself supplies no muscles. After it passes around the neck of the fibula, it bifurcates in the superficial and deep peroneal branches. The deep peroneal nerve supplies the anterior compartment muscles, thus controlling dorsiflexion. The superficial peroneal nerve supplies the lateral compartment and is therefore responsible for foot eversion.

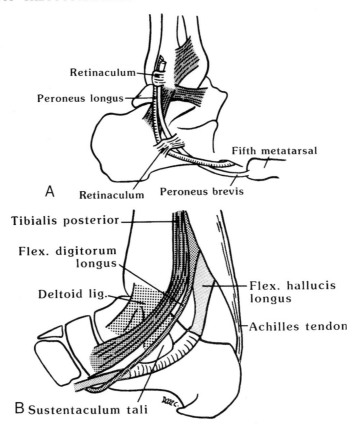

FIGURE 14–7 ■ Tendons. *A,* Lateral view of the tendons of the peroneus brevis and the peroneus longus muscles. These muscles evert the foot. They lie in a common synovial sheath behind the lateral malleolus. The peroneus longus crosses the lateral aspect of the cuboid and the sole and attaches to the lateral sides of the bases of the first metatarsal and the medial cuneiform. The peroneus brevis tendon passes around the lateral malleolus, anterior to the peroneus longus, and inserts on the base of the fifth metatarsal. *B,* Medial view. The posterior tibial tendon, in a separate sheath, passes around the medial malleolus, anterior to the tendon of the flexor digitorum longus. It functions to invert the foot. The tendon of the flexor hallucis longus passes under the sustentaculum tali.

(From Weissman BNW, Sledge CB: Orthopedic Radiology. Philadelphia, WB Saunders Company, 1986, p 592; reprinted by permission.)

BIOMECHANICS

Despite their somewhat complex anatomy, the foot and ankle are well adapted to function in three important roles: (1) a rigid lever, (2) a flexible shock absorber, and (3) a self-correcting structure compensating for irregular terrain. The ankle joint is essentially a hinge joint allowing about 70 degrees of total motion—20 degrees of dorsiflexion and 50 degrees of plantar flexion. The ankle allows the body to move forward relative to the ground, this being accomplished as the tibia "rolls over" the talus (Fig. 14–9).

Within the foot proper, the subtalar joint is most important. The foot at heel strike is somewhat flexed; it becomes progressively more rigid through toe off, functioning as a rigid lever, and then reverts to flexibility through the swing phase. This sequence is accomplished primarily through the subtalar joint and secondarily through the midfoot articulations. At heel strike, the calcaneus is everted and the subtalar joint somewhat mobile. At mid-stance through toe off the calcaneus progressively inverts and the subtalar joint becomes less mobile. As a secondary phenomenon of this process, the articular surfaces of the talonavicular and calcaneonavicular joints progress from parallelism (with heel everted) to a nonparallel relationship (with the heel inverted). This results in "locking" of the midfoot. Thus a rigid lever is created preparing the foot for toe off. Assisting in this endeavor is the "windlass effect" (Fig. 14–10). As the toes begin to dorsiflex, the plantar structures of the foot, especially the plantar fascia, become increasingly taut. This tends to elevate the arch of the foot as it progresses from heel strike to toe off.

As is obvious, any injury or pathologic state that affects these joints or soft tissue structures will alter the biomechanics of the foot and, in doing so, will alter the gait cycle.

Normally weight is shared equally (50/50) between the forefoot (metatarsal heads) and the os calcis. In the forefoot, half of the load is taken through the head of the first metatarsal and the remainder is shared by the lateral four metatarsal heads. Trauma and surgery can alter the normal weight-bearing mechanism and frequently create a painful syndrome.

EXAMINATION OF THE FOOT

History

Without doubt, the most common reason patients seek evaluation of this region is for pain. The painful foot is a somewhat ubiquitous

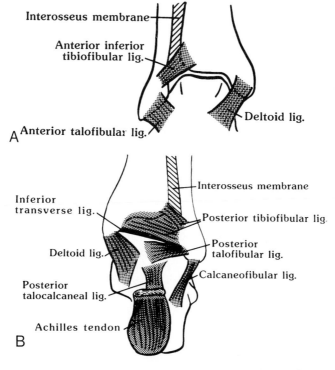

FIGURE 14–8 ■ The tibiofibular syndesmosis. The syndesmosis consists of the interosseous membrane, the anterior and the posterior inferior tibiofibular ligaments, and the inferior transverse ligament. *A,* Anterior view. *B,* Posterior view.

(From Weissman BNW, Sledge CB: Orthopedic Radiology. Philadelphia, WB Saunders Company, 1986, p 594; reprinted by permission.)

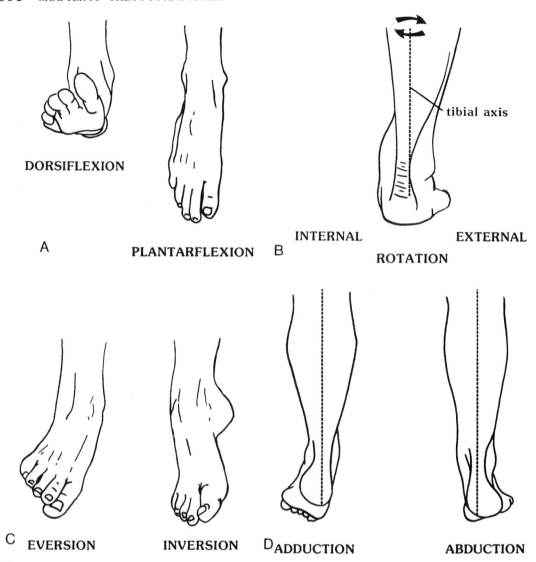

FIGURE 14–9 ■ Motions of the foot and ankle. *A, Plantar flexion* and *dorsiflexion* refer to movement of the foot downward or upward. *Supination* and *pronation* refer to rotation of the foot internally or externally around the longitudinal axis of the foot. *B, Internal* and *external rotation* of the foot refer to motion around the vertical axis of the tibia. *C, Eversion* directs the sole laterally, whereas *inversion* refers to rotation of the foot until the sole is directed medially. *D, Adduction* and *abduction* describe motion of the forefoot toward or away from the midline.

(From Weissman BNW, Sledge CB: Orthopedic Radiology. Philadelphia, WB Saunders Company, 1986, p 606; reprinted by permission.)

problem, and one that requires careful evaluation if the correct etiology is to be determined. The pain can be static without weight bearing or static with weight bearing. The pain can likewise be only kinetic—that is, associated with walking. An effort should be made to characterize the pain as to: (1) its location, (2) its character (dull aching, sharp lancinat-

ing, burning), (3) its temporal relationship, (4) what makes it better, (5) what makes it worse, (6) its relationship to walking and standing, and (7) its relation to shoes.

Occasionally the complaints will be related to gait dysfunction, in which case an attempt to characterize the abnormality should consider: (1) the type of limp (antalgic, "drop foot," Trendelenburg), (2) the need for external aids, (3) the impact on activity, and (4) the effect of shoeing.

Physical Examination

The physical examination of the foot is essential to establish a diagnosis, but one must remember that a physical examination of the shoe may be equally helpful. Despite the sense of frustration one feels when confronted by a patient with a shopping bag full of shoes, it is well worth a careful look at the soles, outer and inner, for evidence of abnormal wear patterns or kinetic damage suggesting an abnormal gait pattern.

Perhaps most difficult is determining what findings fall within the range of normal. The foot in weight bearing should demonstrate a central heel, straight flexible toes, no fixed contractures, and a reasonable longitudinal arch maintained by normal muscle balance. When examined while not bearing weight, the foot should be supple, with acceptable ranges of motion in all joints. The skin should be carefully inspected for areas of increased pressure as reflected by corns, calluses, and cornified skin. Skin color and temperature are important components of the circulatory assessment, as is the integrity of the pulses. Neurologically, the sensory as well as the motor modalities should be assessed to ensure integrity.

Finally, careful evaluation of the longitudinal arch should be carried out in the weight-bearing, as well as the non-weight-bearing foot. If one finds the medial border of the foot in contact with the ground, the term "supple flatfoot" or "pronated foot" is used. Etiologically this results from ligamentous laxity such as that seen in Marfan's or Down's syndrome or simply occurs as a heritable trait. This foot will be flat when bearing weight, but when not bearing weight the arch reappears.

The so-called rigid flatfoot shows *no* change with weight bearing and usually is associated with an intrinsic bony deformity such as tarsal coalition or congenital vertical talus. The joints will demonstrate limited range of motion. In addition, peroneal muscle spasm is often appreciable.

Laboratory Evaluation

Blood Tests

Only a few blood tests have clinical relevance specific to foot and ankle problems. A complete blood count (CBC), sedimentation, and levels of rheumatoid factor and uric acid should routinely be obtained in patients with obscure atraumatic pain in these areas. The

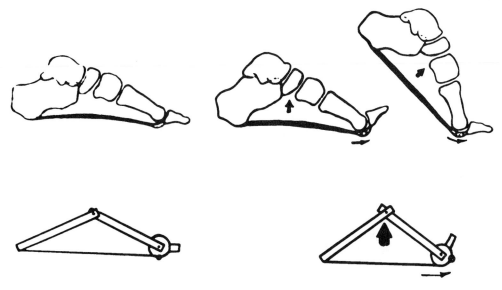

FIGURE 14–10 ■ Plantar aponeurosis and windlass mechanism provide stability to the longitudinal arch of the foot when the first metatarsophalangeal joint is forced into dorsiflexion and its secondarily plantar flexes the first metatarsal.

(From Mann RA: The great toe. Orthop Clin North Am 20[4]:520, 1989; reprinted by permission.)

results will give a clue to infections or inflammatory disease, as well as gout, which classically affects the foot.

Routine Radiography

It is important to ask for appropriate studies—ankle films will not show the foot and vice versa. The standard three views of the ankle include the anteroposterior (AP), lateral, and internal oblique ("mortise") view. The latter is taken by internally rotating the lower extremity so as to place the transmalleolar axis in the coronal plane, thereby disclosing the anatomic configuration of the ankle mortise in its most favorable light.

The foot typically is viewed in AP, lateral, and oblique projections. The latter, or Sloman, view is particularly helpful when looking for certain tarsal coalitions and injuries in the midfoot. Although radiographs are often taken while not bearing weight, weight-bearing views give additional information about the integrity of the arch, as well as static changes that occur with the imposition of body weight.

Special Studies

Tomograms are used to carefully evaluate the complex areas of the midfoot and hindfoot for occult trauma or deformity. The *computerized tomography (CT) scan* (Fig. 14–11) seems especially valuable to assess the subtalar and midfoot joints. Tarsal coalitions, fractures of the os calcis, and midfoot fracture-dislocations are particularly well studied by this technique. On *bone scans* although nonspecific, the bone-seeking isotope, technetium polyphosphate can identify areas of bone activity that occur in the presence of tumor or infection. *Magnetic resonance imaging* (MRI) currently remains a technology in search of indication as it relates to foot and ankle disease. The cost effectiveness is an open question, since other techniques currently available appear adequate to assess most afflictions in this region.

Computer software now exists to carefully study abnormal stress distribution across the plantar surface of the foot (*foot plate analysis*) as well as evaluate gait disturbances. *Gait analysis* has proven particularly helpful in evaluating the pathologic gait in patients with cerebral palsy.

The diabetic patient, as well as the individual with chronic arterial insufficiency, frequently develops significant foot pathology.

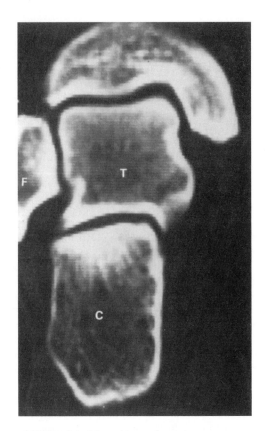

FIGURE 14–11 ■ Normal anatomy seen on computerized tomography: coronal section through the ankle and subtalar joint. C indicates calcaneus; F, fibula; T, talus.

(From Weissman BNW, Sledge CB: Orthopedic Radiology. Philadelphia, WB Saunders Company, 1986, p 632; reprinted by permission.)

Doppler evaluation of blood flow can frequently assist in decision making in these patients.

DISEASES OF THE FOOT AND ANKLE

This overview of the pathologic states that affect the foot and ankle is discussed by diagnostic category. This is not meant to be an exhaustive catalog of every affliction, but rather a representative sampling of the more common disease states that mandate medical care.

Trauma

Ankle Fractures

Ankle fractures are discussed in detail in Chapter 4. Fractures and dislocations that relate to

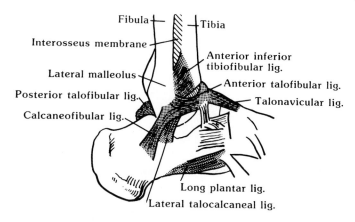

Fibula

Tibia

Interosseus membrane

Anterior inferior tibiofibular lig.

Lateral malleolus

Anterior talofibular lig.

Posterior talofibular lig.

Talonavicular lig.

Calcaneofibular lig.

Long plantar lig.

Lateral talocalcaneal lig.

FIGURE 14–12 ■ The lateral collateral ligament. The anterior talofibular, posterior talofibular, and calcaneofibular portions of the lateral collateral ligament are shown.

(From Weissman BNW, Sledge CB: Orthopedic Radiology. Philadelphia, WB Saunders Company, 1986, p 593; reprinted by permission.)

the specific anatomic and functional peculiarities of the foot are discussed later in this section.

Ankle Sprains

Ligamentous disruptions, partial and complete, are common about the ankle. The most common ligament to be injured is the anterior talofibular (Fig. 14–12). Partial injuries can be treated with either a cast, ankle taping, or splinting. Complete ligament disruption, especially of the deltoid, may require surgical repair.

Chronic Instability

Many patients who have had repeated ligamentous injuries to the ankle will, with each insult, lose more and more of the normal "check rein" effect of these ligaments. The net result is an ankle that is chronically unstable. This instability can be demonstrated by stress testing with radiographs (Figs. 14–13 and 14–14). These patients typically complain of repeated inversion sprains with the slightest provocation. Simple things such as walking on the beach or uneven terrain, or stepping from a curb, are ample challenge to the stretched lateral ligaments, and the ankle sprains.

Initial local care, such as nonsteroidal anti-inflammatory drugs (NSAIDs), ice, and splinting, are adequate to control acute symptoms. A program of aggressive lateral muscle strengthening exercises may minimize recurrences; if the condition is severe enough, de-

finitive treatment relies on a surgical reconstruction for the lateral side of the ankle. Although several procedures are described, most use the tendon of the peroneus brevis to reconstruct the lateral ankle ligaments. Long-term results are dependably good.

Fractures in the Forefoot

Most fractures in the forefoot (toes and metatarsals) are simply treated by reduction if displaced, and taping, splinting, or stiff-soled shoes. One metatarsal fracture of special note occurs at the base of the fifth metatarsal. This bony process is avulsed by the peroneus brevis tendon, which attaches to the tuberosity. These

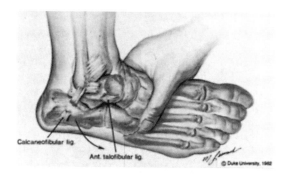

Calcaneofibular lig.

Ant. talofibular lig.

© Duke University, 1982

FIGURE 14–13 ■ Inversion stress testing, or the talar tilt.

(From Lasseter TE Jr, Malone TR, Garrett WE Jr: Injury to the lateral ligaments of the ankle. Orthop Clin North Am 20[4]:631, 1989; reprinted by permission.)

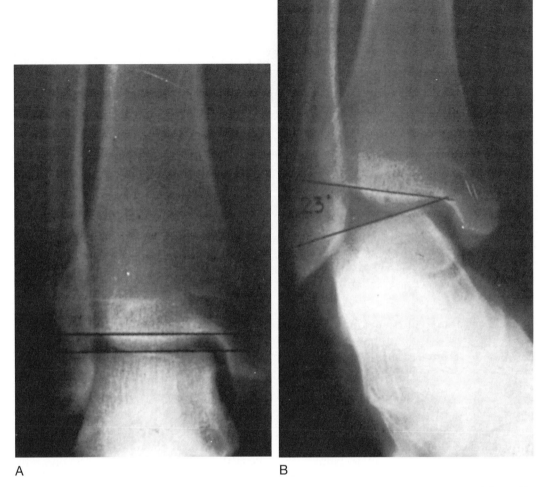

A   B

FIGURE 14–14 ■ *A,* Anteroposterior view of the ankle prestress. *B,* Anteroposterior view of the ankle with inversion stress reveals marked lateral ligament injury.

(From Lasseter TE Jr, Malone TR, Garrett WE Jr: Injury to the lateral ligaments of the ankle. Orthop Clin North Am 20[4]:632, 1989; reprinted by permission.)

are benign injuries, simply treated in a stiff shoe. They should not be confused with a fracture more distal in the shaft of the fifth metatarsal (Jones' fracture), which is actually a stress fracture and requires more aggressive cast immobilization or open reduction with fixation, lest nonunion occur.

The more common stress fracture in the foot occurs in the neck/shaft of the second metatarsal and is referred to as a "March" fracture. These can be simply treated in a stiff shoe once the diagnosis is established. This frequently requires sequential radiographs since it usually takes 3 to 4 weeks for the bony callus to form, permitting the radiographic diagnosis to be made.

Fractures of the Hindfoot

Fractures of the Talus. This bone, as previously mentioned, forms the keystone of the foot. It is the most proximal bone of the foot articulating in the ankle joint. It is also important to remember that this bone is covered with articular cartilage over 60 percent of its surface (Fig. 14–15). Because of this unique anatomic fact, and because there are no muscle attachments to the talus, its blood supply is quite tenuous (Fig. 14–16). The blood supply enters the talus at the neck and travels retrograde into the body and the dome.

In many ways, the talus is similar to its embryologic homolgue, the scaphoid in the wrist. Fractures of the talus typically occur through the neck and result from an acute dorsiflexion injury. The anterior lip of the tibia acts as the anvil against which the talar neck fractures. Depending on the intensity of the force, these fractures can be nondisplaced or displaced, and the proximal segment (body and dome) may or may not be dislocated. Standard radiographic techniques, in conjunction with CT scans are usually adequate to demonstrate the extent of the fracture (Fig. 14–17).

Once the diagnosis has been made, the treatment is generally based on the amount of displacement and the extent of subluxation. Remembering the tenuous blood supply, it becomes essential to restore normal talar anatomy. The greatest concern with these frac-

tures is the development of avascular necrosis of the proximal segment. Just as the blood supply to the carpal scaphoid is retrograde, so it is in the talus; hence one should anticipate necrosis of the proximal segment. Timely anatomic restoration of the bone and rigid fixation of this structure are the best approaches to preclude this disastrous complication. Despite all efforts being made, the incidence of avascular necrosis has been reported to be as high as 80 percent in severely displaced fracture-dislocations of the talus. If this untoward event occurs, osteoarthritis of the ankle is a common sequela.

Fractures of the Calcaneus.   Located below the talus and poised to accept ground contact, this somewhat block-shaped bone is composed al-

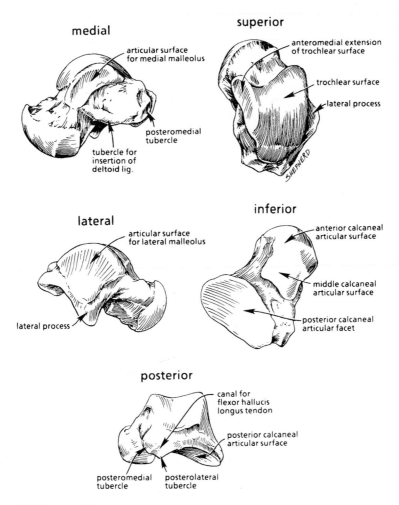

FIGURE 14–15 ■ Important anatomic structures of the talus.

(From Adelaar RS: The treatment of complex fractures of the talus. Orthop Clin North Am 20[4]:692, 1989; reprinted by permission.)

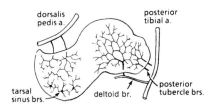

FIGURE 14–16 ■ Extraosseous and intraosseous circulation of the talus.

(From Adelaar RS: The treatment of complex fractures of the talus. Orthop Clin North Am 20[4]:693, 1989; reprinted by permission.)

most entirely of cancellous bone. It is covered by a very thin shell of cortical bone. Despite this seemingly fragile anatomy, the os calcis accepts full load bearing at heel strike. Fractures of this bone typically result from a fall from a height, classically a ladder, with direct impact over the tuberosity of the os calcis. This results in failure through the cancellous bone.

These patients typically present with severe pain and swelling. Standard radiographs plus a tangential heel view, plus CT scanning, will fully define the anatomy of this injury. It is extremely important to be cognizant of the fact that vertical load can be transmitted above the level of the heel. For that reason, if the patient complains of any back pain whatsoever, or as a routine part of evaluating a calcaneal fracture, radiographs of the lumbar spine should be obtained. There is a relatively high association of lumbar spine fractures with fractures of the calcaneus.

Treatment for these fractures remains somewhat controversial. The options, however, include the immediate use of a compression dressing, followed by an elastic stocking and stiff-soled shoe; a compression dressing followed by 6 to 8 weeks of short leg casting with or without closed reduction of the fracture; and open reduction and internal fixation of the fracture. The major concern is the late stiffness that ordinarily follows these injuries. Typically, the fractures enter the subtalar joint and are therefore intra-articular (Fig. 14–18). The subtalar joint, as a result, frequently becomes stiff and occasionally develops osteoarthritic changes. There is a current trend toward aggressive operative treatment of these fractures so that early motion of the subtalar joint can be initiated.

Injuries of the Midfoot

Typically, severe injury to the midfoot can produce a number of bony and ligamentous disruptions. In general, the term "Lisfranc fracture-dislocation" is used to describe a multiplicity of injuries. The unique anatomic feature of the metatarsal-tarsal relationship is the fact that the base of the second metatarsal is set, or "keyed" into the cuneiforms, thereby locking the metatarsal-tarsal joint. When a forceful inversion or eversion injury is applied, classically while playing racquet sports or horseback riding, the Lisfranc articulation will be disrupted. One of the more common configurations is to fracture the base of the second metatarsal and dislocate the remaining tarsometatarsal joints.

The major clinical problem is that these injuries tend to be subtle, and are occasionally

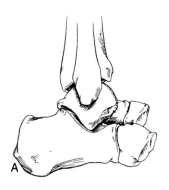 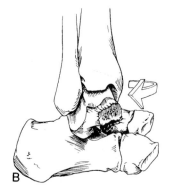 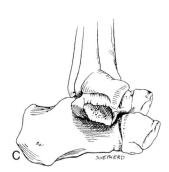

FIGURE 14–17 ■ Classification of talus neck fractures: *A,* Class I; *B,* Class II; *C,* Class III.

(Modified from Hawkins LG: Fractures of the neck of the talus. J Bone Joint Surg 52A:991–1002, 1970.)

(From Adelaar RS: The treatment of complex fractures of the talus. Orthop Clin North Am 20[4]:696, 1989; reprinted by permission.)

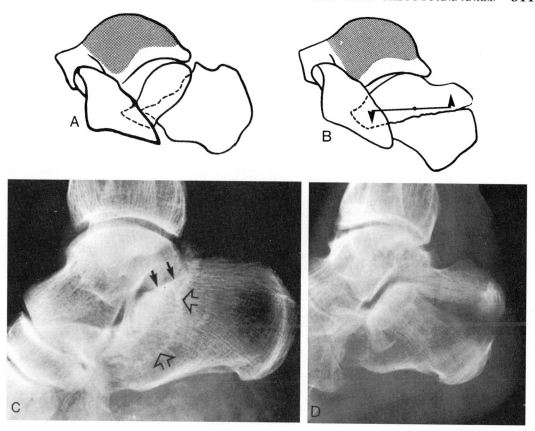

FIGURE 14–18 ■ The Essex-Lopresti classification of fractures. Fractures involving the subtalar joint are subdivided into joint depression *(A)* and tongue *(B)* types. Severe examples are shown. *C,* Joint depression fracture. There is depression of the subtalar articular surface *(arrows)*, with flattening of Böhler's angle. Overlapping and impacted fracture lines are seen *(open arrows)*. *D,* Tongue-type fracture. The horizontal fracture line extends into the posterior portion of the subtalar joint. (*A* and *B* after Essex-Lopresti P: Br J Surg 39:395, 1952.)

(From Weissman BNW, Sledge CB: Orthopedic Radiology. Philadelphia, WB Saunders Company, 1986, p 644; reprinted by permission.)

overlooked on routine radiographs. Awareness of their existence and careful radiographic analysis will usually permit diagnosis. Treatment generally involves closed reduction with percutaneous pinning, or open reduction with pinning if acceptable reduction cannot be achieved closed (Fig. 14–19). Virtually all patients who sustain a significant Lisfranc fracture-dislocation will develop late stiffness in the midfoot and frequently complain of pain when walking on uneven ground.

Infections

The bones of the foot, as well as their associated joints, can be involved in standard musculoskeletal septic processes, such as osteomy-elitis and septic arthritis. Below are listed five of the more classic infectious processes that are somewhat unique to the foot and ankle.

Puncture Wounds

In a world in which most people enjoy being barefoot, the problem of puncture wounds to the foot is ubiquitous. Glass, nails, and plant and animal parts are just a few of the things that frequently penetrate the sole of the foot. The popular use of sneakers has introduced a new therapeutic challenge. The insole of sneakers seems to be a favorite habitat of the *Pseudomonas* organism. Puncture wounds such as those made by nails, which penetrate the sole of a sneaker and enter the foot, frequently produce a septic metatarsophalangeal joint with an

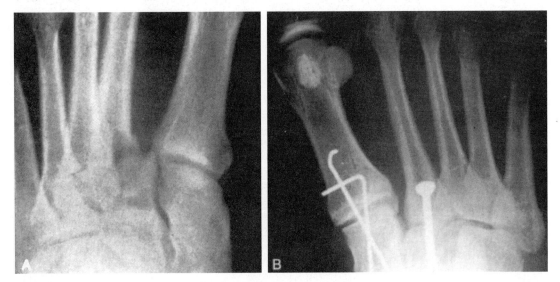

FIGURE 14–19 ■ *A,* Closed reduction was attempted for this type B-2 Lisfranc fracture pattern. *B,* Persistent subluxation of the first metatarsal base that was not evident initially prompted open reduction with a combination of internal fixation techniques.

(From Myerson M: The diagnosis and treatment of injuries to the Lisfranc joint complex. Orthop Clin North Am 20[4]:633, 1989; reprinted by permission.)

adjacent osteomyelitis in the metatarsal head. These wounds often will culture *Pseudomonas aeruginosa*. This has become such a common problem that it is referred to as "Nike syndrome" (Fig. 14–20).

The patients frequently will present late with a swollen, cellulitic foot. The (CBC) and sedimentation rate will occasionally be abnormal. Standard radiographs and a technetium bone scan will usually confirm the diagnosis. Whenever there is bone or joint involvement, aggressive surgical debridement, including removal of all of the necrotic tissue and sequestered bone, is mandatory for satisfactory resolution. Obviously, appropriate antibiotic coverage is required until the infection has been adequately eradicated.

Paronychia

Infections of the medial or lateral nail fold, especially of the great toe, are extremely common. Usually these are seen in association with an abnormally growing nail. The nail penetrates the thickened skin of the lateral nail fold, introducing pyogenic bacteria. Subsequently, the soft tissues about the fold become abscessed and a paronychia develops. This has been referred to as an acute ingrown toenail. Many patients have this problem chronically and suffer from repeated paronychial infec-

tions. The diagnosis is rarely in question. Under local anesthesia, excision of the lateral one third of the nail is usually adequate to decompress the abscess in the acute situation. For patients with chronic paronychial infections,

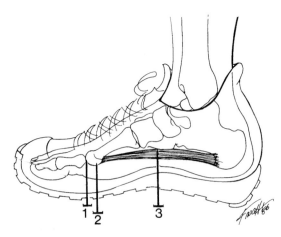

FIGURE 14–20 ■ Puncture injury sites. *1,* Metatarsophalangeal joint. *2,* Cartilage of metatarsal head. *3,* Plantar fascia.

(From Clinton JE: Puncture wounds by inanimate objects. *In* Gustilo RB, Gruninger RP, Tsukayama DT [eds]: Orthopaedic Infection: Diagnosis and Treatment. Philadelphia, WB Saunders Company, 1989, p 300; reprinted by permission.)

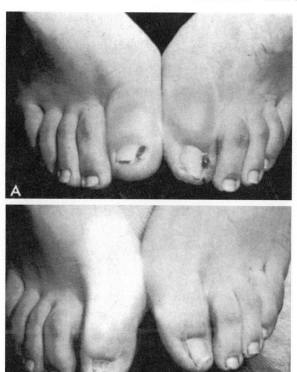

FIGURE 14–21 ■ *A,* Bilateral infected ingrowing of both edges of the big toenails. The toenail of the right big toe was practically completely separated from its bed and was avulsed. The operation, which was performed under a local anesthetic, consisted of bilateral resection of all onychogenic tissue in the longitudinal grooves.

B, Sixteen months after surgery.

(From Lapidus PW: The toenails. *In* Jahss M [ed]: Disorders of the Foot, vol I. Philadelphia, WB Saunders Company, 1982, p 929; reprinted by permission.)

more aggressive nail excisions, even including nail ablation, may be required for control (Fig. 14–21).

Mycotic Infection (Athlete's Foot)

Redness and cracking of the skin found in the web space between small toes is a common dermatologic condition affecting the forefoot. Because this condition is acquired typically in locker rooms or other areas in which the floor is chronically damp, the term "athlete's foot" is often given to it. Usually these are superficial mixed fungal infections and respond extremely well to commercially available preparations. In more chronic or resistant cases, clotrimazole (Lotrimin) cream is usually effective.

Maduromycosis

The maduromycosis organism *(Madurella)* is endemic in subtropical and tropical locales. Many individuals in those areas spend the better part of their time barefoot. Puncture wounds introduce the fungal organism typically into the sole of the foot, generally in the area of the midfoot. A mycotic osteomyelitis (Fig. 14–22) subsequently develops and produces rather sweeping and destructive changes throughout the tarsus. The diagnosis frequently requires biopsy of the area and,

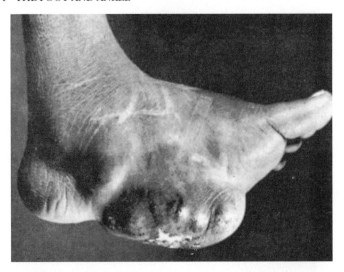

FIGURE 14–22 ■ Maduromycosis: granulomatous mycotic abscess with multiple sinuses on the sole of the foot.

(From Selvapandian AJ: Infections of the foot. *In* Jahss M [ed]: Disorders of the Foot, vol II. Philadelphia, WB Saunders Company, 1982, p 1411; reprinted by permission.)

once the diagnosis is confirmed, aggressive antifungal treatment, usually via the intravenous route, is required for control. Unfortunately, this particular fungal organism is somewhat resistant to many currently available agents.

Diabetic Foot Infections

The diabetic foot presents a unique substrate for bacterial growth. The organism most often enters the foot through cutaneous defects. Frequently, these defects are patient induced, as the diabetic with poor eyesight attempts to perform a pedicure. The other common reason for bacterial entry is small blisters that develop on the toes (Fig. 14–23) or dorsum of the insensate forefoot. Abscesses, ulcers (Fig. 14–24)—both acute and chronic—septic arthritis, and osteomyelitis are frequently the end result. Aggressive treatment of any infection in the diabetic foot is mandatory for salvage. It goes without saying that, for treatment of the diabetic foot infection to be successful, the patient must be under strict diabetic control. Hospitalization for elevation and intravenous antibiotics is almost always necessary. In addition, these infections are often polymicrobial and frequently mandate either multiple antibiotics or a very broad-spectrum antibiotic.

Tumors

A complete discussion of soft tissue and bone tumors that can involve the foot is well beyond the scope of this chapter. There are, however, a

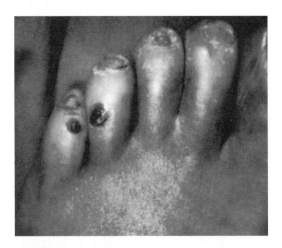

FIGURE 14–23 ■ This diabetic patient had recently obtained new shoes. The two small, dorsal ulcers were exquisitely painful. Note the blanching of the toes distal to the ulcers.

(From Harrelson JM: Management of the diabetic foot. Orthop Clin North Am 20[4]:606, 1989; reprinted by permission.)

a popular site for the development of xanthomas. Particularly in patients with hereditary hyperlipidemias, large fatty masses can be palpated in the area of the Achilles tendon. They occasionally will cause pressure symptoms that can best be dealt with by excision.

Bone Tumors

Any primary benign or malignant neoplasm of bone can occur in the tarsals or metatarsals. A few, however, are more common than others. The *enchondroma* is somewhat typical in short tubular bones, making the foot a favored location for this lesion. It is a benign cartilage tumor and occasionally is associated with pathologic fracture. The *chondromyxoid fibroma* (Fig. 14–25) is another benign cartilage tumor that has a modest predilection for the bones of

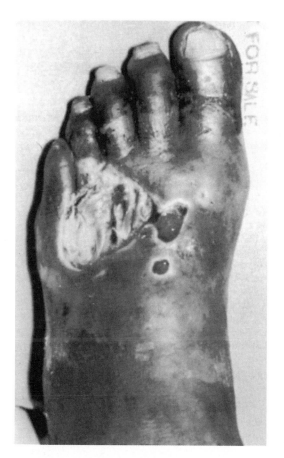

FIGURE 14–24 ■ One day of new shoe wear produced the ulcers seen over the fifth metatarsal head and lateral sides of the fourth and fifth toes.

(From Harrelson JM: Management of the diabetic foot. Orthop Clin North Am 20[4]:606, 1989; reprinted by permission.)

few specific lesions that have a particular predilection for the foot, and those are mentioned here.

Soft Tissue Lesions

The anterolateral ankle is a common site for the development of a ganglion cyst. Similarly, a soft tissue lipoma may occasionally be seen in this area. Both of these lesions are benign, and the decision regarding excision is based on symptoms. The plantar surface of the foot will frequently be the site of thickening, as noted by palpation. Large, firm, mildly tender nodules can occasionally be palpated along the plantar fascia. These fibromas are benign, and again their removal rests on the symptoms that they cause. The area around the Achilles tendon is

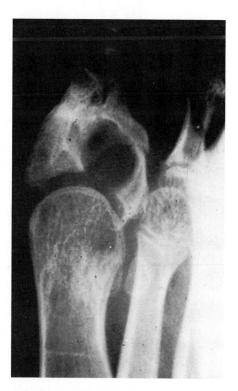

FIGURE 14–25 ■ Chondromyxoid fibroma. This lesion has a tendency for localization in small bones of the hands and feet. A sharply circumscribed defect in the proximal phalanx of the great toe is shown here.

(From Bogumill GP: Orthopaedic Pathology: A Synopsis with Clinical and Radiographic Correlation. Philadelphia, WB Saunders Company, 1984, p 447; reprinted by permission.)

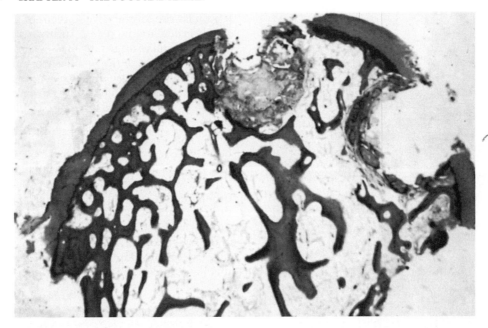

FIGURE 14–26 ■ Gout. Histologic appearance of the margin of a tophus exhibiting acellular material surrounded by foreign-body giant cells. The deposition of urate salts in the tissue and the proteinaceous material produced in response to them elicit a foreign-body reaction. Crystals have been removed in the preparation of the sections.

(From Bogumill GP: Orthopaedic Pathology: A Synopsis with Clinical and Radiographic Correlation. Philadelphia, WB Saunders Company, 1984, p 281; reprinted by permission.)

the foot. It also can be managed by curettage of the lesion. More aggressive treatment is rarely required.

The calcaneus is an occasional site for a *bone cyst*. Because of the size of this lesion, pathologic fracture through it occasionally occurs. Indeed, this may be the presenting complaint that allows diagnosis. Many believe that this bone cyst is in some way different than the unicameral bone cyst occurring more typically in other long bones. Treatment usually requires curettage and bone grafting, since injection therapy with steroids is rarely successful in this particular bone.

Metastatic disease to the small bones of the foot is exceedingly uncommon. In point of fact, acral metastasis to the hands or feet is a very rare event. When seen, one should suspect the lung as the primary site of the patient's disease.

Metabolic Diseases

Within this diagnostic category, there is essentially only one disease of major import in the foot or ankle: The foot has maintained a place of historic importance in the description of gouty arthritis. This inborn error of metabolism has for many years been heralded clinically by the development of an acute arthritic attack localized in the first metatarsophalangeal joint. The clinical presentation of a male with acute nontraumatic onset of a red, hot, exquisitely painful forefoot should be considered as a case of gout until proven otherwise.

The diagnosis is generally easy to make on clinical grounds alone. The deposition of sodium urate crystals into the synovial membrane around these joints produces an intense chemical synovitis (Fig. 14–26). Supportive laboratory studies, including a sampling of blood for uric acid level and an aspiration of the joint, are required for confirmation of the diagnosis. Hyperuricemia alone is not adequate confirmation; rather, the finding of negatively birefringent crystals in the joint aspirate is necessary.

One should initiate treatment immediately without waiting for confirmatory diagnosis. The use of a fast-acting NSAID will usually produce some symptomatic resolution within 24 hours. Septic arthritis must be ruled out before the use of corticosteroids is indicated.

Vascular Disease

Diabetes, as well as chronic arterial insufficiency, are both very able to wreak destructive changes throughout the foot. More often than not, severe vascular compromise results in local or regional dry gangrene, mandating amputation of the involved portion of the extremity. In addition, diabetes has become the most common cause of neuropathic arthropathy in this country today. It will be remembered that the loss of proprioception is the pathway to joint destruction. Typically, the midfoot is involved with the "Charcot" changes (Figs. 14–27 and 14–28). Severe degenerative joint disease with loss of bony mass, joint subluxations, severe joint erosions, and deformity result from this neurovascular event.

One other vascular lesion of note is osteochondritis dissecans of the talus (Fig. 14–29). Unlike in the knee, trauma is the generally accepted etiology of this lesion. These lesions frequently are preceded by the history of an ankle sprain or sprains. The patient presents with chronic, dull, aching pain either medially or laterally about the ankle. Routine radiographs and tomograms (Fig. 14–30) or MRI will usually show a small fragment of necrotic bone poised on the dome of the talus. Treatment for small in situ lesions, as well as displaced lesions that have become loose bodies, is currently arthroscopic débridement of the involved area. The approach to larger in situ lesions remains somewhat controversial.

Arthritis/Inflammatory Lesions

Osteoarthritis

Degenerative joint disease can certainly involve any of the joints of the foot or ankle. Typically, it is a sequela of prior trauma. Osteoarthritis of the ankle, most commonly secondary to a previous fracture-dislocation, can be particularly disabling for the patient. In the early stages, anti-inflammatories, ankle-foot orthoses, and appropriate shoeing are adequate conservative treatment. Once the pain is such that the patient requires external aids, surgical intervention can be considered. The standard surgical treatment remains the ankle arthrodesis. Total ankle replacement, although available and helpful in the rheumatoid patient with a low-demand ankle, has not proved effective in the long-term management of the osteoarthritic ankle. Most believe that the reason for this is the demands made on the

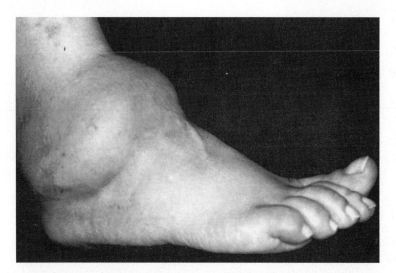

FIGURE 14–27 ■ Charcot's arthropathy. Clinical photograph of ankle region demonstrating pronounced enlargement and distortion from neuropathic joint changes following minor injury 20 years earlier. There is no evidence of neurologic disease or diabetes mellitus. The ankle is mildly painful.

(From Bogumill GP: Orthopaedic Pathology: A Synopsis with Clinical and Radiographic Correlation. Philadelphia, WB Saunders Company, 1984, p 190; reprinted by permission.)

prosthesis in the otherwise normal patient with localized arthritis.

Hallux Rigidus. Degenerative osteoarthritic changes of the first metatarsophalangeal joint, including dorsal spurs and joint space narrowing, are a common cause of great toe pain (Fig. 14–31). Frequently, these patients are young and have developed the disease secondary to chronic trauma. Aggressive joggers are particularly at risk. Chronic pain, swelling, and positive radiographs permit easy diagnosis. Nonsurgical treatment is occasionally beneficial. Intra-articular steroids, NSAIDs, rest, and stiff-soled shoes frequently bring about acceptable relief. Surgical treatment mandated by severe pain depends on the activity status of the patient. Joggers tend to do better with a joint fusion; other more sedentary individuals may be satisfied with an arthroplasty.

Rheumatoid Arthritis

There is no diarthrodial joint in the body that is immune to the ravages of this disease (Fig. 14–32). It is not uncommon that the small joints of the foot herald this disease. These patients frequently have involvement of the small joints of the forefoot and present with generally swollen, red, and painful feet. Medical treatment is generally adequate to control symptoms in the early stages. Surgical treatment must be coordinated with overall patient management.

Reiter's Syndrome

The young male with Reiter's syndrome (urethritis, uveitis, arthritis) will occasionally present with pain in the forefoot or, even more specifically, a small toe. Atraumatic swelling,

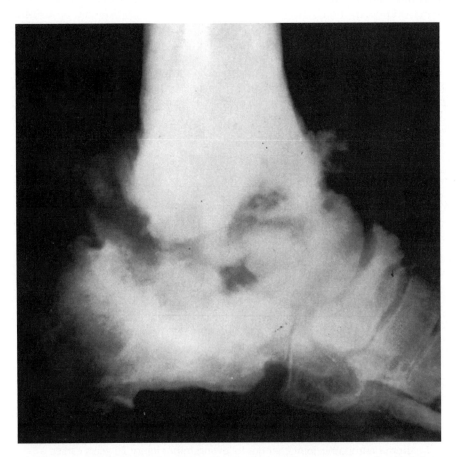

FIGURE 14–28 ■ Charcot's arthropathy. Radiographic appearance of ankle joint in patient with syphilis exhibiting fragmentation of bone and deposition within the hypertrophied synovium.

(From Bogumill GP: Orthopaedic Pathology: A Synopsis with Clinical and Radiographic Correlation. Philadelphia, WB Saunders Company, 1984, p 198; reprinted by permission.)

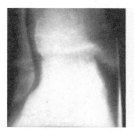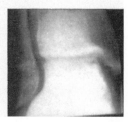

FIGURE 14–29 ■ Anteroposterior radiograph of osteochondritis dissecans of the talus. Note the radiolucent area surrounding the piece of bone.

(From Trott AW: Developmental disorders. *In* Jahss M [ed]: Disorders of the Foot, vol I. Philadelphia, WB Saunders Company, 1982, p 205; reprinted by permission.)

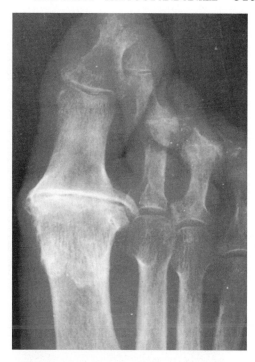

FIGURE 14–31 ■ Hallux Rigidus. The posteroanterior view of the great toe metatarsophalangeal joint show the marked cartilage loss, flattening of articular surfaces, and hypertrophic lipping that resulted in severe loss of motion.

(From Weissman BNW, Sledge CB: Orthopaedic Radiology. Philadelphia, WB Saunders Company, 1986, p 662; reprinted by permission.)

redness, and tenderness of a lesser toe should encourage one to consider this diagnosis. Radiographs may occasionally show some changes, but comprehensive diagnosis and

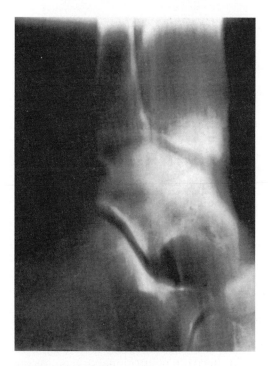

FIGURE 14–30 ■ Lateral tomogram of osteochondritis dissecans of the talus to delineate the lesion in the dome of the talus.

(From Trott AW: Developmental disorders. *In* Jahss M [ed]: Disorders of the Foot, vol I. Philadelphia, WB Saunders Company, 1982, p 205; reprinted by permission.)

treatment generally require rheumatologic consultation.

Overuse Syndromes

A whole host of soft tissue inflammatory lesions can result from overuse, or asymmetric, unbalanced movement of the foot and ankle. Only a few examples have been selected for consideration.

Inflammatory Tendinitis.   The anterior and posterior tibial tendons are particularly prone to develop an inflammatory tendinitis. Often the patients do not recall injury. However, a change of footgear will frequently alter the normal posture of the foot in gait or stance. It should be remembered that the various muscle-tendon groups balance the foot in inversion and eversion. Any alteration of this balance will stretch one or the other of the tendon groups, causing it to become overused and irritated.

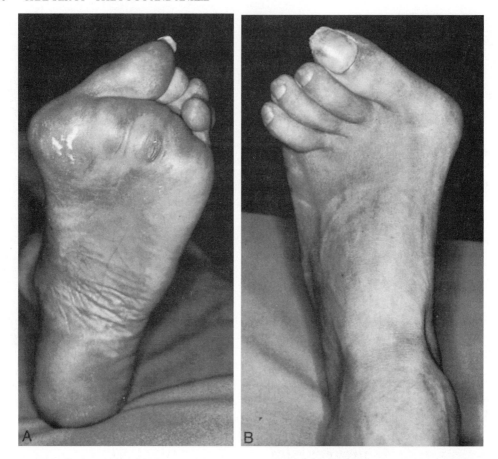

FIGURE 14–32 ■ Plantar *(A)* and dorsal *(B)* views of the foot of a patient with rheumatoid arthritis with characteristic dislocation of all toes, which tend to drift off into marked hallux valgus with dorsal displacement of the phalanges onto the metacarpals. The metacarpal heads become very prominent in the sole of the foot, and large, painful callosities are common.

(From Bogumill GP: Orthopaedic Pathology: A Synopsis with Clinical and Radiographic Correlation. Philadelphia, WB Saunders Company, 1984, p 229; reprinted by permission.)

The diagnosis is usually based on local tenderness, pain with resisted activity of the tendon in question, and a strong clinical suspicion. Radiographic studies are rarely helpful. Treatment is generally divided into three components. First, NSAIDs or intrasheath steroid injections are frequently helpful to decrease the acute inflammation, in conjunction with icing or heat. Second, altering the moments of force about the painful area is best accomplished with a simple orthotic. Third, restrengthening the injured area should be delayed until pain is decreased, at which time strengthening and stretching exercises for the painful muscle-tendon unit are prescribed.

Achilles Tendinitis. Although the patient rarely gives a history of trauma, the Achilles tendon is frequently the site of small, low-grade collagen disruptions. These minor traumatic events may become somewhat cumulative, producing a clinical tendinitis or, indeed, a frank tendon rupture. These Achilles tendon syndromes probably represent nothing more than a spectrum of attritional disease. As outlined above for tibial tendinitis, Achilles tendinitis can be managed in a similar fashion. If frank rupture of the tendon has occurred, this mandates much more aggressive treatment.

The patient with an Achilles tendon rupture presents with inability to plantar flex the foot. If the patient is examined prone and the calf is "squeezed," the normal response is for the foot to plantar flex. If tendinous continuity has been lost, the foot will not plantar flex, and the patient has a positive Thompson test. Once the diagnosis is established, either prolonged casting in the gravity equinus position or surgical repair are the treatments of choice.

Plantar Fasciitis.   The most common cause of the painful heel in adults is plantar fasciitis. This inflammatory condition of the plantar fascia, and its overlying bursa at the attachment to the calcaneal tuberosity, is frequently seen in the same group of patients who typically develop gall bladder disease—specifically, overweight females in middle age, who typically have a somewhat pronated foot. Frequently, the patient complains of a stabbing pain in the heel when it first contacts the ground on arising in the morning. As the patient ambulates, the pain lessens slightly. Clinical tenderness is always found over the tuberosity of the calcaneus, and frequently a contracture of the Achilles tendon is apparent. Radiographs often show a small calcaneal spur (Fig. 14–33) to

be present, which many believe is not the primary pathologic event, but rather a secondary phenomenon caused by chronic attritional changes in the plantar fascia.

Initial conservative treatment includes stretching of the heel cord, orthotics to correct the pronation, and anti-inflammatories or direct steroid injection for the inflammation. Surgical treatment should be reserved for the few patients with severe, recurrent symptoms. The surgical treatment includes incision of the plantar fascia and excision of the heel spur. The procedure is occasionally complicated by residual scar tissue and tender neuromas, which preclude an excellent result.

Neurologic and Developmental Diseases

Neurologic Diseases

Numerous diseases that affect the nerve and muscle components of the lower extremities will certainly impact on the foot and ankle. A selection of examples will demonstrate how systemic neurologic disease or local peripheral

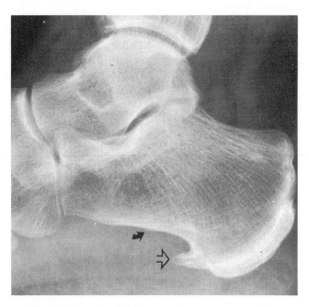

FIGURE 14–33 ■ Calcaneal spurs. The normal plantar spur *(open arrow)* has smooth margins, no sclerosis or erosion, and no adjacent soft tissue swelling. Very small spurs are present at the insertions of the long plantar ligament *(arrow)* and the Achilles tendon.

(From Weissman BNW, Sledge CB: Orthopaedic Radiology. Philadelphia, WB Saunders Company, 1986, p 637; reprinted by permission.)

nerve problems will cause foot and ankle symptoms.

Polio. Destruction of the anterior horn cells by the polio virus typically produces a lower motor neuron lesion. These patients developed flaccid muscles to portions of the foot and ankle. The paralysis is rarely complete and frequently leaves some of the musculature intact. This creates a relative imbalance between agonist and antagonist muscles, resulting in deformity. The foot typically is in equinus because the dorsiflexors are weakened or paralyzed, and occasionally claw toes and cavus deformity (high arch) of the foot are secondary phenomena. In the United States today, more polio residua are now being seen because of the influx of immigrants from third-world countries. Corrective surgical procedures are available to realign the foot and reestablish the normal plantigrade position.

Spastic Foot. Cerebral palsy and stroke victims suffer from spasticity of certain muscle groups. This also creates an unbalanced situation. However, it is critical to recognize that the imbalance is between spastic and more spastic muscle, unlike polio, in which the imbalance is between paralyzed and normal muscle. The spastic foot can take on many different configurations, including commonly equinus, as a result of hyperactivity of the triceps surae group. Abnormal hindfoot version and forefoot deformity are similarly common. The scope of this chapter does not allow for a complete discussion of the spastic foot.

Plantar Neuroma. One of the most common causes of forefoot pain in the adult is the formation of a neuroma at the bifurcation of the common digital sensory nerve between two adjacent rays. Typically, the common sensory branch divides at the level of the metatarsal head. Frequently, pressure of the metatarsal heads, as they juxtapose on weight bearing, will trap the nerve and cause the formation of a traumatic neuroma. Typically, these patients complain of forefoot pain. Their pain usually is mechanical in that it is worse with standing, especially in shoes. Oftentimes one can obtain a history of pain relief by shoe removal.

Vertical compression of the web space, as well as transverse compression of the entire transverse arch, will frequently exaggerate the lancinating pain in the forefoot. Radiographs are always negative, which is important since a stress fracture of the metatarsal neck must be considered in the differential diagnosis. Treatment for this common problem initially might include metatarsal pads under the sole of the foot and injection of steroid around the neuroma, which may be diagnostic as well as therapeutic. Excision is indicated if the conservative modalities fail.

Tarsal Tunnel Syndrome. Like the carpal tunnel in the wrist, there is a tarsal tunnel behind the medial malleolus. The tibial nerve passes through this fibrous canal on its way into the foot. Unlike carpal tunnel syndrome in the upper extremity, some question the existence of tarsal tunnel syndrome. Nevertheless, this diagnosis can be considered in the patient who presents with burning pain on the sole of the foot, perhaps some weakness of intrinsic musculature with a negative history for trauma, and negative radiographs. Electromyography and nerve conduction studies are essential for confirmation of this diagnosis. Once confirmed, decompression of the tunnel surgically is the best treatment approach.

Reflex Sympathetic Dystrophy. Abnormal firing of the sympathetic fibers in the peripheral nerves entering the foot and ankle has been implicated as an etiologic mechanism for the development of this bizarre and clinically troublesome syndrome. Reflex sympathetic dystrophy is not truly a causalgia since no damage to a peripheral nerve is generally found. Rather, this syndrome follows usually minor trauma to the extremity in a predisposed patient. The implication of an abnormal psychologic overlay has always been suggested when this syndrome is described. However, it must be remembered that organic findings are indeed present. The typical patient is a somewhat hysterical woman, or a man following a work-related accident, who sustains a trivial bony or ligamentous injury to the foot and 2 to 3 months later develops severe pain, swelling, redness, and increased perspiration of the extremity. The associated radiographic osteopenia is called Sudeck's atrophy (Fig. 14–34). The findings all suggest abnormal sympathetic outflow.

The treatment, as might be imagined, is exceedingly difficult and controversial. Emotional support, physical therapy, antidepressants, β-blocking agents and short-term use of immobilizing devices all have been employed with variable success. Indeed, lumbar sympathetic blockade and lumbar sympathectomy are occasionally considered for these patients. Perhaps most important is to treat the patient

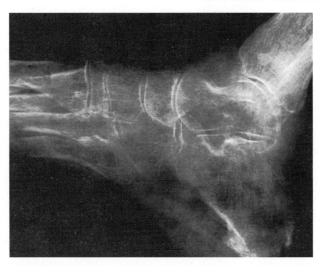

FIGURE 14–34 ■ Radiographic view of Sudeck's atrophy exhibiting severe osteoporosis of feet. High-speed flow shows greatest effects in the metaphyseal area, in which there are many trabeculae with greater surface area exposed to osteoclastic activity. Diaphyseal manifestations are nonspecific and seen in many other conditions.
(From Bogumill GP: Orthopaedic Pathology: A Synopsis with Clinical and Radiographic Correlation. Philadelphia, WB Saunders Company, 1984, p 162; reprinted by permission.)

aggressively. These patients require careful and regular follow-up and constant encouragement if any headway is to be made in improving this very painful condition.

Developmental Static Foot Deformities

Probably the most important group of diseases that affect the foot fall within this category. The normal plantigrade foot—that is, one that is flat on the ground with all contact points in their appropriate location—is somewhat of an idealized concept. It is probably fair to say that no two feet are identical. However, the pressures created about the standing and walking foot, particularly by shoeing, will frequently alter the normal plantigrade configuration of the foot. Women, because of the mandates of fashion, are generally the greatest sufferers within this category.

Hallux Valgus. Better known as bunion deformity, the development of this abnormality is most often ascribed to abnormal forefoot pressure creating a valgus thrust on the great toe. With time and constant strain, the structures about the forefoot deform, creating a bunion deformity. There are three classic abnormali-

ties described in any bunion and they occur to varying degrees (Fig. 14–35):

1. The *exostosis* itself is occasionally pointed out by the patient to be the bunion. Typically, there is a red, tender, and painful bursa overlying the bony exostosis.

2. *Hallux valgus*—a big toe deviates in a lateral direction. It also frequently rotates or pronates. This deformity occurs in conjunction with stretching and laxity of the medial capsule of the first metatarsophalangeal joint.

3. *Metatarsus primus varus*—the first metatarsal is frequently deviated medially, thus increasing the angle created at the first metatarsophalangeal joint, as the big toe deviates laterally. It is important to note that the angulation of the first metatarsal is considered the genetic component of a bunion deformity and is the basis for adolescent bunion development.

Numerous secondary phenomena occur coincident with the formation of the deformity. Subluxation of tendons and sesamoid bones, development of deformities of the small toes, and disturbances of the plantar skin can all be associated with the development of a bunion.

It has been said that if an individual never wore shoes, he or she would never develop a bunion. This statement certainly indicates that pressure from the shoe, typically in an adult, is a major etiologic component in the development of hallux valgus. Therefore, decompression of the forefoot by widening the toe box and lowering the heel may delay the progression of deformity. Once established, chronic pain and progressive difficulty in shoe fitting become the clinical hallmarks of this disease. The radiographs are helpful in determining the angles about the deformity, the presence of associated joint arthritis, and associated deformity elsewhere in the foot.

Surgical treatment for bunions is generally mandated by severe pain and inability to fit shoes. There are well over 100 different operative procedures available for bunion correction. In principle, they all accomplish three things to varying degrees: (1) most simply, removal of the bony exostosis, or bunion; (2) realignment of the great toe in a more neutral axis; and (3) alignment of the first ray. The technical aspects of implementation are not germane to this discussion. The prognosis for bunion surgery is generally very good, depending on the exact surgical technique selected. It is important to point out to patients that postoperatively they will need to dramatically modify their footwear.

Bunionette. A similar bony exostosis can form along the lateral border of the foot at the fifth metatarsophalangeal joint. This has been referred to as a bunionette or tailor's bunion. It frequently makes shoeing difficult because it widens the forefoot. If conservative modalities

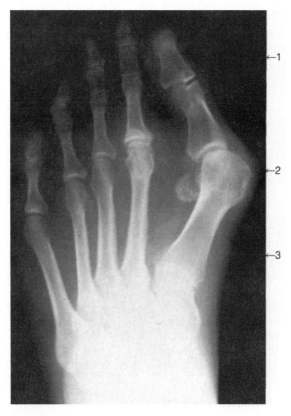

FIGURE 14–35 ■ Classic abnormalities in a bunion: *1,* the exostosis; *2,* hallux valgus; and *3,* metatarsus primus varus.

(From Mann RA: The great toe. Orthop Clin North Am 20[4]:524, 1989; reprinted by permission.)

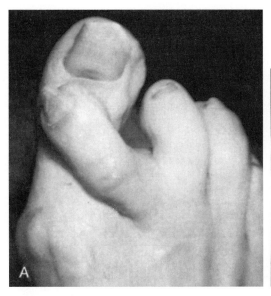

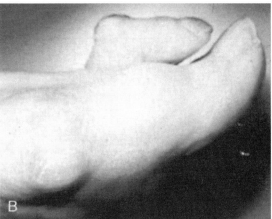

FIGURE 14–36 ■ *A,* Medial deviation of the second toe may be associated with development of acute pain in the second intermetatarsal space. *B,* Hyperextension of the second metatarsophalangeal joint may be associated with plantar capsular pain.

(From Coughlin MJ: The crossover second toe deformity. Foot Ankle 8:29–39, 1987; reprinted by permission.)

such as pads and stretching of the toe box are inadequate, surgical correction may be considered as an option.

Hammer Toe Deformity. The flexion deformity seen at the proximal interphalangeal joint of the lesser toes is often referred to as a hammer toe deformity. Frequently, this is seen in association with a hyperextension deformity at the metatarsophalangeal joint and the distal interphalangeal joint (Fig. 14–36). These small toe deformities usually develop either secondary to muscle imbalance or as a result of abnormal pressure from an adjacent digit, such as a hallux valgus of the great toe. In planning treatment, it is important to determine whether the deformity is flexible or fixed, and manipulation of the digit will frequently resolve this question. If flexible, taping, strapping, and padding may offer some early protection against progression. However, once fixed deformity has developed, and dermatologic changes such as corns or calluses are seen, indicating excessive pressure, surgical intervention is usually required. The surgical goal is to resect a segment of bone usually including the proximal interphalangeal joint and straighten the toe using a wire for fixation. Results from this type of surgery are excellent.

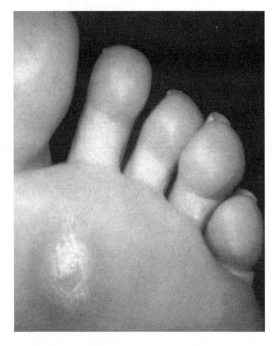

FIGURE 14–37 ■ Intractable plantar keratosis under second metatarsal head.

(From Gould JS: Painful feet. *In* McCarty DJ [ed]: Arthritis and Allied Conditions: A Textbook of Rheumatology, ed 11. Philadelphia, Lea & Febiger, 1989, p 1406; reprinted by permission.)

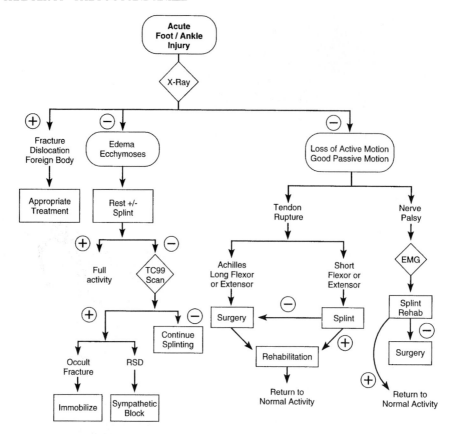

FIGURE 14–38 ■ Algorithm for diagnosis and treatment of foot and ankle pain with acute injury.

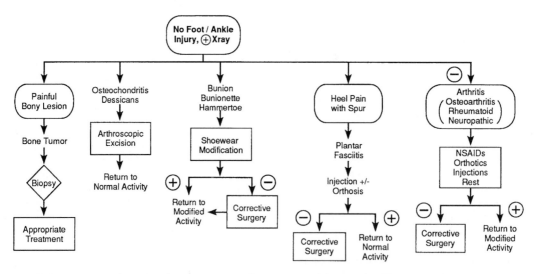

FIGURE 14–39 ■ Algorithm for diagnosis and treatment of foot and ankle pain with no injury and positive radiograph.

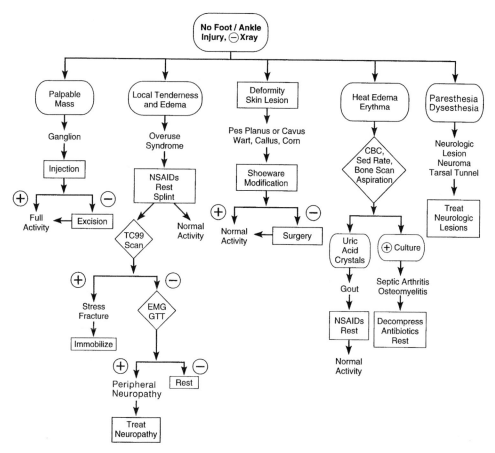

FIGURE 14–40 ■ Algorithm for diagnosis and treatment of foot and ankle pain with no injury and negative radiograph.

Metatarsalgia. As the term implies, pain under a metatarsal head on the plantar surface of the foot is a common presenting complaint. Most typically the pain, tenderness, and thickened callus will be found underneath the head of the second metatarsal (Fig. 14–37). This is not surprising if one remembers that the second metatarsal is generally the longest. The problem is compounded if the patient has a congenitally short first metatarsal. This latter condition is referred to as Morton's foot. Some atrophy of the fatty tissue on the plantar surface of the foot is anticipated with normal aging and unfortunately can accentuate this syndrome. Initial treatment using metatarsal pads or bars is usually successful. However, for intractable pain, consideration should be given to surgical treatment. This usually involves an osteotomy of the metatarsal in question to correct its prominence on the plantar surface of the foot.

Corns and Calluses

Thickening and cornification of the skin, when seen in the foot, particularly about the toes, has come to be known as a corn or a callus. Depending on the location, one term tends to be more favored over the other; essentially the pathologic process is the same. The trigger for the development of these dermatologic findings is excessive pressure over a bony prominence. As noted in previous sections discussing hammer toes and metatarsalgia, pathologic bony prominences focus abnormal pressure. As a result of this abnormal pressure, a callus may develop on the plantar surface of the foot, under a prominent metatarsal head, or a corn may develop over the proximal interphalangeal joint of a small toe, overlying a hammer toe. In any event, the basic mechanism (increased pressure) is the same, and the result is also similar. Because of the pressure on the skin, there is thickening and keratinization of the skin initially in an effort to protect the relatively tender skin from the applied load. Over time, as the thickening becomes progressive and dominant, the areas of cornified skin become problems in and of themselves.

Initial treatment may be as simple as soaking the foot, followed by an abrasion of the thickened area using either a pumice stone or a sharp blade. Local measures such as this are frequently successful for protracted periods to control symptoms. In addition to local skin care, protection of these areas from the implied load by the use of pads, such as metatarsal pads behind the painful plantar callosity or small corn pads for use on the dorsum of the toes, have proved helpful.

Ultimately, local measures may not suffice to control symptoms and surgical intervention to relieve the painful pathologic bony prominences may be necessary. The specific surgical procedure must be tailored to the specific pathologic bony abnormality.

SUMMARY

As can be appreciated, numerous diseases impact on the foot and ankle. Nevertheless, foot pain remains the most common presenting complaint. Deformity and gait disturbances will occasionally bring the patient to the physician for care. The algorithm in Figures 14–38 through 14–40 attempts to structure the diagnostic and treatment approach to these patients. The initial division is based on a history of trauma. If the determination is made that the patient has had no injury, the evaluation of the painful foot and ankle will follow a categorization based on whether or not the symptoms are mechanical or nonmechanical in type.

SUGGESTED READINGS

Fleming LL (ed): Management of Foot Problems. Orthop Clin North Am 20(4), 1989.

Johnson K. Surgery of the Foot and Ankle. New York, Raven Press, 1989.

Mann R (ed): Surgery of the Foot, ed 5. St. Louis, CV Mosby, 1986.

GLOSSARY

abscess: a collection of purulent material which usually consists of bacteria, both alive and dead, and the byproducts of local infection including viable and nonviable neutrophils, lymphocytes, and lysosomal enzymes. The presence of neutrophils within an abscess often results in a localized inflammatory reaction which can become systemic and life threatening if allowed to persist.

acute osteomyelitis: bacterial colonization of bone or bone marrow with signs of acute inflammation and periostitis. Radiographic changes are usually present within the first 6 weeks.

adjuvant therapy: therapy which is administered to assist in the treatment of a neoplasm. Adjuvant therapy can include radiation therapy or chemotherapy and usually is utilized to improve the results of a primary type of treatment (i.e., surgery).

allograft: tissue for transplantation which is acquired from donated cadaveric sources. Musculoskeletal allografts are generally processed by either deep freezing or dehydration utilizing freeze-drying techniques. Sterilization is generally performed with either gamma radiation, aseptic acquisition in an operating room setting, or treatment with ethylene oxide.

ankylosis: spontaneous bony fusion of a joint.

antalgic gait: a type of limp characterized by shortening the stance phase of gait, in an attempt to relieve pain on weight-bearing.

apophysis: secondary ossification center which develops in response to tension, and ultimately forms a process for muscular attachment.

arthrodesis: fusion performed surgically between two articulating bones by removal of the joint cartilage, removal of cortical bone, bone grafting, and immobilization.

arthrofibrosis: restricted joint motion due to formation of dense scar tissue around the articulation (contracture).

arthroplasty: an operation to improve function and relieve pain caused by arthritis in a peripheral joint. Joint resection or replacement, as well as interposition between joint surfaces, are forms of arthroplasty.

arthroscopy: a procedure to inspect, and operate on, the contents of a joint through a small portal utilizing a fiber-optic light source and specialized viewing and operative instruments.

benign: a neoplasm which has local capability for growth, with well-differentiated cells that are not capable of vascular or lymphatic invasion. Benign neoplasms can be either latent, with limited local growth, or aggressive, with growth proceeding in a destructive manner.

biopsy: the acquisition of material from a lesion, whether it be neoplastic or infectious, for diagnostic review. An adequate biopsy requires obtaining enough material for complete pathological review to arrive at a definitive diagnosis.

bone cement: polymethylmethacrylate (PMMA), used as a filler to enhance the fixation of total joint components.

bone graft: bone used to promote fracture healing, reconstruct a defect in bone, or enhance fusion by providing an organic matrix, osteoblasts, and hormonal factors that contribute to osteogenesis.

calcification: the deposition of calcium within a cartilaginous matrix. This occurs secondary to mineralization of an existing lobule of cartilage which may appear punctate, comma shaped, or popcorn-like on radiographs.

callus: reparative tissue at the site of a fracture that evolves and matures, leading to fracture healing.

cancellous bone: mature bone found in the epiphysis and metaphysis of long bones, and in flat bones, comprised of a three-dimensional lattice of trabecular bone that is less densely packed than cortical bone.

chondrocyte: cartilage matrix-producing cells which rely on nutrition from synovial fluid and not blood vessels. These cells are often arranged in lacunae which are arranged in rather distinct layers.

chronic osteomyelitis: a chronic infection of bone, usually involving the presence of an involucrum or sequestrum, in addition to radiographic changes within the bone. Sclerosis surrounding chronic sites of radiolucency on radiographs and a sinus tract may be present. Chronic osteomyelitis generally requires at least 6 weeks in order to demonstrate radiographic changes.

Codman's triangle: a region at the periphery of a bone tumor which is formed secondary to the deposition of reactive bone underneath the periosteum. As the periosteum lays down new bone in response to stress, the bony trabecular patterns in this region are usually at a right angle to the underlying cortical bone. A Codman's triangle usually represents a rapidly growing tumor or osteomyelitis, with elevation of the periosteum off of the bone secondary to neoplastic tissue, bone edema, or purulent material.

comminution: disruption of a fractured bone into more than two fragments.

compartment syndrome: an increase in the resting pressure in a contained fibro-osseous compartment, such as the forearm or leg, resulting sequentially in decreased lymphatic drainage, decreased venous drainage, loss of arterial inflow, and finally death to the muscle contained in the affected compartment. Sequelae include contracture, pain, and severe functional disability.

computerized axial tomography/computerized tomography (CAT/CT scan): an imaging modality which utilizes computer-generated analysis and imaging resulting from multi-planar exposure through either an extremity or the spine. These scans provide clinicians with excellent axial representation of body segments that were previously not available. Tissue density is graded based on Hounsfield units with dense structures being represented by a bright or white image.

contracture: fixed loss of motion in one direction caused by hypertrophy and shortening of periarticular soft-tissue structures such as tendon, ligament, or capsule.

cortical bone: mature, organized, densely packed bone, making up the periphery of flat bones and the diaphysis of long bones.

crepitus: audible or palpable grinding, usually located in a peripheral joint, with motion.

curettage: the mechanical removal of neoplastic or infectious tissue from a primary site. This generally involves entering a lesion and scraping its contents from within its lesional cavity, and has the potential for leaving residual disease, at the microscopic level, in the periphery. This type of "intralesional resection" is generally utilized for benign neoplasms.

cyst: a fluid-filled cavity which results from the production of fluid from a surrounding glandular membrane. The majority of cysts in orthopaedic terminology, such as a simple bone cyst or aneurysmal bone cyst are not true cysts, since the fluid does not directly result from the surrounding mesenchymal tissue present in the wall lining, but from the passive accumulation of fluid within the marrow cavity of bone.

debridement: the removal of infected or devitalized bone, muscle, and skin. The purpose of debridement is to remove any material that can serve as a substrate which harbors bacteria and to enable antibiotics, via parental or local routes, to reach colonies of bacteria.

delayed union: failure of a fracture to heal within the desired and expected time frame, with the potential still present for eventual union.

developmental: pertaining to growth and differentiation.

diarthrodial joint: a joint which consists of connections between two rigid parts of the musculoskeletal system which is lined by synovial tissue, lubricated by synovial fluid, and demonstrates appreciable ranges of motion. The ends of bones in diathrodial joints are usually covered with hyaline cartilage.

diaphysis: the tubular midportion of a long bone, consisting primarily of cortical bone.

dislocation: loss of normal articular congruity of a joint, with no contact between opposing articular surfaces.

dysostosis: an isolated disruption of normal bone growth with no identifiable etiology.

dysplasia: intrinsic defect in normal bone growth, which may be localized or generalized.

dystrophy: alteration in bone growth due to extrinsic defect, typically an endocrine abnormality.

electromyography (EMG): recording of the variations of electric potential or voltage from skeletal muscle. The EMG/nerve conduction velocity test is useful in determining the site of injury of a peripheral nerve or nerve root, and in identifying peripheral neuropathy caused by metabolic abnormalities.

enchondral ossification: bone formation following the template of a cartilaginous matrix.

enchondroma: a benign tumor of bone, with a cartilaginous matrix, commonly occurring in the hand.

epiphysis: a secondary ossification center, adjacent to the physis, which develops in response to compression and is covered by articular cartilage.

external fixation: the use of an extracorporeal device to stabilize a part of the skeleton, usually following an open fracture.

fracture: a cortical disruption, ranging from incomplete and non-displaced to completely displaced.

fracture healing: the process of biologic repair of a fracture in response to hormonal, biochemical, and mechanical factors. Fracture healing encompasses the phases of inflammation, soft callus, hard callus, and remodeling.

free tissue transfer: one-stage transplantation of distant autogenous composite tissue from a donor site to a recipient site. Free tissue transfer can involve transplantation of muscle, fasciocutaneous tissue, or bone with or with out attached soft tissue. This type of transfer requires immediate revascularization, utilizing microsurgical anastomosis of graft and recipient site arteries and veins.

frozen section: the preparation of pathological sections from fresh tissue, used primarily in the operating room for rapid diagnosis which may impact on surgical decision making.

ganglion: a soft, mucin-filled cyst arising from a tendon, tendon-sheath, or joint capsule. Most common about the hand and wrist, and more common in women.

gigantism (overgrowth): hypertrophy of a single digit or entire limb, primarily involving soft tissues. Causes include neurofibromatosis, tumor, or vascular anomaly.

haversian bone: cortical bone composed of vascular channels surrounded by mature (lamellar) bone.

herniated nucleus pulposus (HNP): Extrusion of gelatinous nucleus pulposus through the anulus fibrosus, into the spinal canal or neural foramen. When an HNP results in nerve root compression, radicular pain, numbness, or weakness may be seen. Herniated disc, ruptured disc.

hydroxyapatite: the calcium mineral crystal component of bone.

internal fixation: the use of an implant to stabilize the skeleton, usually after a fracture.

involucrum: newly formed reactive bone, usually occurring at the interface between diseased bone and healthy tissue. An involucrum consists of viable bone which is the opposite of a sequestrum, which is composed of dead bone.

joint reaction force: the force across a joint that results from a combination of weight bearing and muscular contraction.

kyphosis: forward bending of the spine, when viewed from the side, which is normal in the thoracic spine.

laminectomy: removal of a lamina from its superior to its inferior margin, performed as surgical treatment for spinal stenosis or HNP. Laminotomy or hemilaminectomy refer to partial removal of the lamina.

lordosis: backward bending, or "sway," of the spine when viewed from the side. Lordosis is normal in the neck and low back.

low back strain: nonspecific term referring to acute onset of pain in the low back, occasionally radiating into the buttocks, with associated muscle spasm. Low back sprain, lumbago.

magnetic resonance imaging (MRI): an imaging modality utilizing resonance phenomenon resulting in the absorption and/or emission of electromagnetic energy by nuclei or electrons in a static magnetic field. Magnetic resonance imaging requires unpaired electrons that are excited by exposure to a magnetic field with a particular signal being emitted once that field is removed. Differences in density of tissues are then represented on images as varying shades of gray, black, or white, depending on their concentration of hydrogen. The modality is extremely useful in the evaluation of musculoskeletal tumors, as well as disorders of the spine, knee, shoulder, and foot.

malignancy: a neoplasm consisting of undifferentiated or dedifferentiated cells which have the active capability of vessel invasion, transport, and establishment of a secondary site of neoplastic growth in a distant organ.

malunion: healing of a fracture in a nonanatomic position.

membranous bone formation: bone formation occurring directly from a fibrous, mesenchymal, connective tissue template.

metaphysis: the transition segment of a long bone from the enlarged end (epiphysis) to the tubular shaft (diaphysis). The funnel-shaped metaphysis is usually made up of abundant cancellous bone, and during growth, woven bone.

metastasis: the deposition to secondary sites of neoplastic cells from a primary neoplasm.

myelopathy: noninflammatory dysfunction of the spinal cord resulting in long-tract signs and symptoms, most commonly caused by mechanical compression in the cervical spine.

neoadjuvant therapy: the application of adjuvant treatment, usually chemotherapy or radiation, prior to a primary procedure in an attempt to facilitate surgical removal of the primary tumor.

neuroma: a nodule, frequently painful, developing in a nerve that has been partially or completely lacerated or traumatized.

nonunion: failure of a fracture to heal within the upper range of time expected, with sequential radiographic documentation of a lack of any progression towards healing.

nonsteroidal anti-inflammatory drugs (NSAIDs): these agents are in widespread use to treat arthritis as well as a variety of soft-tissue injuries and for pain relief. Gastrointestinal side effects are common.

open fracture: a fracture which has come into contact with the outside, extracorporeal environment. Implications primarily relate to an increased risk of infection and impaired fracture healing secondary to soft-tissue injury.

ossification: the deposition of mineral along osteoid matrix, produced by either normal (fracture healing) or malignant osteoblasts (osteosarcoma).

osteoarthritis: noninflammatory degeneration of a diarthrodial joint characterized by loss of articular cartilage, effusion, crepitus, deformity, and pain. Radiographic changes include loss of joint space, subchondral sclerosis, cyst formation, and periarticular osteophytes.

osteoblast: a type of differentiated mesenchymal cell that is essential for the process of osteogenesis or ossification. Osteoblasts alone can produce the organic intercellular substance or matrix which makes up bone tissue, called osteoid.

osteoclasis: to manually fracture a bone, usually to correct malposition.

osteoclast: bone resorbing cell.

osteocyte: histologically and possibly biochemically inert osteoblast, usually present in bone which is not undergoing any active remodeling or repair.

osteoid: organic component of bone.

osteomalacia: metabolic disorder of bone characterized by inadequate mineralization of normal osteoid. Less common than osteoporosis, causes include Ca^{++} deficiency and renal disease.

osteomyelitis: infection involving bone. (See acute and chronic osteomyelitis)

osteoporosis: pathologic condition of bone characterized by a decrease in bone matrix with normal mineralization of the matrix that is present. Causes include postmenopausal estrogen deficiency, steroid usage, immobilization, and bed rest. Fractures of the spine, hip, wrist, and shoulder are common.

osteotomy: surgical cutting and realignment of bone to change the mechanical environment of adjacent joints, posture, or appearance.

pannus: hyperplastic, hypertrophic synovium seen in the inflammatory arthritides. Source of degradative enzymes.

paraesthesia: a "pins and needles" or "tingling" sensation in an extremity, typically along the distribution of a peripheral nerve or nerve root.

pathologic fracture: a fracture occurring in bone that is of abnormal quality, either from metabolic changes (e.g., osteoporosis), tumor, or infection.

periosteum: thick fibrous tissue covering of a bone.

physis (epiphyseal plate, growth plate): a highly specialized cartilaginous structure, at each end of long bones, through which longitudinal growth of the bone occurs. The physis regresses and closes at the end of active skeletal growth.

polydactyly: the presence of an extra digit, either partial or complete. Most common in the hand, polydactyly may occur on either the ulnar or radial side.

prosthesis: a mechanical replacement for a removed portion of either bone or soft tissue. Prostheses include endoprostheses, which are internal replacements (joints, valves, etc.), and exoprostheses as would be used following an amputation.

radial club hand: congenital absence of all or part of the radius, resulting in a near-normal hand attached to, but radially deviated on, the forearm.

radicular pain: pain traveling down the extremity in a dermatomal distribution, often associated with paraesthesia. Pain should typically extend distal to the elbow or knee to be considered radicular.

radiculopathy: noninflammatory dysfunction of a spinal nerve with abnormal neurologic findings, most commonly secondary to a herniated nucleus pulposus or spinal stenosis.

referred pain: sclerotomal pain in a region that shares a common embryologic origin with the diseased region, such as the trapezius and shoulders for cervical disc pathology or the buttocks and posterior thighs for the lumbar spine.

remodeling: continuous process whereby older bone is removed and replaced with new bone, usually in response to mechanical stresses.

rheumatoid arthritis: inflammatory arthritis characterized by morning stiffness, swelling of peripheral joints, subcutaneous nodules, pain, and deformity.

rheumatoid factor: a blood marker that is usually, but not always, present in patients with rheumatoid arthritis. Some patients who do not have rheumatoid arthritis may have a positive rheumatoid factor.

rotation tissue transfer: soft tissue, such as muscle, or bone which is transplanted for wound coverage from one local site to another without transecting the blood supply to the transplanted tissue.

scintigraphy: a sensitive but nonspecific imaging modality for the diagnosis and staging of various orthopaedic problems. The standard "bone scan" utilizes technetium 99m, a gamma-emitting radioisotope with a half-life of 6 hours, coupled with methylene diphosphonate, a bone-seeking mineral material. Positive bone scans usually demonstrate increased uptake in areas of bony repair or destruction caused by neoplasm, fracture, infection, inflammation, or arthritis.

sclerosis: a rim of host bone reaction around the periphery of a lesion, or in an area of degeneration, which appears white (radiopaque) on radiographs.

scoliosis: coronal plane curvature, typically associated with rotation, leading to asymmetric rib or flank prominence. Common etiologies are idiopathic, neuromuscular, and congenital.

segmental instability: abnormal motion pattern between adjacent vertebrae resulting in excessive motion under physiologic loads and causing, in some individuals, characteristic mechanical back or neck pain.

septic arthritis: the presence of bacteria or their byproducts within a diarthrodial joint.

sequestrum: a microscopic or macroscopic island of necrotic bone found at the nidus of an infection within viable bone. Often, sequestered fragments are surrounded by purulent material and infected granulation tissue and occur secondary to devitalization of cortical bone.

spinal fusion: arthrodesis of two or more adjacent vertebrae for painful or unstable conditions of the spine including spinal deformity, trauma, or degenerative segmental instability. Bone graft or bone-graft substitute is utilized and internal fixation may be used. Fusion may be performed anteriorly (interbody) or posterolaterally (intertransverse).

spinal stenosis: narrowing of the spinal canal or neural foramen resulting in compression of the cord or nerve roots. Causes include congenital narrowing, degenerative changes, and spondylolisthesis.

spondylolysis: defect of the pars interarticularis, most commonly a stress fracture that occurs during childhood. May be associated with back pain and lead to spondylolisthesis.

spondylolisthesis: the forward slippage of a vertebrae on the one below it (most commonly L5 on S1). The most common types are isthmic (secondary to spondylolysis), degenerative (caused by degenerative instability of the disc and facet joints) or postsurgical.

sprain: partial or complete injury to a ligament resulting from excessive stretching.

straight-leg raising (SLR) test: with the patient supine or seated, simultaneous hip flexion and knee extension places the sciatic nerve on stretch. Reproduction of ipsilateral sciatica (not back pain) constitutes a positive SLR sign.

subluxation: partial dislocation of a joint, with some retained contact of the articular surfaces.

syndactyly: webbing of the fingers, usually resulting from congenital failure of formation, and commonly seen with other congenital abnormalities.

synostosis: congenital fusion, either partial or complete, of adjacent bones. Synostosis is far more common in the upper than in the lower extremity, and may involve the elbow, carpus, metatarsals, or phalanges.

synovectomy: removal of the synovium (lining surface of a diarthrodial joint), for inflammatory conditions such as rheumatoid arthritis or infection.

synovial membrane: a soft glandular tissue which lines diarthrodial joints and produces synovial fluid. The synovial membrane has a rich capillary network and serves both in phagocytosis of foreign debris and the production of synovial fluid.

tension sign: a physical finding produced by placing the involved nerve root on stretch to assess for mechanical compression. A positive tension sign requires reproduction of pain, in a dermatomal distribution, down the extremity.

Trendelenburg gait: a type of limp, caused by ineffective hip abduction, marked by swaying the torso over the effected hip on weight-bearing.

Trendelenburg sign: an abnormal drooping of the pelvis, on single-leg stance, away from the effected side due to ineffective hip abduction secondary to neurologic or mechanical factors, or pain.

ulnar club hand: congenital absence of all or part of the ulna, resulting in a near-normal hand attached to, but ulnarly deviated on, the forearm.

valgus: malalignment of an extremity, in the coronal plane, with the apex of the deformity pointing to the midline ("knock-knees").

varus: malalignment of an extremity, in the coronal plane, with the apex of the deformity pointing away from the midline ("bow-legs").

volar: the palmar surface of the hand and forearm.

Wolff's Law: physiologic phenomenon whereby new bone forms in response to mechanical stress and resorbs in the absence of it ("form follows function").

woven bone: immature bone found in the embryo and newborns, fracture callus, tumors, and osteogenesis imperfecta or Paget's disease.

zone of transition: the boundary between what is perceived as normal bone and lesional tissue on radiographs. The zone of transition can be very sharply defined, indicative of a slow-growing process (benign tumor), or very poorly defined, indicative of an aggressive process (neoplasm or infection).

INDEX

Note: Page numbers in *italic* refer to illustrations; those followed by t refer to tables.